Handbook of Eating Disorders and Obesity

Handbook of Eating Disorders and Obesity

Editor: Carlyle Bennet

AMERICAN
MEDICAL PUBLISHERS
www.americanmedicalpublishers.com

AMERICAN
MEDICAL PUBLISHERS
www.americanmedicalpublishers.com

Cataloging-in-Publication Data

Handbook of eating disorders and obesity / edited by Carlyle Bennet.
p. cm.
Includes bibliographical references and index.
ISBN 978-1-63927-680-6
1. Eating Disorders. 2. Obesity. 3. Metabolism--Disorders. 4. Eating disorders--Treatment.
5. Eating disorders--Prevention. 6. Weight loss. 7. Reducing diets. I. Bennet, Carlyle.
RC552.E18 H36 2023
616.852 6--dc23

American Medical Publishers,
41 Flatbush Avenue,
1st Floor, New York,
NY 11217, USA

ISBN 978-1-63927-680-6 (Hardback)

Contents

Preface

In my initial years as a student, I used to run to the library at every possible instance to grab a book and learn something new. Books were my primary source of knowledge and I would not have come such a long way without all that I learnt from them. Thus, when I was approached to edit this book; I became understandably nostalgic. It was an absolute honor to be considered worthy of guiding the current generation as well as those to come. I put all my knowledge and hard work into making this book most beneficial for its readers.

An eating disorder refers to a type of mental disorder, which occurs due to abnormal eating behaviors affecting mental or physical health negatively. There are various types of eating disorders such as bulimia nervosa, avoidant/restrictive food intake disorder (ARFID), anorexia nervosa, pica, binge eating disorder, rumination syndrome and a group of other feeding or eating disorders. The treatment of eating disorders differs from disorder to disorder, and includes reducing excessive exercise, counseling, reduction of efforts to eliminate food, and dietary advice. Obesity is the state where excess body fat gets accumulated in the body, which results in negative impacts on human health. It is measured through body mass index (BMI) in which a person's weight is divided by the square of the person's height. It is a major cause of disability and also leads to various diseases and conditions like obstructive sleep apnea, osteoarthritis, cardiovascular diseases, certain types of cancer and type 2 diabetes. The readers would gain knowledge that would broaden their perspective about eating disorders and obesity through this book. It unravels the recent studies on these disorders. This book will prove to be immensely beneficial to students and researchers in this field of study.

I wish to thank my publisher for supporting me at every step. I would also like to thank all the authors who have contributed their researches in this book. I hope this book will be a valuable contribution to the progress of the field.

Editor

The Homeostatic Theory of Obesity: An Empirical Verification of the Circle of Discontent with an Assessment of its Relationship to Restrained and Uncontrolled Eating among Children and Adolescents

Kamila Czepczor-Bernat [1,*], Anna Brytek-Matera [2] and Paweł Matusik [3]

1 Faculty of Psychology in Katowice, SWPS University of Social Sciences and Humanities, 40-326 Katowice, Poland
2 Institute of Psychology, University of Wroclaw, 50-527 Wroclaw, Poland; anna.brytek-matera@uwr.edu.pl
3 School of Medicine in Katowice, Department of Pediatrics and Pediatric Endocrinology, Medical University of Silesia, 40-752 Katowice, Poland; pmatusik73@gmail.com
* Correspondence: kamila.czepczor-bernat@uwr.edu.pl

Abstract: The purpose of the present study was to provide an empirical verification of the Circle of Discontent with an assessment of its relationship to restrained and uncontrolled eating among children and adolescents. This study examined whether our results confirm a new hypothesized model. The total sample comprised 282 children and adolescents (148 girls and 134 boys; 141 participants with normal body weight and 141 with obesity). The mean age was 12.23 years (SD = 2.80), and the average BMI (body mass index) was 23.29 kg/m^2 (SD = 6.27). The following were used: Positive and Negative Affect Scale for Children, Children's Body Image Scale, Figure Rating Scale, Three-Factor Eating Questionnaire and Eating Disorders in Youth. The obtained values of the model fit indices proved the goodness of fit. Our findings show that obesity accompanies body dissatisfaction and uncontrolled and restrictive eating. Moreover, the higher the level of restrictive eating, the lower the level of uncontrolled eating. The relationships between body dissatisfaction, negative affect and restrictive eating, as well as that between uncontrolled eating and high-energy consumption, are significant and positive. Other relationships are non-significant. The above-mentioned relationships established in the Circle of Discontent, as well as relationships of restrained and uncontrolled eating with variables described in the circle, were confirmed. Based on our results, preventive strategies and psychological interventions can be created and may include changes in body image, eating behaviors and emotional functioning.

Keywords: childhood obesity; the homeostatic theory of obesity; the circle of discontent; children; adolescents; body dissatisfaction; negative affect; restrictive eating; uncontrolled eating; high-energy consumption

1. Introduction

Obesity has become a global epidemic in developed, as well as developing countries [1,2]. In Poland, the prevalence of obesity is worryingly high [3,4]. A recent study showed that the prevalence of obesity (with 95% CI) in the 7–18 age group was 4.3–8.8% among boys and 2.7–4.2% among girls [3].

Obesity is considered a multi-factorial disease, and multi-component interventions are more effective than single-component interventions in reducing body weight [1,4]. It is therefore important to consider obesity from an interdisciplinary theory- and evidence-based perspective. One such approach is the Homeostatic Theory of Obesity [5]. This model was created by Marks [5] and is based on a homeostatic theory of physical and mental health and illness. Marks [5] assumes that obesity is at least in part an effect of homeostatic imbalance in psychological functioning. By providing considerable scientific evidence, Marks created the Homeostatic Theory of Obesity, in which the Circle of Discontent (COD) is considered particularly important. This vicious circle describes the relationship between obesity, high-energy consumption, negative affect and body dissatisfaction. One of the variables listed in the model, related to the Circle of Discontent, is restraint (identified by restrictive eating). All these interrelationships have been widely researched in many studies [5]. Based on these new outcomes [6–13], a new variable (uncontrolled eating) and new relationships (between uncontrolled and restrictive eating and other variables) were added to the model (Figure 1). These studies show that body mass index (BMI) [7,10] and high-energy consumption [6,9,12] increase as uncontrolled eating increases. Moreover, a high level of restrictive eating is accompanied by a low level of uncontrolled eating [13] and a high level of body dissatisfaction [8,10,11].

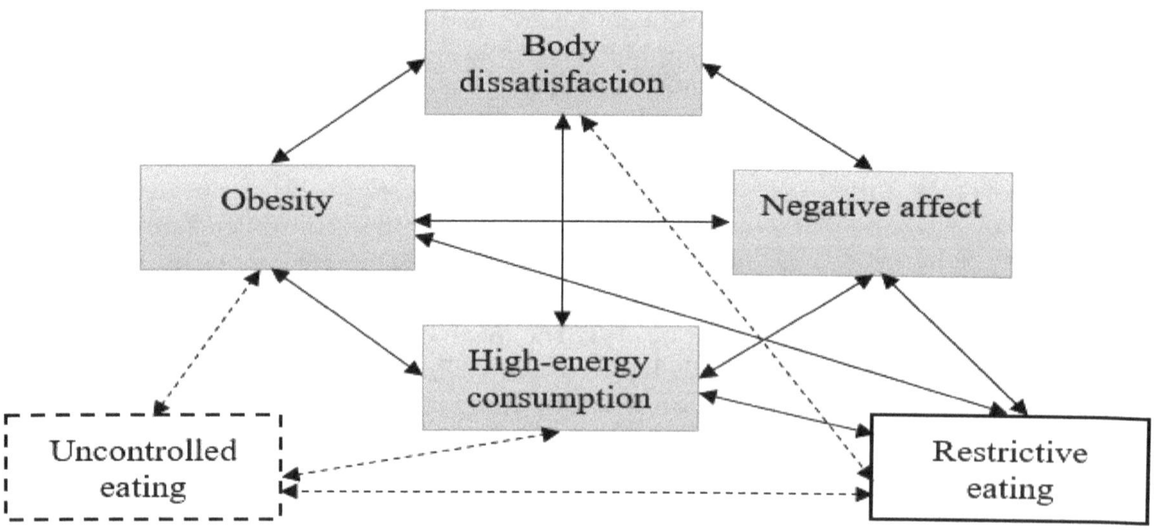

Figure 1. The Circle of Discontent (COD) and its relationship to restrained and uncontrolled eating among children and adolescents: a hypothesized model. the variables from the Circle of Discontent; a variable from Homeostatic Theory of Obesity whose relationship with COD was described by Marks; a new variable (proposed to be tested by the authors); relationships described by Marks; new relationships (proposed to be tested by the authors).

Based on Marks' theory [5] and the other studies mentioned above, it was assumed that all relations (except for restrictive eating and uncontrolled eating as well as restrictive eating and high-energy consumption) are positive.

To the best of our knowledge, the model has not yet been empirically verified in research. Therefore, the purpose of the present study was to provide an empirical verification of the Circle of Discontent with an assessment of its relationship to restrained and uncontrolled eating among children and adolescents. This study examined whether our results confirm a new hypothesized model.

2. Materials and Methods

2.1. Participants

We focused on children and adolescents because obesity in these groups is a growing public health problem—the prevalence of obesity increased several times among both girls and boys between 1975 and 2016 [2]. Moreover, in obese children and adolescents, an increased risk of being obese in adulthood has been observed [1]. Seeking new information on obesity can help increase effectiveness in preventing and treating obesity at an early stage of development.

Information about the study was passed on to parents and their children by doctors, nutritionists and teachers. Three hundred twenty-two participants applied for the study (Figure 2).

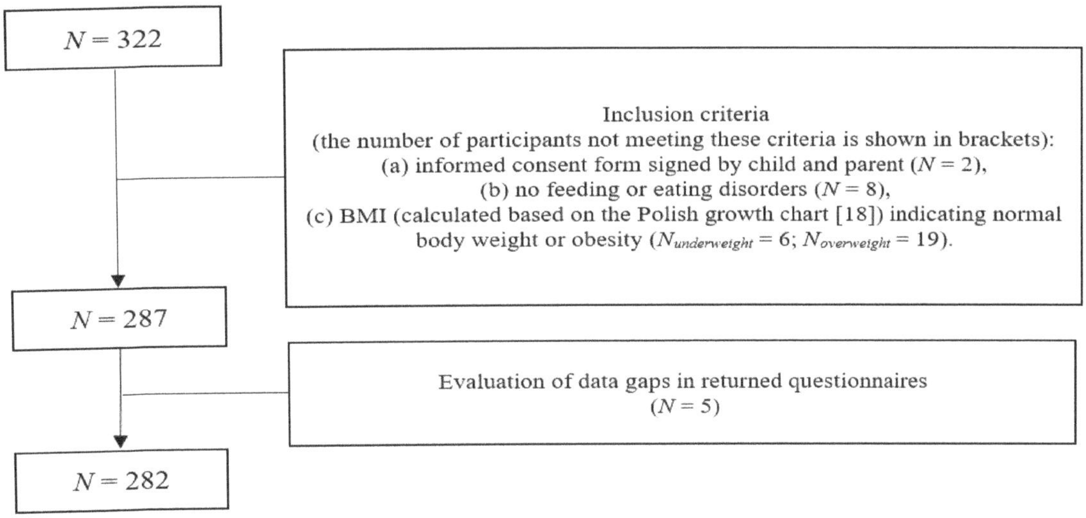

Figure 2. Flow chart of participants.

The total sample comprised 282 children and adolescents (148 girls and 142 boys; 141 participants with normal body weight and 141 with obesity). The mean age was 12.23 years ($SD = 2.80$), and the average BMI was 23.29 kg/m^2 ($SD = 6.27$). Based on the percentile analysis (BMI) [14], the participants were divided into two groups: normal body weight and obesity. Table 1 shows the characteristics of the participants.

Table 1. Characteristics for the two BMI categories.

	Normal Body Weight **N = 141**	**Obesity** **N = 141**	
	N (%)		***p***
Sex 1			
Female	76 (53.90)	72 (51.06)	>0.05
Male	65 (46.10)	69 (48.94)	
	M (SD)		
Age	11.72 (2.74)	12.73 (2.77)	>0.05
Weight	46.80 (17.84)	71.06 (22.47)	<0.001
Height	153.24 (17.15)	159.44 (15.34)	<0.01
BMI 2	19.26 (4.31)	27.32 (5.26)	<0.001
BMI z-score 3	0.25 (1.38)	2.34 (0.96)	<0.001

[1] The number of boys and girls in the two body mass index (BMI) groups did not differ significantly, χ^2 (1, $N = 282$) = 0.23; $p > 0.05$. [2] The "OLAF" and "OLA" projects (the Polish growth chart—percentile analysis) were used to calculate children's and adolescents' body mass index [14] [3] WHO AnthroPlus was used [15].

2.2. Measures

Questionnaires that already had Polish validation and the reliability of which had been assessed at an earlier stage of the project (the first stage of longitudinal research, the National Science Centre, Poland, no. 2017/25/N/HS6/00004) were used.

2.2.1. Negative Affect: Positive and Negative Affect Scale for Children (PANAS-C)

The Positive and Negative Affect Scale for Children (PANAS-C) is a self-report instrument measuring negative affect (NA) and positive affect (PA) among children and adolescents [16]. In the present study, a shorter 10-item Polish version was used, including (a) NA: "sad", "scared", "miserable", "afraid", and "mad"; (b) PA: "happy", "cheerful", "proud", "joyful", and "lively" [16]. The participants were asked, "How often have you felt this way during the past few weeks?" and responded on a 5-point scale (from 1—"not much or not at all" to 5—"a lot") [16,17]. The higher the scores are, the higher the intensity of negative and positive affect. Cronbach's alpha reliability (internal consistency) coefficients were (a) NA: 0.70 and (b) PA: 0.84.

2.2.2. Body Dissatisfaction: Children's Body Image Scale (Children) and Figure Rating Scale (Adolescents)

These scales are self-applied tools assessing the level of body dissatisfaction based on the discrepancy between one's ideal and real self [18–20]. These questionnaires contain seven hand-drawn children's and adolescents' silhouettes (from the thinnest to the fattest) [18–20]. The participants were asked to answer two questions: (a) one's real self: "Mark the red circle as you look now" and (b) one's ideal self: "Mark the green circle to show how you would like to look". We calculated body dissatisfaction by subtracting the number of the silhouette indicated as "one's real self" from the number of the silhouette indicated as "one's ideal self".

2.2.3. Uncontrolled and Restrictive Eating: Three-Factor Eating Questionnaire (TFEQ-R13)

This is a brief 13-item Polish version of a self-report measure [21]. This questionnaire assesses three types of maladaptive eating: (a) uncontrolled eating—"I am always hungry; therefore, I cannot stop eating until I empty my plate"; (b) restrictive eating—"I take small portions on purpose in order to control my body mass"; (c) emotional eating—"I eat when I feel nervous". In the first twelve items, the participants responded on a 4-point scale (from 1—"definitely false" to 4—"definitely true"). The last item (13) used an 8-point scale (from 1—"eating whatever you want, whenever you want it" to 8—"constantly limiting food intake and never 'giving in'"). This answer was recorded on a 4-point scale (1–2 into 1; 3–4 into 2; 5–6 into 3; 7–8 into 4). The higher the score, the higher the maladaptive eating style. In the current sample, Cronbach's α (internal consistency) was (a) uncontrolled eating: 0.76; (b) restrictive eating: 0.87; (c) emotional eating: 0.88.

2.2.4. Anthropometrical Status Based on BMI (Normal Body Weight vs. Obesity) and High-Energy Consumption: Sociodemographic Survey and Clinical Diagnosis

The sociodemographic survey included questions about sex, age, weight, height and high-energy consumption. In the case of younger children, parents helped with the measurement of weight and height. BMI was calculated based on self-report data. However, the diagnosis of obesity had to be confirmed by a doctor and/or dietitian. The participants were divided into two groups based on the percentile analysis (the calculation of children's and adolescents' body mass index using the Polish growth chart—the "OLAF" and "OLA" projects) [14]; thus, the variable included in the analyzed model was dichotomous—normal body weight (cut off points: 10–85th BMI percentile) vs. obesity (cut off point: above 95th BMI percentile). Additionally, to assess the level of high-energy consumption, the participants were asked "How often do you eat high-calorie snacks during the day (e.g., sweets, fast food, chips, salt sticks)?" (responses ranged from 1—"once a day or less often" to 6 "six or more times a day").

2.2.5. Feeding and Eating Disorders: Eating Disorders in Youth—Questionnaire (EDY-Q)

This brief self-report 14-item tool was used to exclude children and adolescents with symptoms of feeding and eating disorders [22]. This questionnaire was created based on the Diagnostic and Statistical Manual of Mental Disorders, Fifth Edition (DSM-5) [23].

2.3. *Procedure*

The participants were recruited in primary schools and centers specializing in the treatment of obesity (inpatient/outpatient) in the Opolskie and Silesian voivodeships between2018 and 2019. Before the participants completed the questionnaires, consent was obtained from them and their parents. No compensation was offered to the participants. The study was approved by the local ethics committee (no. 50/03/2017).

2.4. *Data Analysis*

The Statistical Package for Social Sciences version 25.0 with AMOS was used to verify the Circle of Discontent and its relationship to restrained and uncontrolled eating among children and adolescents. The proposed conceptual model was tested using structural equation modelling [24]. The generalized least squares (GLS) technique was used to estimate the parameters in our model. Moreover, bootstrapping was performed (number of bootstrap samples = 200).

The overall goodness of fit was assessed by the chi-square statistic (χ^2), degrees of freedom (df), comparative fit index (CFI), root mean square error of approximation (RMSEA) and standardized root mean square residual (SRMR). A chi-square with a p-value greater than 0.05 and χ^2/df less than 2 suggested goodness of fit, as did CFI greater than 0.95, RMSEA less than 0.06 (with pclose > 0.05) and SRMR less than 0.08 [24]. Moreover, the Bayesian information criterion (BIC) and Akaike information criterion (AIC) indicated that the hypothesized models were substantially nearer to saturated than the independent models.

3. Results

3.1. *Descriptive Statistics and Correlations*

Descriptive statistics and correlations (Pearson's r) are shown in Table 2.

Table 2. Correlations between analyzed variables.

	2	3	4	5	6
1. Negative affect	0.177 **	0.075	0.172 **	0.032	0.009
2. Body dissatisfaction		0.008	0.487 ***	0.559 ***	0.102
3. Uncontrolled eating			−0.125 *	0.154 **	0.168 **
4. Restrictive eating				0.505 ***	−0.073
5. Obesity [1]					0.087
6. High-energy consumption [2]					

* $p < 0.05$, ** $p < 0.01$, *** $p < 0.001$; [1] dichotomous variable: normal body weight vs. obesity; [2] "How often do you eat high-calorie snacks during the day (e.g., sweets, fast food, chips, salt sticks)?". Participants were asked to respond to the following question by marking their response either: 1—"once a day or less often", 2—"two times a day", 3—"three times a day", 4—"four times a day", 5—"five times a day", 6—"six or more times a day".

3.2. *Empirical Verification of the Circle of Discontent and its Relationship to Restrained and Uncontrolled Eating Among Children and Adolescents*

The goodness-of-fit statistics are presented in Table 3. We determined the goodness of fit between the hypothesized model (Figure 1) and our data and the obtained values of the model fit indices proved the goodness of fit [24].

Table 3. Fit index.

χ^2	*df*	*p*	χ^2/df	RMSEA [1]	*pclose*	SRMR	CFI	AIC [2]	BIC [3]
1.60	2	0.449	0.80	0.00	0.655	0.02	0.99	39.60	40.57

[1] with approximately 90% confidence (0.00; 0.111); [2] saturated model: 42.00, independent model: 148.44; [3] saturated model: 43.07, independent model: 148.74.

Based on Table 3, we conclude that the hypothetical relationships match the data well. Therefore, our results provide a basis for accepting the hypothetical model presented in Figure 1. Figure 3 captures the results (unstandardized estimates) with respect to the set of relations hypothesized by the researchers.

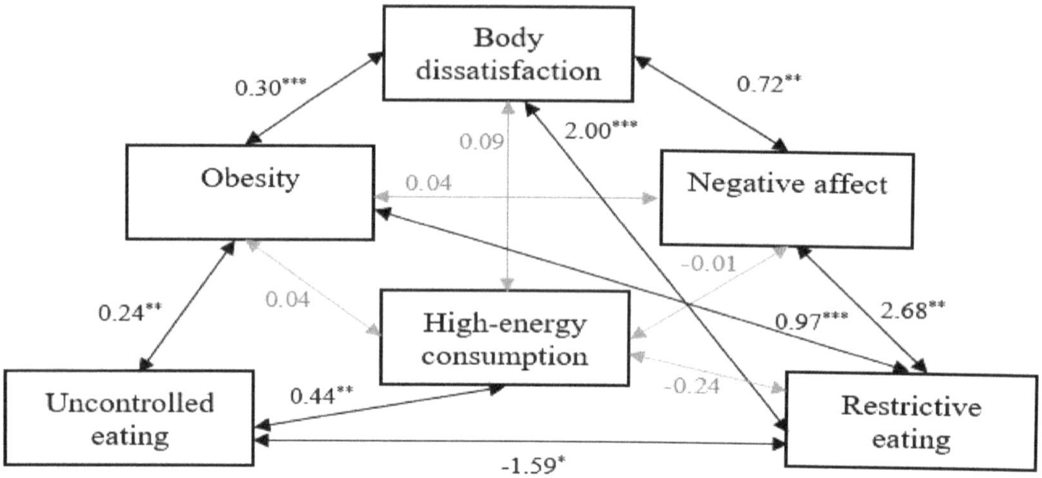

Figure 3. The Circle of Discontent and its relationship to restrained and uncontrolled eating among children and adolescents: a statistical model. * $p < 0.05$, ** $p < 0.01$, *** $p < 0.001$. The values for unstandardized coefficients are shown above the arrows. ⟷ a significant relationship; ⟷ a non-significant relationship.

With regard to Figure 3, obesity accompanies body dissatisfaction and uncontrolled and restrictive eating. Moreover, the higher the level of restrictive eating, the lower the level of uncontrolled eating. The relationships between body dissatisfaction, negative affect and restrictive eating, as well as that between uncontrolled eating and high-energy consumption, are significant and positive. Other relationships are non-significant. Being obese is not related to the experience of negative affect and high-energy consumption. In addition, body dissatisfaction is not significantly associated with high-energy consumption, nor is high-energy consumption associated with negative affect and restrictive eating.

Additional information about the outcomes can be found on the website https://drive.google.com/open?id=10JfSwZRKss2ds5nk9nnaHa8n-DF3O0Ne.

4. Discussion

In the present study, we empirically verified the Circle of Discontent with an assessment of its relationship to restrained and uncontrolled eating among children and adolescents. To our knowledge, our evaluation is the first assessment of the relations assumed in the Homeostatic Theory of Obesity using structural equation modelling. Several key findings were revealed in the present work. Most of the relationships described in the hypothesized model are significant and consistent with the assumed direction.

Being obese co-occurs with experiencing body dissatisfaction and maladaptive eating behaviors in the form of uncontrolled and restrictive eating. Moreover, the association between restrictive eating and uncontrolled eating is significant and negative. The current findings are in line with previous studies demonstrating significant relationships between the above-mentioned variables [5,7,13]. A possible explanation for our outcomes is the current ideal of beauty. Numerous studies presented in Marks' article [5] indicate that the current ideal of beauty is associated with having a thin silhouette [25]. Therefore, if there is a discrepancy between the current body weight and the ideal, there may be social pressure to change the appearance and strong body dissatisfaction. As a consequence, behaviors are undertaken to reduce body weight (e.g., restrictive eating) [5,25]. On the one hand, as everyone knows, these behaviors often do not have the desired effect because a restrictive diet often increases the risk of overeating (e.g., "masking hypothesis") [5,26,27]. On the other hand, not all studies confirm the negative impact of restrictions on overeating [28,29] or show that this relationship is negative [13]. Therefore, further research into these relationships is necessary.

Consistent with previous findings [5,6,8–11], our findings indicate that the subsequent relationships between body dissatisfaction, negative affect and restrictive eating, as well as that between uncontrolled eating and high-energy consumption, are significant and positive. Therefore, as predicted by Marks [5], a high level of body dissatisfaction is associated with the experience of a high intensity of negative affect, and the source of these emotions can be difficulty in controlling eating behavior, a large discrepancy between current and ideal body weight, and discrimination on the basis of physical appearance and body weight. Negative affect can trigger emotional eating, which, if it becomes a constant way of regulating emotions, may lead to weight gain [5,30]. Therefore, people often use dietary restraint to prevent weight gain and reduce the level of body dissatisfaction, negative affect and uncontrolled eating [5,30]. Dietary restrictions are a particularly important method of weight control for people with a high level of uncontrolled eating because they often consume more total energy, snacks and desserts than controlled eaters [9,30,31]. This is because a tendency towards uncontrolled eating is associated with the consumption of high-calorie foods (e.g., sweets, chocolate, fast food), which can also lead to weight gain [32–34].

Other relationships have not been confirmed. Obesity is not associated with the experience of negative affect and high-energy consumption. In addition, the analysis shows that body dissatisfaction is not significantly related to high-energy consumption, nor is high-energy consumption associated with negative affect and restrictive eating. Interestingly, Marks [5] assumes that all these relationships are significant and positive (except for restrictive eating and high-energy consumption). However, we can find studies both confirming these assumptions [32,33,35–37], and contradicting them or showing that the relationship among the variables is weak [38,39]. Still, other studies indicate the need to include moderators and mediators (e.g., sex, stress, size of image on food packaging targeting children) of the relationships we analyze [40–42].

It should be noted here that almost all relationships between high-energy consumption and other variables are non-significant. Consideration should therefore be given to conducting a future study using a different questionnaire that will more validly and reliably assess high-energy consumption (more information is provided in the paragraph on limitations). Moreover, many of the studies presented in this article have been conducted in the adult population (and not among children and adolescents). Therefore, caution should be exercised in drawing conclusions. Future research can help clarify current inconsistencies in the literature.

Given the high costs of obesity and comorbidities in terms of healthcare expenditure, prevention strategies are much needed [43]. When planning actions, keep in mind that childhood obesity is a complex issue [4,44]. Interestingly, one of the reports of the World Health Organization on obesity among Polish children indicates the need to carry out activities directed at improving the mental functioning of obese children [4]. Therefore, for the effectiveness of such activities to be as high as possible, it is necessary to integrate knowledge from many disciplines (including medicine, dietetics, physiotherapy, psychology) [4].

4.1. Strengths

To eliminate the impact of a subjective assessment of obesity, children and adolescents with a diagnosis of obesity confirmed by a doctor and/or dietitian participated in the study. First empirical verification of the relations assumed in the Homeostatic Theory of Obesity, an evaluation of obesity as a complex issue and knowledge that can be helpful in a multidisciplinary approach to obesity are the strong points of this study.

4.2. Limitations

Our study has some limitations that should be taken into consideration in interpreting outcomes and planning further studies. First, due to the cross-sectional design of the study, causality cannot be inferred, and longitudinal studies are required. Second, the size of the sample in the present study (based on the standards for structural equation modelling; [24]) is relatively small. Third, our analysis assesses only a selected fragment of relations assumed in the Homeostatic Theory of Obesity (the Circle of Discontent) together with an assessment of the relationship to restrained and uncontrolled eating among children and adolescents. Fourth, the study does not include emotional eating, which, as it turned out, could be important for interpreting the relationship between negative affect and restrictive eating. Therefore, we plan (in the third stage of our research, no. 2017/25/N/HS6/00004) to evaluate all relationships between the variables described in the Homeostatic Theory of Obesity, taking into account both the new relationships presented in this study and a much larger number of participants as well as incorporating emotional eating into the model. Fifth, we used a measure of high-energy consumption based on a single item about the frequency of eating high-calorie snacks during the day. In the future, a valid and reliable questionnaire (e.g., Food Frequency Questionnaire) may be used. This will provide information on the frequency and/or portion size of different types of food and beverages (typically over the past month or year). Sixth and last, because in our study BMI was calculated based on self-reported data, it would be worth applying an objective assessment of weight and height to all participants using bioelectrical impedance analysis to estimate body composition.

5. Conclusions

Most of the relationships established in the Circle of Discontent, as well as relationships of restrained and uncontrolled eating with variables described in the circle, are confirmed among children and adolescents. The following relationships are significant and consistent with our assumptions: (a) positive relationships: (1) obesity and body dissatisfaction, (2) obesity and uncontrolled eating, (3) obesity and restrictive eating, (4) body dissatisfaction and negative affect, (5) body dissatisfaction and restrictive eating, (6) negative affect and restrictive eating, (7) uncontrolled eating and high-energy consumption; and (b) negative relationship: (1) uncontrolled eating and restrictive eating. As suggested in the Discussion and Limitations sections, the main findings of our research and all limitations should be included in the next stages of the study.

Based on our research, we might create prevention strategies and psychological interventions that involve: (a) decreasing body dissatisfaction; (b) reducing high-energy consumption and maladaptive eating styles (uncontrolled and/or restrictive eating); (c) decreasing negative emotions and increasing adaptive emotional regulation. This information can be combined with knowledge already available in the fields of medicine, dietetics and related disciplines. In the light of these and other findings, there can be little doubt that the addition of psychological components to interventions would lead to improvements in the functioning of children and adolescents with obesity. These proposed interventions can help to slow the obesity epidemic.

The mechanism of obesity development is still being explored [1]. A biopsychosocial approach is based on the belief that the causes of obesity are attributable to genetic, nutritional and environmental factors [4,45–47]. Our and previous research shows that an increased body mass index can also be associated with psychological factors (e.g., increased body dissatisfaction, restrictive eating and uncontrolled eating) [6,8–11]. The above-mentioned factors often form a vicious circle that hinders effective behavioral control and weight loss [4]. It is therefore necessary to create prevention strategies and psychological interventions that take this information into account.

Author Contributions: Conceptualization, K.C.-B. and A.B.-M.; methodology, K.C.-B. and A.B.-M.; validation, K.C.-B. and A.B.-M.; formal analysis, K.C.-B. and A.B.-M.; investigation, K.C.-B. and P.M.; writing—original draft preparation, K.C.-B., A.B.-M. and P.M.; writing—review and editing, K.C.-B., A.B.-M. and P.M.; visualization, K.C.-B.; supervision, A.B.-M.; project administration, K.C.-B.; funding acquisition, K.C.-B. All authors have read and agreed to the published version of the manuscript.

Acknowledgments: I am extremely grateful to Zenobia Majewska (Junior High School Complex in Branice) for her support of this research. I would also like to express my sincere appreciation to Aleksandra Musioł (Primary School No. 17 in Katowice).

Abbreviations

AIC	Akaike information criterion
BIC	Bayesian information criterion
BMI	body mass index
CFI	comparative fit index
COD	Circle of Discontent
df	degrees of freedom
DSM-5	Diagnostic and Statistical Manual of Mental Disorders, Fifth Edition
EDY-Q	Eating Disorders in Youth—Questionnaire
GLS	generalized least squares
M	mean
N	sample size
NA	negative affect
p	probability value
PA	positive affect
PANAS-C	Positive and Negative Affect Scale for Children
RMSEA	root mean square error of approximation
SD	standard deviation
SRMR	standardized root mean square residual
TFEQ-R13	Three-Factor Eating Questionnaire
χ^2	chi-square statistic

References

1. Sahoo, K.; Sahoo, B.; Choudhury, A.K.; Sofi, N.Y.; Kumar, R.; Bhadoria, A.S. Childhood obesity: Causes and consequences. *J. Fam. Med. Prim. Care* **2015**, *4*, 187–192. [CrossRef]
2. World Health Organization 2020. Obesity and Overweight. Available online: https://www.who.int/news-room/fact-sheets/detail/obesity-and-overweight (accessed on 3 June 2020).
3. Kułaga, Z.; Grajda, A.; Gurzkowska, B. The prevalence of overweight and obesity among polish school-aged children and adolescents. *Przegl. Epidemiol.* **2016**, *70*, 641–651. [PubMed]
4. World Health Organization. Reducing Childhood Obesity in Poland by Effective Policies. 2017. Available online: http://www.euro.who.int/__data/assets/pdf_file/0011/350030/Reducing-childhood-obesity-in-Poland_final_WEB.pdf?ua=1 (accessed on 3 June 2020).
5. Marks, D.F. Homeostatic theory of obesity. *Health Psychol. Open* **2015**, *2*, 2055102915590692. [CrossRef] [PubMed]
6. Ames, S.L.; Kisbu-Sakarya, Y.; Reynolds, K.D.; Boyle, S.; Cappelli, C.; Cox, M.G.; Dust, M.; Grenard, J.L.; Mackinnon, D.P.; Stacy, A.W. Inhibitory control effects in adolescent binge eating and consumption of sugar-sweetened beverages and snacks. *Appetite* **2014**, *81*, 180–192. [CrossRef]

7. Czepczor-Bernat, K.; Brytek-Matera, A. Children's and mothers' perspectives of problematic eating behaviours in young children and adolescents: An exploratory study. *Int. J. Environ. Res. Public Health* **2019**, *16*, 2692. [CrossRef] [PubMed]
8. Figueiredo, R.A.O.; Simola-Ström, S.; Isomaa, R.; Weiderpass, E. Body dissatisfaction and disordered eating symptoms in Finnish preadolescents. *Eat. Disord.* **2019**, *27*, 34–51. [CrossRef]
9. Ledoux, T.; Adamus-Leach, H.; O'Connor, D.P.; Mama, S.; Lee, R.E. The association of binge eating and neighbourhood fast-food restaurant availability on diet and weight status. *Public Health Nutr.* **2015**, *18*, 352–360. [CrossRef]
10. Ribeiro-Silva, R.C.; Fiaccone, R.L.; Conceição-Machado, M.E.P.D.; Ruiz, A.S.; Barreto, M.L.; Santana, M.L.P. Body image dissatisfaction and dietary patterns according to nutritional status in adolescents. *J. Pediatr. (Rio J.)* **2018**, *94*, 155–161. [CrossRef]
11. Rodgers, R.F.; McLean, S.A.; Marques, M.; Dunstan, C.J.; Paxton, S.J. Trajectories of body dissatisfaction and dietary restriction in early adolescent girls: A latent class growth analysis. *J. Youth Adolesc.* **2016**, *45*, 1664–1677. [CrossRef] [PubMed]
12. Agras, W.S.; Robinson, A. *The Oxford Handbook of Eating Disorders*, 2nd ed.; Oxford Univesity Press: New York, NY, USA, 2018; pp. 155–186.
13. Booth, C.; Spronk, D.; Grol, M.; Fox, E. Uncontrolled eating in adolescents: The role of impulsivity and automatic approach bias for food. *Appetite* **2018**, *120*, 636–643. [CrossRef] [PubMed]
14. Instytut "Pomnik-Centrum Zdrowia Dziecka". Siatki centylowe dzieci i młodzieży w wieku 3–18 lat [Centile Grids of Children and Adolescents Aged 3–18 Years]. Available online: http://www.czd.pl/index.php?option=com_content&view=article&id=1717&Itemid=538 (accessed on 3 June 2020).
15. WHO. AnthroPlus Software. Available online: https://www.who.int/growthref/tools/en/ (accessed on 3 June 2020).
16. Laurent, J.; Cantanzaro, S.; Joiner, T.E.J.; Rudolph, K.D.; Potter, K.I.; Lambert, S.; Osborne, S.; Gathright, T. A measure of positive and negative affect for children: Scale development and preliminary validation. *Psychol. Assess.* **1999**, *11*, 326–338. [CrossRef]
17. Wróbel, M.; Finogenow, M.; Szymańska, P.; Laurent, J. Measuring positive and negative affect in a school-based sample: A polish version of the PANAS-C. *J. Psychopathol. Behav. Assess.* **2019**, *41*, 598–611. [CrossRef]
18. Childress, A.C.; Brewerton, T.D.; Hodges, E.L.; Jarrell, P.M. The Kids' Eating Disorders Survey (KEDS): A study of middle school students. *J. Am. Acad. Child. Adolesc. Psychiatry* **1993**, *32*, 843–850. [CrossRef] [PubMed]
19. Stunkard, A.; Sorensen, T.; Schulsinger, F. Use of the Danish Adoption Register for the study of obesity and thinness. *Res. Publ. Assoc. Res. Nerv. Ment. Dis.* **1983**, *60*, 115–120. [PubMed]
20. Truby, H.; Paxton, S.J. Development of the Children's body image scale. *Br. J. Clin. Psychol.* **2002**, *41*, 185–203. [CrossRef] [PubMed]
21. Dzielska, A.; Mazur, J.; Małkowska-Szkutnik, A.; Nelcz, H. Adaptacja polskiej wersji kwestionariusza Three-Factor Eating Questionnaire (TFEQ-13) wśród młodzieży szkolnej w badaniach populacyjnych. *Probl. Hig. Epidemiol.* **2009**, *90*, 362–369.
22. Hilbert, A.; van Dyck, Z. Eating Disorders in Youth Questionnaire English Version. Available online: http://ul.qucosa.de/api/qucosa%3A14486/attachment/ATT-0/ (accessed on 3 June 2020).
23. American Psychiatric Association. *DSM-5: Diagnostic and Statistical Manual of Mental Disorders*, 5th ed.; American Psychiatric Publishing: Arlington, VA, USA, 2013.
24. Byrne, B. *Structural Equation Modeling with AMOS. Basic Concepts, Applications, and Programming*, 2nd ed.; Routledge: New York, NY, USA; London, UK, 2010.
25. Cruz-Sáez, S.; Pascual, A.; Salaberria, K.; Echeburúa, E. Normal-weight and overweight female adolescents with and without extreme weight-control behaviours: Emotional distress and body image concerns. *J. Health Psychol.* **2015**, *20*, 730–740. [CrossRef]
26. Marcus, M.D.; Wing, R.R.; Lamparski, D.M. Binge eating and dietary restraint in obese patients. *Addict. Behav.* **1985**, *10*, 163–168. [CrossRef]
27. Polivy, J.; Herman, C.P. Distress and eating: Why do dieters overeat? *Int. J. Eat. Disord.* **1999**, *26*, 153–164. [CrossRef]
28. De Lauzon-Guillain, B.; Romon, M.; Musher-Eizenman, D.; Heude, B.; Basdevant, A.; Charles, M.A.; Fleurbaix-Laventie Ville Santé Study Group. Cognitive restraint, uncontrolled eating and emotional eating: Correlations between parent and adolescent. *Matern. Child. Nutr.* **2009**, *5*, 171–178. [CrossRef]
29. Johnson, F.; Wardle, J. Dietary restraint, body dissatisfaction, and psychological distress: A prospective analysis. *J. Abnorm. Psychol.* **2005**, *114*, 119–125. [CrossRef] [PubMed]

30. Rossy, L. *The Mindfulness-Based Eating Solution: Proven Strategies to End Overeating, Satisfy Your Hunger, and Savor Your Life*; New Harbinger Publications: Oakland, CA, USA, 2016.

31. Theim, K.R.; Tanofsky-Kraff, M.; Salaita, C.G.; Haynos, A.F.; Mirch, M.C.; Ranzenhofer, L.M.; Yanovski, S.Z.; Wilfley, D.E.; Yanovski, J.A. Children's descriptions of the foods consumed during loss of control eating episodes. *Eat. Behav.* **2007**, *8*, 258–265. [CrossRef] [PubMed]

32. Emond, J.A.; Longacre, M.R.; Titus, L.J.; Hendricks, K.; Drake, K.M.; Carroll, J.E.; Cleveland, L.P.; Dalton, M.A. Fast food intake and excess weight gain over a 1-year period among preschool-age children. *Pediatr. Obes.* **2020**. [CrossRef] [PubMed]

33. Greenberg, J.A.; Manson, J.E.; Buijsse, B.; Wang, L.; Allison, M.A.; Neuhouser, M.L.; Tinker, L.; Waring, M.E.; Isasi, C.R.; Martin, L.W.; et al. Chocolate-candy consumption and 3-year weight gain among postmenopausal U.S. women. *Obesity (Silver Spring)* **2015**, *23*, 677–683. [CrossRef] [PubMed]

34. Larson, N.; Story, M. A review of snacking patterns among children and adolescents: What are the implications of snacking for weight status? *Child. Obes.* **2013**, *9*, 104–115. [CrossRef] [PubMed]

35. Honicky, M.; Cardoso, S.M.; de Lima, L.R.A.; Ozcariz, S.; Vieira, F.; de Carlos Back, I.; Moreno, Y. Added sugar and trans fatty acid intake and sedentary behavior were associated with excess total-body and central adiposity in children and adolescents with congenital heart disease. *Pediatr. Obes.* **2020**, *15*, e12623. [CrossRef]

36. Kivimäki, M.; Head, J.; Ferrie, J.E.; Shipley, M.J.; Brunner, E.; Vahtera, J.; Marmot, M.G. Work stress, weight gain and weight loss: Evidence for bidirectional effects of job strain on body mass index in the Whitehall II study. *Int. J. Obes. (Lond.)* **2006**, *30*, 982–987. [CrossRef]

37. Shroff, M.R.; Perng, W.; Baylin, A.; Mora-Plazas, M.; Marin, C.; Villamor, E. Adherence to a snacking dietary pattern and soda intake are related to the development of adiposity: A prospective study in school-age children. *Public Health Nutr.* **2014**, *17*, 1507–1513. [CrossRef]

38. Njike, V.Y.; Smith, T.M.; Shuval, O.; Edshteyn, I.; Kalantari, V.; Yaroch, A.L. Snack food, satiety, and weight. *Adv. Nutr.* **2016**, *7*, 866–878. [CrossRef]

39. Zhu, Z.; He, Y.; Wang, Z.; He, X.; Zang, J.; Guo, C.; Jia, X.; Ren, Y.; Shan, C.; Sun, J.; et al. The associations between sugar-sweetened beverage intake and cardiometabolic risks in Chinese children and adolescents. *Pediatr. Obes.* **2020**, e12634. [CrossRef]

40. McGale, L.S.; Smits, T.; Halford, J.C.G.; Harrold, J.A.; Boyland, E.J. The influence of front-of-pack portion size images on children's serving and intake of cereal. *Pediatr. Obes.* **2020**, *15*, e12583. [CrossRef] [PubMed]

41. Wouters, S.; Jacobs, N.; Duif, M.; Lechner, L.; Thewissen, V. Negative affective stress reactivity: The dampening effect of snacking. *Stress. Health* **2018**, *34*, 286–295. [CrossRef] [PubMed]

42. Wouters, S.; Jacobs, N.; Duif, M.; Lechner, L.; Thewissen, V. Affect and between-meal snacking in daily life: The moderating role of gender and age. *Psychol. Health* **2018**, *33*, 555–572. [CrossRef] [PubMed]

43. Malik, V.; Willett, W.; Hu, F. Global obesity: Trends, risk factors and policy implications. *Nat. Rev. Endocrinol.* **2013**, *9*, 13–27. [CrossRef] [PubMed]

44. Dobbs, R.; Sawers, C.; Thompson, F.; Manyika, J.; Woetzel, J.; Child, P.; McKenna, S.; Spatharo, A. Overcoming Obesity: An Initial Economic Analysis. Available online: https://www.mckinsey.com/~{}/media/McKinsey/Business%20Functions/Economic%20Studies%20TEMP/Our%20Insights/How%20the%20world%20could%20better%20fight%20obesity/MGI_Overcoming_obesity_Full_report.ashx (accessed on 3 June 2020).

45. Skrypnik, D.; Bogdański, P.; Zawiejska, A.; Wender-Ożegowska, E. Role of gestational weight gain, gestational diabetes, breastfeeding, and hypertension in mother-to-child obesity transmission. *Pol. Arch. Intern. Med.* **2019**, *129*, 267–275. [CrossRef]

46. Skrypnik, D.; Bogdański, P.; Skrypnik, K.; Mądry, E.; Karolkiewicz, J.; Szulińska, M.; Suliburska, J.; Walkowiak, J. Influence of endurance and endurance–strength training on mineral status in women with abdominal obesity. *Medicine* **2019**, *98*, e14909. [CrossRef]

47. Szulińska, M.; Skrypnik, D.; Ratajczak, M.; Karolkiewicz, J.; Madry, E.; Musialik, K.; Walkowiak, J.; Jakubowski, H.; Bogdański, P. Effects of endurance and endurance-strength exercise on renal function in abdominally obese women with Renal Hyperfiltration: A prospective randomized trial. *Biomed. Environ. Sci.* **2016**, *29*, 706–712. [CrossRef]

2

Does Metabolically Healthy Obesity Exist?

Araceli Muñoz-Garach [1,2,*], Isabel Cornejo-Pareja [1] and Francisco J. Tinahones [1,2]

1 Department of Endocrinology and Nutrition, Virgen de la Victoria Hospital, Málaga University, Málaga 29010, Spain; isabelmaria_cornejo@hotmail.com (I.C.-P.); fjtinahones@hotmail.com (F.J.T.)
2 CIBER Fisiopatologia Obesidad y Nutricion (CIBEROBN), Instituto de Salud Carlos III, Madrid 28029, Spain
* Correspondence: aracelimugar@gmail.com

Abstract: The relationship between obesity and other metabolic diseases have been deeply studied. However, there are clinical inconsistencies, exceptions to the paradigm of "more fat means more metabolic disease", and the subjects in this condition are referred to as metabolically healthy obese (MHO).They have long-standing obesity and morbid obesity but can be considered healthy despite their high degree of obesity. We describe the variable definitions of MHO, the underlying mechanisms that can explain the existence of this phenotype caused by greater adipose tissue inflammation or the different capacity for adipose tissue expansion and functionality apart from other unknown mechanisms. We analyze whether these subjects improve after an intervention (traditional lifestyle recommendations or bariatric surgery) or if they stay healthy as the years pass. MHO is common among the obese population and constitutes a unique subset of characteristics that reduce metabolic and cardiovascular risk factors despite the presence of excessive fat mass. The protective factors that grant a healthier profile to individuals with MHO are being elucidated.

Keywords: metabolically healthy obesity; metabolic syndrome; adipose tissue; inflammation

1. Introduction

Obesity is a major health problem and an important risk factor for the development of diseases such as diabetes mellitus. The mechanism by which obesity leads to the development of insulin resistance still needs to be elucidated. There is a large body of epidemiological evidence on the relationship between obesity and other metabolic diseases. However, there are clinical inconsistencies that are exceptions to the paradigm of "more fat, more metabolic disease". There are subjects with long-standing obesity and morbid obesity who can be considered healthy despite a high degree of obesity. This phenomenon was described 15 years ago [1], and these subjects were referred to as metabolically healthy obese (MHO).

There is great inconsistency in the definitions of MHO, with a high degree of variability surrounding the prevalence of this phenotype, which has been estimated to be between 10% and 34% depending on the criteria used [2–5]. MHO appears to be more prevalent in women than in men and its prevalence appears to decrease with age in both sexes [6]. At the same time, there are individuals who, despite having "normal" weight, have an increased risk of disease.

Historically, the primary concern regarding obesity was the concurrent metabolic and cardiovascular risk. In recent years, there has been increased awareness of those individuals who do not fit into this traditional phenotype. This suggests that fat storage is not the only determinant in the association between obesity and insulin resistance, and the term "adiposopathy" is beginning to be used.

Existing guidelines also fail to individualize the management of MHO or metabolically unhealthy/abnormal obese (MUO) patients. This is further complicated because of a gap in the recognition and appropriate management of those normal-weight individuals who demonstrate high metabolic risk profiles.

2. Definition of Metabolically Healthy Obesity

Most studies suggest the definition of MHO (body mass index (BMI) $\geqslant$ 30 kg/m^2) to be obesity without the presence of metabolic diseases such as type 2 diabetes (T2DM), dyslipidemia or hypertension [1,7,8]. To date there are no accepted criteria for identifying MHO [7] individuals. The identification of individuals with MHO is hampered by the absence of a standardized definition of the condition. Several approaches were used to identify or define the MHO phenotype. The most referenced are:

1. Hyperinsulinemic-euglycemic clamp [8–10].
2. The upper quartile of glucose disposal rate [10].
3. The upper quartile of an index of insulin sensitivity after an oral glucose tolerance test [11,12].
4. Less than two of the following cardiometabolic disorders (systolic blood pressure $\geqslant$130 mmHg, diastolic blood pressure $\geqslant$85 mmHg, triglycerides $\geqslant$1.7 mmol/L or $\geqslant$150 mg/dL, fasting glucose $\geqslant$5.6 mmol/L, homeostasis model assessment of insulin resistance (HOMA-IR) $\geqslant$5, ultrasensitive C-reactive protein (CRP) $\geqslant$0.1 mg/L, HDL cholesterol $\leqslant$1.03 mmol/L or 40 mg/dL in men and $\leqslant$1.3 mmol/L or 50 mg/dL in women [3,13].
5. Less than three metabolic syndrome criteria [14].
6. Subjects with BMI above 30 kg/m^2 and HDL cholesterol levels of at least 40 mg/dL in the absence of T2DM and hypertension [15].

Other inflammatory markers (CRP or degree of leukocytosis) have been suggested for inclusion in the definition of MHO [16,17].

An additional marker that is increasingly important in the context of the MHO phenotype is liver fat content. The prevalence of non-alcoholic fatty liver disease appears to be significantly lower in patients with MHO compared with MUO individuals [12]. According to our current knowledge, the classification of "metabolically benign obesity" or "metabolically healthy obesity" only refers to metabolic or cardiovascular complications and does not consider that obesity may be associated with other non-metabolic complications such as orthopedic problems, pulmonary complications, or other physiological conditions. Considering that the descriptions of MHO are inconsistent, the elucidation of the factors or mechanisms underlying this protective profile is far from complete although some works are trying to establisha standard definition of MHO [18].

3. Underlying Mechanisms That Explain the Existence of MHO

3.1. *Subclinical Inflammation*

Inflammation promotes insulin resistance. Greater adipose tissue inflammation is closely associated with increased metabolic risk for T2DM, cardiovascular disease, and fatty liver disease, whereas obese adults without adipose tissue inflammation exhibit reduced metabolic risk.

There is growing evidence to suggest that subclinical inflammation may be the underlying mechanism that determines whether or not an individual is MHO [16]. Subclinical inflammation is associated with insulin resistance, and CRP has emerged as one of the best predictors of vascular inflammation, metabolic syndrome and cardiovascular disease [19]. There is a strong correlation between circulating CRP levels and anthropometric markers and body composition, and CRP has been proposed as a screening tool to assess the risk of the metabolic syndrome in youth [20]. In adulthood, the MHO phenotype is associated with low levels of complement component 3, CRP, alpha necrosis tumor factor (TNF-α), interleukin 6 (IL-6), and a low number of white blood cells, supporting the concept of a more favorable inflammatory state compared to non-MHO subjects [21].

On the other hand, anti-inflammatory adipokines, such as adiponectin, IL-4, IL-10, IL-13, IL-1 receptor antagonist, and transforming growth factor beta are abundant within the adipose tissues of lean individuals, whereas obese adipose tissue is dominated by the release of pro-inflammatory adipokines, including leptin, resistin, TNF-a, IL-6, IL-18, retinol-binding protein 4, lipocalin 2, angiopoietin-like protein 2, CC-chemokine ligand 2, CXC-chemokine ligand 5, and nicotinamide phosphoribosyltransferase [22].

Other systemic inflammation markers or adipose tissue inflammation markers are free fatty acids (FFA) and the number and activation status of peripheral leukocytes. Thus obese patients with T2DM have higher circulating levels of IL-6, FFA and glycerol and a greater absolute number of peripheral leukocytes compared with non-diabetic obese subjects [23,24]. Similarly, our group found that morbidly obese subjects without metabolic disease had a low degree of insulin resistance and identical adipose tissue inflammation markers as those of non-obese subjects, with no infiltration of macrophages and elevated values of TNF-α and IL-6 expression in visceral adipose tissue [25]. All these results suggest that MUO patients show a higher degree of both systemic and local fat inflammation compared with MHO individuals [23].

3.2. Expansion Capacity of Adipose Tissue

Previously, to explain the transition from normal adipose tissue to that which leads to metabolic abnormalities, studies proposed the "adipose tissue expandability hypothesis". This postulated that once adipocytes reached a threshold capacity for storage, they begin to promote insulin resistance with lipotoxicity and adipokine release. This was supported by knockout studies with PPARγ, lipodystrophy models, and alterations in adipokine secretion following saturation of adipose tissue. Investigating this fact led to further characterization of genetic contributors to the pathways of adipogenesis (SFRP1, Wnt, S14), apoptosis (TRAIL, TWEAK, BCL2, CASP3/7), and angiogenesis (VEGF-A, -B,-C,-D). To improve the understanding of adipose tissue in the context of MHO patients, Tinahones *et al.* looked at genes associated with both lipolysis and lipogenesis and BMI, insulin, and HOMA-IR. They found a positive correlation in PPARγ, DGAT1, AQP7, GK, ATGL, HSL, and perilipin and BMI, insulin, and HOMA-IR in both subcutaneous and visceral fat tissues. Additionally, they demonstrated a negative correlation between genes—ACC1, PEPCK, ACSS2, FABP4—and the aforementioned measures of metabolic risk.

A fairlysolid theory attributes the differences between MHO and MUHO subjects to the different capacity for adaptation to excess energy in adipose tissue [26]. When increased fat storage is required, fat tissue needs to increase its storage capacity and can increase the size of adipocytes or increase their number [27]. In addition, this increase in the overall amount of fat must be accompanied by increased vascularization [28]. In those subjects in whom adipose tissue has difficulty expanding in the healthiest way, which is increasing cellularity, metabolic disease does appear [29]. That is what we see in MHO who keep the proper storage capacity. But the loss of expansion capacity can even occur in patients with normal weight, so this theory would explain the existence of metabolically unhealthy lean subjects [30]. Furthermore, the lack of expansion capacity of adipose tissue has been linked to the loss of its main lipogenic function, and the appearance of lipotoxic products in adipose tissue [31].

Traditionally it was thought that there was little cell turnover in adipose tissue in adulthood. Today it is known that adipose tissue is capable of hyperplasia throughout life, and stem/progenitor cells are responsible for this adipose tissue hyperplasia [27,32,33]. Pre-adipocytes found in the vascular stroma are progenitor cells that differentiate into mature adipocytes through a complex program of gene expression [33–36]. Another variable that is directly related to the total number of fat cells is cell death, which may occur by necrosis, autophagy or apoptosis [37,38]. These studies have also alluded to reduced adipocyte hypertrophy, fibrosis and stress as potential contributors to this presentation. Therefore, there are four factors that are directly related to the ability for adipose tissue expansion and functionality: (1) lipogenesis; (2) adipogenesis via the newly formed progenitor cells; (3) apoptotic and anti-apoptotic pathways; and (4) angiogenesis.

Our group, in collaboration with other groups, has shown that metabolically healthy subjects have higher lipogenic [39,40] and angiogenic [41,42] capacity than metabolically unhealthy patients. Furthermore, there is also considerable evidence that adipogenesis and the functionality of mesenchymal cells to become new adipocytes is higher in metabolically healthy subjects because they exhibit mesenchymal cells in the stroma of adipose tissue with a greater capacity to differentiate both bone and fat tissue and a lower senescence [36]. This increased ability to form new adipocytes in the MHO individuals is an observation contributed by our group which clearly shows that the apoptosis of adipocytes increases with obesity, and this has a direct relationship with the degree of adipose tissue inflammation [43].

Adipose tissue is a key regulator of inflammation, and inflammation is involved in the onset and development of atherosclerosis, metabolic syndrome, and T2DM. Although the results of these initial studies suggest that MHO is characterized by a lower inflammatory cytokine environment than MUO, further studies are necessary to better identify the adipose tissue hormones that promote a healthy metabolic profile in obese adults.

There are several adipose tissue compartments and they have different connections with metabolic diseases. Visceral and intrahepatic fat has a direct association with obesity, while subcutaneous fat is not associated with metabolic disease [44]. A plausible hypothesis is that the healthiest way to accumulate fat is through subcutaneous fat expansion but when this capacity is decreased or lost it must resort to other compartments and metabolic diseases occur. Could the MHO phenotype be defined as a group of obese patients with predominantly subcutaneous fat deposits and with little or no visceral and intrahepatic fat? These questions and more still need to be answered.

3.3. *Other Possible Mechanisms*

A new potential factor to explain the differences between MHO and MUO could be circulating microRNA [45]. Insulin resistance in peripheral organs, such as the liver, can develop due to toxic stimulus, initiating secretion of microRNAs associated with insulin resistance, which are incorporated into muscle and fat cells, inducing insulin resistance in these tissues [46].

A study revealed that 20% of patients with a BMI above 40 kg/m^2 had adiponectin levels above the average of subjects with normal BMI, and these adiponectin levels above a certain threshold increase the probability of being metabolically healthy, even after correcting for the confounding effects of age, insulin and waist circumference [15]. This suggests that adiponectin plays a crucial role in the pathogenesis of metabolic complications associated with obesity as patients with the MHO phenotype have similar levels of adiponectin as those found in normal-weight subjects [15]. Furthermore, individuals with the MHO phenotype have a lower visceral fat, liver fat, and muscle fat content than obese subjects without MHO or obese people with insulin resistance, suggesting that the MHO phenotype is associated with improved ability to capture FFA in adipose tissue [12]. These differences in body composition between MHO patients and non-MHO patients are consistent between genders [3].

Finally, lifestyle factors such as level of physical activity or cardiorespiratory condition also appear to play a key role in distinguishing whether or not an individual is MHO. MHO subjects show higher levels of physical activity compared to MUO individuals and have a more favourable lifestyle [14,47,48]. Likewise, occupational physical activity or leisure time physical activity also appears to be important, since the two exercise regimens are differentially associated with obesity and insulin resistance [49].

4. Do Metabolically Healthy Obese Subjects Improve after an Intervention?

The decisive feature of MHO is the absence of visceral fat accumulation. Until definitive data emerges linking genetic predisposition to MHO, currently recommended lifestyle modifications appear beneficial. Thus, promoting lifestyle modifications directed at minimizing visceral fat accumulation is a fundamental public health measure.

However, it is not completely clear if obese subjects with a MHO phenotype would benefit from traditional lifestyle interventions, which focus on dietary therapy and/or increased physical exercise. Few studies have analyzed the metabolic effects of lifestyle modifications with a restrictive diet and/or exercise in MHO subjects, and their results have been contradictory [50,51]. Supporting the theory that MHO and non-MHO individuals could require a different treatment approach, Karelisy *et al.* showed that MHO individuals reacted differently, from a metabolic viewpoint, to a six-month calorie restricted diet compared to "at-risk" obese people despite achieving similar weight loss [52]. There are some studies that showed combining a Mediterranean diet with moderate to high intensity aerobic training is more effective at improving body composition [53,54]. Although the public health message for all obese patients should continue to promote healthy lifestyle habits, the controversial results of lifestyle interventions in MHO individuals would justify prioritizing, for cost-efficacy reasons, the intensive interventions in metabolically abnormal obese individuals and monitoring MHO subjects for early detection of the development of metabolic abnormalities [55].

Currently, bariatric surgery remains among the best options for patients suffering from severe obesity, with excellent results regarding long-term weight loss and decreases in peripheral and visceral fat depot sizes [56]. More research is needed to study the effects of different therapeutic approaches on the metabolic profile of healthy but obese individuals. Results in this area are essential for understanding the pathophysiology and to implement appropriate metabolically healthy obese and healthy non-obese intervention strategies.

5. Do Metabolically Healthy Obese Subjects Stay Healthy as the Years Pass?

Debate continues concerning whether individuals with MHO are truly healthy. The literature differs regarding the relative risk of disease among this population. MHO individuals are at decreased risk for developing cardiovascular disease compared with MUO individuals [57]. Long-term studies have suggested that MHO is a transient state. For example, among a group of Japanese Americans with MHO, two-thirds developed metabolic syndrome during 10 years of observation, and the metabolic abnormality was independently associated with visceral fat accumulation, female sex, higher fasting plasma insulin concentration, and lower serum HDL associated cholesterol concentration [58]. Consistent with this report, among the 1051 participants in the Pizarra Study, the prevalence of MHO decreased during 11 years of observation [59].

Individuals with MHO are not at increased risk for developing cardiovascular disease compared to metabolically healthy normal weight [MHNW] individuals [60–63]. Studies with longer follow-up periods (>15 years) have reported that MHO individuals were at an increased risk for major cardiovascular disease events as compared to MHNW individuals [64,65]. Recently, analysts conducting a systematic review of the associations between BMI and metabolic status with total mortality and cardiovascular events reported that MHO individuals appear to be at increased risk for cardiovascular events, as compared to MHNW individuals [66]. These researchers concluded that obese individuals are at increased risk for adverse long-term outcomes, even in the absence of metabolic abnormalities, compared with MHNW individuals.

A recent study evaluated the prevalence of elevated plasma high sensitivity CRP (hs-CRP) concentrations and hepatic steatosis in MHO, MHNW, and in metabolically unhealthy normal-weight (MUNW) individuals [67]. They observed that both elevated plasma hs-CRP concentrations and hepatic steatosis are more prevalent among MHO and MUNW individuals than they are among MHNW individuals. However, they are most prevalent among individuals with MHO, suggesting that obesity in the absence of metabolic risk factors is not entirely benign but is associated with subclinical vascular inflammation. Another recent study reported that 42% of their subjects with MHO developed the metabolic syndrome within 10 years [68], again suggesting that MHO is not without increased health risks. However, the identification of predictors, biological determinants, and mechanisms underlying MHO, determining whether MHO represents a transient phenotype that is affected by aging, behavioral, and environmental factors, and accurately calculating the true health risks associated with MHO remain viable topics for diligent study through properly designed and conducted longitudinal studies.

The Bogalusa Heart Study examined 1098 individuals, both children (5–17 years) and adults (24–43 years), who participated in the study between 1997 and 2002. Participants with the MHO phenotype during childhood were more likely to maintain MHO status in adulthood. Despite the level of obesity and fat mass continuing to increase throughout childhood and adulthood, this group of MHO individuals showed a generally comparable cardiometabolic profile with non-obese children and adults. In addition, the carotid intima-media thickness did not differ in adulthood among previous MHO children and non-obese children. These results are very important because they show that the MHO phenotype that starts in childhood and continues into adulthood may have a very favourablecardiometabolic risk profile [69]. Even more importantly, there is increasing evidence showing that the metabolic profile of MHO individuals is almost indistinguishable from that of lean individuals [4,7,70].

To date it is not at all clear whether the MHO phenotype decreases morbidity and mortality associated with obesity. MHO patients have a lower prevalence of risk factors for the development of certain diseases. For example, the intima-media thickness as a risk marker of atherosclerosis is significantly different between individuals with the MHO phenotype and metabolically healthy non-obese patients [5,12,70]. However, a recent meta-analysis has evaluated eight studies comparing mortality data from any cause or cardiovascular events in six groups of patients defined by BMI category (n = 61,386) and metabolic comorbidities, with a 10-year follow up. Analyses revealed that MHO individuals had an increased risk (relative risk (RR): 1.24) compared with MHNW subjects, but this was only detected in studies of 10 or more years of follow-up. In addition, all metabolically unhealthy subjects, regardless of their weight, had an increased risk compared with healthy lean individuals. Curiously in metabolically unhealthy patients, the normal-weight individuals had a higher risk (RR: 3.13), followed by overweight (RR: 2.70) and finally obese subjects (RR: 2.65) [71]. Similar results were published, indicating that both MHO and MUO individuals ultimately had a higher risk of mortality [72].

This evidence, too, is conflicting, with the underlying question being whether MHO presentations simply represent an early snapshot along the timeline of metabolic health. One group found that nearly 50% of MHO patients transitioned to metabolically unhealthy phenotypes when followed longitudinally for 10 years. Therefore, at present, it is not clear whether MHO individuals will remain such with the passage of time, or if their cardiovascular morbidity and mortality is comparable to that of non-obese subjects.

6. Conclusions

MHO is common among the obese population and constitutes a unique subset of characteristics that reduce metabolic and cardiovascular risk factors despite the presence of excessive fat mass. The protective factors that grant a healthier profile to individuals with MHO are being elucidated.

Despite the knowledge that visceral fat deposition is the seminal factor that ultimately causes insulin resistance and the detrimental inflammatory and hormonal profile that contributes to increased risk for cardiovascular disease, it remains unknown whether MHO has genetic predisposing factors, and whether MHO ultimately succumbs to insulin resistance and the metabolic syndrome.

Acknowledgments: This work was supported in part by grants from Instituto de Salud Carlos III (PI12/0235) and Consejería de Innovacion, Ciencia y Empresa de la Junta de Andalucía (CTS-8181). This study has been co-funded by FEDER funds. A.M.G. is the recipient of a postdoctoral grant (Rio Hortega CM 14/00078) from the Spanish Ministry of Economy and Competitiveness. All sources of funding of the study should be disclosed.

Author Contributions: A.M.G. and F.T. wrote the manuscript. I.C.P. helped with final revisions and writing the manuscript. M.R. reviewed the manuscript.

References

1. Sims, E. Are there persons who are obese, but metabolically healthy? *Metabolism* **2001**, *50*, 1499–1504. [CrossRef] [PubMed]
2. Roberson, L.; Aneni, E.; Maziak, W.; Agatston, A.; Feldman, T.; Rouseff, M.; Tran, T.; Blaha, M.J.; Santos, R.D.; Sposito, A.; *et al.* Beyond BMI: The "Metabolically healthy obese" phenotype & its association with clinical/subclinical cardiovascular disease and all-cause mortality—A systematic review. *BMC Public Health* **2014**, *14*, 1–12.

3. Wildman, R.; Muntner, P.; Reynolds, K.; McGinn, A.; Rajpathak, S.; Wylie-Rosett, J.; Sowers, M.R. The obese without cardiometabolic risk factor clustering and the normal weight with cardiometabolic risk factor clustering: Prevalence and correlates of 2 phenotypes among the US population (NHANES 1999–2004). *Arch. Intern. Med.* **2008**, *168*, 1617–1624. [CrossRef] [PubMed]
4. Pajunen, P.; Kotronen, A.; Korpi-Hyövälti, E.; Keinänen-Kiukaanniemi, S.; Oksa, H.; Niskanen, L.; Saaristo, T.; Saltevo, J.T.; Sundvall, T.; Vanhala, M.; *et al.* Metabolically healthy and unhealthy obesity phenotypes in the general population: The FIN-D2D survey. *BMC Public Health* **2011**, *1*, 754–762. [CrossRef] [PubMed]
5. Shea, J.; Randell, E.; Sun, G. The prevalence of metabolically healthy obese subjects defined by BMI and dual-energy X-ray absorptiometry. *Obesity (Silver Spring)* **2011**, *19*, 624–630. [CrossRef] [PubMed]
6. Van Vliet-Ostaptchouk, J.; Nuotio, M.; Slagter, S.; Doiron, D.; Fischer, K.; Foco, L.; Gaye, A.; Gögele, M.; Heier, M.; Hiekkalinna, T.; *et al.* The prevalence of metabolic syndrome and metabolically healthy obesity in Europe: A collaborative analysis of ten large cohort studies. *BMC Endocr. Disord.* **2014**, *14*, 9–22. [CrossRef] [PubMed]
7. Karelis, A. Metabolically healthy but obese individuals. *Lancet* **2008**, *372*, 1281–1283. [CrossRef]
8. Blüher, M. The distinction of metabolically 'healthy' from 'unhealthy' obese individuals. *Curr. Opin. Lipidol.* **2010**, *21*, 38–43. [CrossRef] [PubMed]
9. Brochu, M.; Tchernof, A.; Dionne, I.; Sites, C.K.; Eltabbakh, G.H.; Sims, E.A.; Poehlman, E.T. What are the physical characteristics associated with a normal metabolic profile despite a high level of obesity in postmenopausal women? *J. Clin. Endocrinol. Metab.* **2001**, *86*, 1020–1025. [PubMed]
10. Karelis, A.; Faraj, M.; Bastard, J.; St-Pierre, D.; Brochu, M.; Prud'homme, D.; Rabasa-Lhoret, R. The metabolically healthy but obese individual presents a favorable inflammation profile. *J. Clin. Endocrinol. Metab.* **2005**, *90*, 4145–4150. [CrossRef] [PubMed]
11. Kantartzis, K.; Machann, J.; Schick, F.; Rittig, K.; Machicao, F.; Fritsche, A.; Häring, H.-U.; Stefan, N. Effects of a lifestyle intervention in metabolically benign and malign obesity. *Diabetologia* **2011**, *54*, 864–868. [CrossRef] [PubMed]
12. Stefan, N.; Kantartzis, K.; Machann, J.; Schick, F.; Thamer, C.; Rittig, K.; Balletshofer, B.; Machicao, F.; Fritsche, A.; Häring, H.U. Identification and characterization of metabolically benign obesity in humans. *Arch. Intern. Med.* **2008**, *168*, 1609–1616. [CrossRef] [PubMed]
13. Camhi, S.M.; Katzmarzyk, P.T. Differences in body composition between metabolically healthy obese and metabolically abnormal obese adults. *Int. J. Obes. (Lond.)* **2014**, *38*, 1142–1145. [CrossRef] [PubMed]
14. Bobbioni-Harsch, E.; Pataky, Z.; Makoundou, V.; Laville, M.; Disse, E.; Anderwald, C.; Konrad, T.; Golay, A. Frommetabolic normality to cardiometabolic risk factors in subjects with obesity. *Obesity (Silver Spring)* **2012**, *20*, 2063–2069. [CrossRef] [PubMed]
15. Aguilar-Salinas, C.; García, E.; Robles, L.; Riaño, D.; Ruiz-Gomez, D.; García-Ulloa, A.; Melgarejo, M.A.; Zamora, M.; Guillen-Pineda, L.E.; Mehta, R.; *et al.* High adiponectin concentrations are associated with the metabolically healthy obese phenotype. *J. Clin. Endocrinol. Metab.* **2008**, *93*, 4075–4079. [CrossRef] [PubMed]
16. Karelis, A.; Rabasa-Lhoret, R. Obesity: Can inflammatory status define metabolic health? *Nat. Rev. Endocrinol.* **2013**, *9*, 694–695. [CrossRef] [PubMed]
17. Hamer, M.; Stamatakis, E. Metabolically healthy obesity and risk of all-cause and cardiovascular disease mortality. *J. Clin. Endocrinol. Metab.* **2012**, *97*, 2482–2488. [CrossRef] [PubMed]
18. Phillips, C.M.; Dillon, C.; Harrington, J.M.; McCarthy, V.J.C.; Kearney, P.M.; Fitzgerald, A.P.; Perry, I.J. Defining metabolically healthy obesity: Role of dietary and lifestyle factors. *PLoS ONE* **2013**, *8*, e76188. [CrossRef] [PubMed]
19. Sutherland, J.; McKinley, B.; Eckel, R. The metabolic syndrome and inflammation. *Metab. Syndr. Relat. Disord.* **2004**, *2*, 82–104. [CrossRef] [PubMed]
20. DeBoer, M. Obesity, systemic inflammation, and increased risk for cardiovascular disease and diabetes among adolescents: A need for screening tools to target interventions. *Nutrition* **2013**, *29*, 379–386. [CrossRef] [PubMed]
21. Phillips, C.; Perry, I. Does inflammation determine metabolic health status in obese and nonobese adults? *J. Clin. Endocrinol. Metab.* **2013**, *98*, E1610–E1619. [CrossRef] [PubMed]
22. Ouchi, N.; Parker, J.L.; Lugus, J.J.; Walsh, K. Adipokines in inflammation and metabolic disease. *Nat. Rev. Immunol.* **2011**, *11*, 85–97. [CrossRef] [PubMed]

23. VanBeek, L.; Lips, M.; Visser, A.; Pijl, H.; Ioan-Facsinay, A.; Toes, R.; Berends, F.J.; van Dijk, K.W.; Koning, F.; van Harmelen, V. Increased systemic and adipose tissue inflammation differentiates obese women with T2DM from obese women with normal glucose tolerance. *Metabolism* **2014**, *63*, 492–501. [CrossRef] [PubMed]
24. Blüher, S.; Schwarz, P. Metabolically healthy obesity from childhood to adulthood-does weight status alone matter? *Metabolism* **2014**, *63*, 1084–1092. [CrossRef] [PubMed]
25. Barbarroja, N.; López-Pedrera, R.; Mayas, M.D.; García-Fuentes, E.; Garrido-Sánchez, L.; Macías-González, M.; Bekay, R.; Vidal-Puig, A.; Tinahones, F.J. The obese healthy paradox: Is inflammation the answer? *Biochem. J.* **2010**, *430*, 141–149. [CrossRef] [PubMed]
26. Lionetti, L.; Mollica, M.P.; Lombardi, A.; Cavaliere, G.; Gifuni, G.; Barletta, A. From chronic overnutrition to insulin resistance: The role of fat-storing capacity and inflammation. *Nutr. Metab. Cardiovasc. Dis.* **2009**, *19*, 146–152. [CrossRef] [PubMed]
27. De Ferranti, S.; Mozaffarian, D. The perfect storm: obesity, adipocyte dysfunction, and metabolic consequences. *Clin. Chem.* **2008**, *54*, 945–955. [CrossRef] [PubMed]
28. Ledoux, S.; Queguiner, I.; Msika, S.; Calderari, S.; Rufat, P.; Gasc, J.M.; Corvol, P.; Larger, E. Angiogenesis associated with visceral and subcutaneous adipose tissue in severe human obesity. *Diabetes* **2008**, *57*, 3247–3257. [CrossRef] [PubMed]
29. Arner, E.; Westermark, P.O.; Spalding, K.L.; Britton, T.; Rydén, M.; Frisén, J.; Bernard, S.; Arner, P. Adipocyte turnover: Relevance to human adipose tissue morphology. *Diabetes* **2010**, *59*, 105–109. [CrossRef] [PubMed]
30. Virtue, S.; Vidal-Puig, A. It's not how fat you are, it's what you do with it that counts. *PLoS Biol.* **2008**, *6*, e237. [CrossRef] [PubMed]
31. Barbarroja, N.; Rodriguez-Cuenca, S.; Nygren, H.; Camargo, A.; Pirraco, A.; Relat, J.; Cuadrado, I.; Pellegrinelli, V.; Medina-Gomez, G.; Lopez-Pedrera, C.; *et al.* Increased dihydroceramide/ceramide ratio mediated by defective expression of degs1 impairs adipocyte differentiation and function. *Diabetes* **2015**, *64*, 1180–1192. [CrossRef] [PubMed]
32. Spalding, K.L.; Arner, E.; Westermark, P.O.; Bernard, S.; Buchholz, B.A.; Bergmann, O.; Blomqvist, L.; Hoffstedt, J.; Näslund, E.; Britton, T.; *et al.* Dynamics of fat cell turnover in humans. *Nature* **2008**, *453*, 783–787. [CrossRef] [PubMed]
33. Baglioni, S.; Francalanci, M.; Squecco, R.; Lombardi, A.; Cantini, G.; Angeli, R.; Gelmini, S.; Guasti, D.; Benvenuti, S.; Annunziato, F.; *et al.* Characterization of human adult stem-cell populations isolated from visceral and subcutaneous adipose tissue. *FASEB J.* **2009**, *23*, 3494–3505. [CrossRef] [PubMed]
34. Isakson, P.; Hammarstedt, A.; Gustafson, B.; Smith, U. Impaired preadipocyte differentiation in human abdominal obesity: role of Wnt, tumor necrosis factor-alpha, and inflammation. *Diabetes* **2009**, *58*, 1550–1557. [CrossRef] [PubMed]
35. Cleveland-Donovan, K.; Maile, L.A.; Tsiaras, W.G.; Tchkonia, T.; Kirkland, J.L.; Boney, C.M. IGF-I activation of the AKT pathway is impaired in visceral but not subcutaneous preadipocytes from obese subjects. *Endocrinology* **2010**, *151*, 3752–3763. [CrossRef] [PubMed]
36. Roldan, M.; Macias-Gonzalez, M.; Garcia, R.; Tinahones, F.J.; Martin, M. Obesity short-circuits stemness gene network in human adipose multipotent stem cells. *FASEB J.* **2011**, *25*, 4111–4126. [CrossRef] [PubMed]
37. Sorisky, A.; Gagnon, A.M. Clinical implications of adipose tissue remodelling: Adipogenesis and apoptosis. *Can. J. Diabetes* **2002**, *26*, 232–240.
38. Arner, P.; Spalding, K.L. Fat cell turnover in humans. *Biochem. Biophys. Res. Commun.* **2010**, *396*, 101–104. [CrossRef] [PubMed]
39. Ortega, F.J.; Mayas, D.; Moreno-Navarrete, J.M.; Catalán, V.; Gómez-Ambrosi, J.; Esteve, E.; Rodriguez-Hermosa, J.I.; Ruiz, B.; Ricart, W.; Peral, B.; *et al.* The gene expression of the main lipogenic enzymes is downregulated in visceral adipose tissue of obese subjects. *Obesity* **2010**, *18*, 13–20. [CrossRef] [PubMed]
40. Clemente-Postigo, M.; Queipo-Ortuño, M.I.; Fernandez-Garcia, D.; Gomez-Huelgas, R.; Tinahones, F.J.; Cardona, F. Adipose tissue gene expression of factors related to lipid processing in obesity. *PLoS ONE* **2011**, *6*, e24783. [CrossRef] [PubMed]
41. Cao, Y. Adipose tissue angiogenesis as a therapeutic target for obesity and metabolic diseases. *Nat. Rev. Drug Discov.* **2010**, *9*, 107–115. [CrossRef] [PubMed]

42. Tinahones, F.J.; Coín-Aragüez, L.; Mayas, M.D.; Garcia-Fuentes, E.; Hurtado-Del-Pozo, C.; Vendrell, J.; Cardona, F.; Calvo, R.M; Obregon, M.J.; Bekay, E.L.R. Obesity-associated insulin resistance is correlated to adipose tissue vascular endothelial growth factors and metalloproteinase levels. *BMC Physiol.* **2012**, *12*. [CrossRef] [PubMed]
43. Tinahones, F.J.; Coín-Aragüez, L.; Murri, M.; Oliva-Olivera, W.; Mayas Torres, M.D.; Barbarroja, N.; Gomez-Huelgas, R.; Malagón, M.M.; Bekay, E.L.R. Caspase induction and BCL2 inhibition in human adipose tissue: A potential relationship with insulin signaling alteration. *Diabetes Care* **2013**, *36*, 513–521. [CrossRef] [PubMed]
44. Bluher, S.; Markert, J.; Herget, S.; Yates, T.; Davis, M.; Muller, G.; Waldow, T.; Schwarz, P.E. Who should we target for diabetes prevention and diabetes risk reduction? *Curr. Diabetes Rep.* **2012**, *12*, 147–156. [CrossRef] [PubMed]
45. Mitchell, P.S.; Parkin, R.K.; Kroh, E.M.; Fritz, B.R.; Wyman, S.K.; Pogosova-Agadjanyan, E.L.; Peterson, A.; Noteboom, J.; O'Briant, K.C.; Allen, A.; *et al.* Circulating microRNAs as stable blood-based markers for cancer detection. *Proc. Natl. Acad. Sci. USA* **2008**, *105*, 10513–10518. [CrossRef] [PubMed]
46. Zhang, T.; Lv, C.; Li, L.; Chen, S.; Liu, S.; Wang, C.; Su, B. Plasma miR-126 is a potential biomarker for early prediction of type 2 diabetes mellitus in susceptible individuals. *BioMed Res. Int.* **2013**, *2013*, 6. [CrossRef] [PubMed]
47. Ortega, F.; Lee, D.; Katzmarzyk, P.; Ruiz, J.; Sui, X.; Church, T. The intriguing metabolically healthy but obese phenotype: Cardiovascular prognosis and role of fitness. *Eur. Heart J.* **2013**, *34*, 389–397. [CrossRef] [PubMed]
48. Katzmarzyk, P.; Church, T.; Janssen, I.; Ross, R.; Blair, S. Metabolic syndrome, obesity, and mortality: Impact of cardiorespiratory fitness. *Diabetes Care* **2005**, *28*, 391–397. [CrossRef] [PubMed]
49. Larsson, C.; Krøll, L.; Bennet, L.; Gullberg, B.; Råstam, L.; Lindblad, U. Leisure time and occupational physical activity in relation to obesity and insulin resistance: A population-based study from the Skaraborg Project in Sweden. *Metabolism* **2012**, *61*, 590–598. [CrossRef] [PubMed]
50. Arsenault, B.J.; Côté, M.; Cartier, A.; Lemieux, I.; Després, J.P.; Ross, R.; Earnest, C.P.; Blair, S.N.; Church, T.S. Effect of exercise training on cardiometabolic risk markers among sedentary, but metabolically healthy overweight or obese post-menopausal women with elevated blood pressure. *Atherosclerosis* **2009**, *207*, 530–533. [CrossRef] [PubMed]
51. Janiszewski, P.M.; Ross, R. Effects of weight loss among metabolically healthy obese men and women. *Diabetes Care* **2010**, *33*, 1957–1959. [CrossRef] [PubMed]
52. Karelis, A.; Messier, V.; Brochu, M.; Rabasa-Lhoret, R. Metabolically healthy but obese women: Effect of an energy-restricted diet. *Diabetologia* **2008**, *51*, 1752–1754. [CrossRef] [PubMed]
53. Martínez-González, M.A.; Salas-Salvadó, J.; Estruch, R.; Corella, D.; Fitó, M.; Ros, E. PREDIMED INVESTIGATORS. Benefits of the Mediterranean diet: Insights from the PREDIMED Study. *Prog. Cardiovasc. Dis.* **2015**, *58*, 50–60.
54. Dalzill, C.; Nigam, A.; Juneau, M.; Guilbeault, V.; Latour, E.; Mauriège, P.; Gayda, M. Intensive lifestyle intervention improves cardiometabolic and exercise parameters in metabolically healthy obese and metabolically unhealthy obese in dividuals. *Can. J. Cardiol.* **2014**, *30*, 434–440. [CrossRef] [PubMed]
55. Samaropoulos, X.F.; Hairston, K.G.; Anderson, A.; Haffner, S.M.; Lorenzo, C.; Montez, M. A metabolically healthy obese phenotype in Hispanic participants in the IRAS family study. *Obesity (Silver Spring)* **2013**, *21*, 2303–2309. [CrossRef] [PubMed]
56. Buchwald, H.; Avidor, Y.; Braunwald, E.; Jensen, M.D.; Pories, W.; Fahrbach, K. Bariatric surgery: A systematic review and meta-analysis. *JAMA* **2004**, *292*, 1724–1737. [CrossRef] [PubMed]
57. Hinnouho, G.M.; Czernichow, S.; Dugravot, A.; Nabi, H.; Brunner, E.J.; Kivimaki, M. Metabolically healthy obesity and the risk of cardiovascular disease and type 2 diabetes: The Whitehall II cohort study. *Eur. Heart J.* **2015**, *36*, 551–559. [CrossRef] [PubMed]
58. Hwang, Y.C.; Hayashi, T.; Fujimoto, W.Y.; Kahn, S.E.; Leonetti, D.L.; McNeely, M.J. Visceral abdominal fat accumulation predicts the conversion of metabolically healthy obese subjects to an unhealthy phenotype. *Int. J. Obes.* **2015**, *39*, 1365–1370. [CrossRef] [PubMed]
59. Soriguer, F.; Gutierrez-Repiso, C.; Rubio-Martin, E.; Garcia-Fuentes, E.; Almaraz, M.C.; Colomo, N. Metabolically healthy but obese, a matter of time? Findings from the prospective Pizarra study. *J. Clin. Endocrinol. Metab.* **2013**, *98*, 2318–2325. [CrossRef] [PubMed]

60. Song, Y.; Manson, J.E.; Meigs, J.B.; Ridker, P.M.; Buring, J.E.; Liu, S. Comparison of usefulness of body mass index *versus* metabolic risk factors in predicting 10-year risk of cardiovascular events in women. *Am. J. Cardiol.* **2007**, *100*, 1654–1658. [CrossRef] [PubMed]
61. Meigs, J.B.; Wilson, P.W.; Fox, C.S.; Vasan, R.S.; Nathan, D.M.; Sullivan, L.M. Body mass index, metabolic syndrome, and risk of type 2 diabetes or cardiovascular disease. *J. Clin. Endocrinol. Metab.* **2006**, *91*, 2906–2912. [CrossRef] [PubMed]
62. Calori, G.; Lattuada, G.; Piemonti, L.; Garancini, M.P.; Ragogna, F.; Villa, M. Prevalence, metabolic features, and prognosis of metabolically healthy obese Italian individuals: The Cremona Study. *Diabetes Care* **2011**, *34*, 210–215. [CrossRef] [PubMed]
63. Ogorodnikova, A.D.; Kim, M.; McGinn, A.P.; Muntner, P.; Khan, U.; Wildman, R.P. Incident cardiovascular disease events in metabolically benign obese individuals. *Obesity (Silver Spring)* **2012**, *20*, 651–659. [CrossRef] [PubMed]
64. Arnlov, J.; Ingelsson, E.; Sundstrom, J.; Lind, L. Impact of body mass index and the metabolic syndrome on the risk of cardiovascular disease and death in middle-aged men. *Circulation* **2010**, *121*, 230–236. [CrossRef] [PubMed]
65. Flint, A.J.; Hu, F.B.; Glynn, R.J.; Caspard, H.; Manson, J.E.; Willett, W.C. Excess weight and the risk of incident coronary heart disease among men and women. *Obesity (Silver Spring)* **2010**, *18*, 377–383. [CrossRef] [PubMed]
66. Kramer, C.K.; Zinman, B.; Retnakaran, R. Are metabolically healthy overweight and obesity benign conditions? A systematic review and meta-analysis. *Ann. Intern. Med.* **2013**, *159*, 758–769. [CrossRef] [PubMed]
67. Shaharyar, S.; Roberson, L.L.; Jamal, O.; Younus, A.; Blaha, M.J.; Ali, S.S. Obesity and metabolic phenotypes (metabolically healthy and unhealthy variants) are significantly associated with prevalence of elevated C-reactive protein and hepatic steatosis in a large healthy Brazilian population. *J. Obes.* **2015**, *2015*, 178526. [CrossRef] [PubMed]
68. Eshtiaghi, R.; Keihani, S.; Hosseinpanah, F.; Barzin, M.; Azizi, F. Natural course of metabolically healthy abdominal obese adults after 10 years of follow-up: The Tehran Lipid and Glucose Study. *Int. J. Obes.* **2015**, *39*, 514–519. [CrossRef] [PubMed]
69. Li, S.; Chen, W.; Srinivasan, S.; Xu, J.; Berenson, G. Relation of childhood obesity/cardiometabolic phenotypes to adult cardiometabolic profile: The Bogalusa Heart Study. *Am. J. Epidemiol.* **2012**, *176*, S142–S149. [CrossRef] [PubMed]
70. Dvorak, R.; DeNino, W.; Ades, P.; Poehlman, E. Phenotypic characteristics associated with insulin resistance in metabolically obese but normal-weight young women. *Diabetes* **1999**, *48*, 2210–2214. [CrossRef] [PubMed]
71. Park, J.; Kim, S.; Cho, G.; Baik, I.; Kim, N.; Lim, H. Obesity phenotype and cardiovascular changes. *J. Hypertens.* **2011**, *29*, 1765–1772. [CrossRef] [PubMed]
72. Khan, U.; Wang, D.; Thurston, R.; Sowers, M.; Sutton-Tyrrell, K.; Matthews, K. Burden of subclinical cardiovascular disease in "metabolically benign" and "at-risk" overweight and obese women: The Study of Women's Health Across the Nation (SWAN). *Atherosclerosis* **2011**, *217*, 179–186. [CrossRef] [PubMed]

3

Insights into the Experiences of Treatment for An Eating Disorder in Men: A Qualitative Study of Autobiographies

Priyanka Thapliyal [1,*], Deborah Mitchison [2] and Phillipa Hay [1]

1 Translational Health Research Institute, School of Medicine, Western Sydney University, Building 3.G.P9, Locked Bag 1797, Penrith NSW 2751, Australia; p.hay@ westernsydney.edu.au
2 Centre for Emotional Health, Department of Psychology, Macquarie University, Sydney 2109, Australia; deborah.mitchison@mq.edu.au
* Correspondence: p.thapliyal@westernsydney.edu.au

Academic Editors: Amanda Sainsbury and Felipe Q. da Luz

Abstract: Eating disorders are increasingly recognized as a problem for men but help-seeking is low and little is known about their treatment experiences. This paper sought to determine the treatment experiences of men who have suffered from an eating disorder using autobiographical data. Inclusion criteria were autobiographies of men who had experienced an eating disorder and sought any form of treatment for this, written in the English language, published between 1995 and 2015, and available for purchase in 2016. The search resulted in six books that were thematically analyzed. Analysis of data resulted in two broad themes (1. Positive experiences; 2. Negative experiences) with sub-themes. With regards to the first theme, factors such as concern of staff members, therapist's expertise (in treating eating disorders in men), and a collaborative treatment approach were considered favorable for treatment. In contrast to the first theme, apathy of staff members, the authors' own negative preconceptions, treatment providers being perceived as prioritizing financial concerns, perceived as incompetent and judgmental behavior of therapist(s), and time limitations of sessions were considered unfavorable treatment experiences. In this study, the perceived success of treatment depended on therapist's features and the form of treatment provided. Further research examining these is indicated.

Keywords: eating disorder; men; treatment; experiences

---

1. Introduction

Eating disorders include anorexia nervosa (AN), bulimia nervosa (BN) and binge eating disorder (BED). AN is a condition in which an individual practices extreme food restriction to the point of self-starvation and excessive weight loss. By definition the person is underweight for their age and height. Two subtypes are defined: the restrictive/compulsive exercise and binge-eating/purging types [1]. BN is characterized as a condition in which an individual has episodes of overeating accompanied by a sense of loss of control (binge eating). These are followed by repeated compensatory behaviors that include self-induced vomiting, laxative misuse, excessive exercise, fasting, use of diuretics, and/or other medications to prevent weight gain [1]. BED is characterized as having recurrent and distressing binge eating episodes which may be characterized by eating more rapidly than normal, eating until uncomfortably full, eating large amounts even when not hungry, eating alone because of embarrassment and/or feeling disgusted or guilty after eating [1].

Despite the popular view of these as conditions suffered by women, eating disorders are not rare among men. Raevuori et al. [2] recently conducted a review of eating disorders in men. The paper emphasized the revised Diagnostic and Statistical Manual of Mental Disorders (DSM-5) published in 2013 as an important landmark in recognizing BED alongside AN and BN [1], a disorder almost as prevalent in adult men as in women. Further, the elimination of amenorrhea as a criterion improves conceptual inclusiveness of men with a diagnosis of AN. The overall prevalence of eating disorders in male and female Swedish twins born between 1935 and 1958 was 1.20% in women and 0.29% in men [3] and the lifetime prevalence in Finnish twin men born between 1975 and 1979 was 0.24% [4]. Carlat et al. [5] also conducted a review of prevalence literature and concluded that men account for 10–15% of all bulimic patients, and that 0.2% of all adolescent and young adult men meet strict criteria for BN. Similar prevalence figures have been reported for male patients with AN [6,7]. Hudson et al. [8] conducted a large population-based household survey in the US in 2001–2003 and estimated the lifetime prevalence of DSM-IV AN, BN, and BED as 0.3%, 0.5% and 2.0%, respectively, among men. A similar pattern to that seen in women, with BED prevalence higher than BN which in turn is higher in prevalence than AN, has been reported in men [9]. Despite this, men are excluded from the majority of epidemiological and other research studies, reinforcing the perception of eating disorders as a problem predominantly concerning women, and making it less likely for researchers to design future studies representative of men [10].

There may however be differences between men and women in regards to eating disorder epidemiology. For example, as reported by Mitchison et al. [11] the prevalence of extreme dietary restriction and purging behaviors are increasing at a faster rate in men (2008 vs. 1998 odds ratios = 4.9 and 6.2, respectively) compared to women (odds ratios = 1.7 and 0.9, respectively). While treatment approaches are based on interventions developed for women with eating disorders; there are no male-specific treatment guidelines [12]. Although treatment in predominantly "feminine" environments can be successful for men [13], issues of stigmatization and isolation have also been reported [14,15]. Men may have unique needs, including consideration of masculine identity, gender role conflict and emasculation [16,17]. Further, behavioral manifestations may differ (e.g., more emphasis on muscle-building and exercise in general).

Seeking help for an eating disorder is not common in general, however men with AN and BN have said that their willingness to seek professional help has been further thwarted by societal ideals that include notions of gender-specific illnesses [18]. A quantitative study by Ming et al. [19] evaluated service utilization in men with eating disorders in Singapore. The study reported that a significant proportion of men with an eating disorder had never been hospitalized (62.5%) or enrolled in specialized inpatient/outpatient treatment programs (68.1%). The low rate of treatment-uptake was associated with unwillingness among the men in this study to seek help.

In regard to men who do access treatment, a quantitative study [20] has reported on the experiences of 334 men in a residential center (23% binge/purge type, 24% BN, 23% EDNOS including n = 6 with BED). Overall treatment was reported to be effective. The authors surmised that the men's experiences of treatment did not appear to differ to that observed among women, but no specific similarities were reported. There were also distinctive aspects of the program perceived as particularly relevant to men. These included addressing excessive exercise, body image concerns with muscularity, sexual orientation, sexual identity, and spirituality. This study also emphasized the importance of "male only" group therapy to facilitate discussion of eating disorder symptoms that have been viewed as "female" problems.

In a recent systematic review [21] of qualitative studies exploring the treatment experiences of men with eating disorders, only four papers were eligible for review. Of the four included studies [22–25] only two had a primary focus on men's experiences of treatment [23,24]. Common themes that emerged across the studies were most often related to an understanding of the barriers to help-seeking with less about processes once treatment engagement had occurred. Key themes identified included: (1) delays in seeking treatment; (2) clinical features distinctive to men such as drive for muscularity; (3) feminine and other aspects of treatment services; and (4) a lack of consensus in views about the relevance of gender in treatment. Similarly, in some of the studies the participating men described feeling disappointed with the competency of the help they received and also expressed a wish for their maleness to be recognized when in the treatment setting [26,27].

Similar to studies of females [28,29], two studies [26,27] reported that some males perceived their treatment experience as being unsupportive, with professionals lacking time and experience. Men also reported feeling a loss of power and control when in treatment. The males in this review drew attention to a lack of care providers' appreciation of male issues. Male participants with AN or BN reported that female-oriented treatments for eating disorders were not entirely appropriate for them.

General stigmatization of eating disorders also affects men's treatment experiences. Robinson et al. [24] explored the experiences of men using eating disorder services and identified that the biggest challenge they had faced was admitting to themselves and others that they had an eating disorder and that it was a problem. This may be because of the stereotype that eating disorders only affects women. Similarly, a study by Griffiths et al. [30] supported this premise, as males with eating disorders reported that they were being more frequently stigmatized as "less of a man" than women experienced being stigmatized as "less of a woman".

2. Deficits in Previous Research

Whereas quantitative research aims to assess causal relationships between variables, qualitative research understands truth to be evolving, culturally constructed and derived from an interaction between experience and the human mind [31]. Qualitative methods are particularly suited to understanding a lived experience, as they target underlying processes and meaning that cannot be adequately conveyed in surveys or represented by numbers.

Qualitative literature pertaining to men's experiences of eating disorder treatment is scarce. Historically few men have been included as participants in such research designs. In a systematic review and meta-synthesis of qualitative studies [32] on patients' understanding of eating disorder treatment and recovery, the participants were almost exclusively women. Likewise, Bezance and Holliday [33] identified 11 qualitative studies of adolescents' experiences that included only one paper with a single male participant. In the eating disorder field men are either not being represented at all, or at best, studies have included only very small numbers [34–37]. Other limitations of previous qualitative studies include a narrow focus on a specific eating disorders or subset of eating disorders, such as AN [38] or AN and BN only [39]. This is problematic as we know that men are more likely to experience disorders such as BED, and are over-represented in the residual diagnostic category, Other/Unspecified Feeding or ED. To our knowledge there is no qualitative study to date that has focused primarily on treatment experiences of men with an eating disorder.

3. Aims

Eating disorders in men is an under-researched area, particularly with regards to the exploration of male experiences in treatment. The aim of this present study was to explore the experiences of men who ever had any form of treatment for an eating disorder. Given the relatively unexplored nature of this topic, a qualitative approach was deemed most suitable.

4. Methods

4.1. Study Sample: Men's Eating Disorder Autobiographies

The sample consisted of autobiographical accounts written by men who had experienced an eating disorder. Inclusion criteria were that the book should be an autobiography of a man, who had or has had a treatment experience with an eating disorder. Further, the books were to be written in the English language and published between the years 1995 and 2015.

4.2. Autobiographical Literature Search

Autobiography is referred to as a form of "personal document". At the core of personal document research is the life story—an account of one person's life in his or her own words. For example, oral interviews, testaments, literary biographies, and psychological case studies bring life stories into being that would not otherwise have happened in everyday life [40]. On the other hand, personal documents include "any first-person narrative that describes an individual's actions, experiences and beliefs" [41]. Autobiographies provide a complementary and rich source of qualitative data regarding authors' attitudes, beliefs and views of the world. It reflects the author's perspective, which is what most qualitative research is seeking, and it also provides a subjective account of the situation it records. In addition, autobiography as a source of unsolicited data in our view may reduce one element of investigator bias when compared to other commonly used forms of qualitative data, such as participant interviews, in which the investigator chooses the topic and questions to be posed. Aronson [42] analyzed around 270 book length stories, most written in the past 20 years, and concluded that more men than women write about their illness. He concluded that men write out of a desire to help other patients, and to come to terms with their own illnesses, and also for doctors to have a better understanding of their experiences. Thus men may primarily write to express repressed emotions and create awareness about male mental illness, and less often are driven to write their autobiography out of mercenary motivations.

The search for published autobiographies was conducted using Amazon.com and the keywords were ["biography" AND "man" AND "eating disorders"]. The search resulted in twelve books. Further scrutiny of the texts led to the exclusion of six books: one was written by a mother, two were concerned with recovering from obesity rather than an eating disorder, one was about the presentation of illness narratives, one did not mention treatment experience, and one was a collection of motivational stories on staying young. Additional searches of Booktopia and The Book Depository produced 4 and 31 books respectively, of which none were autobiographies of men with an eating disorder.

5. Procedure

The qualitative method employed was thematic analysis, according to the five phases in the Framework method outlined by Ritchie and Spencer [43] and Pope, Zeibland and Mays [44]. This comprised the following stages:

(1) *Familiarization* (reviewing a subsample of the raw data in detail). This involved the first (PT) and second (DM) authors reading the books two times completely to familiarize themselves with the content and to empathize with the authors.

(2) *Identifying a Thematic Framework*. This involved ascertaining all key issues and themes in the books by drawing both from the research aims and from the data itself. PT and DM undertook this separately and then discussed the themes identified until a consensus was reached on an overarching framework.

(3) *Indexing*. This phase was undertaken by PT and involved systematically applying the agreed upon thematic framework to the data by coding sections of text. Any newly emerging themes were identified and discussed at regular meetings with the other authors, and if agreed, added to the framework.

(4) *Charting*. This involved rearrangement of distilled summaries of the data according to the thematic framework. A thematic tree was formed to highlight the main themes that were identified by the first author (PT).

(5) *Mapping and Interpretation*. This involved finding associations between themes and mapping the range and nature of phenomena to find explanations for the findings. This was carried out by PT and DM with regular review by PH.

6. Results

6.1. Characteristics of Sample

The autobiographies of six men that suffered eating disorders formed the data sample. The age of authors ranged from 25 to 50 years. A brief description of each book follows and is also presented in Table 1.

(1) "Born Round" [45] presents a sufferer's account of binge eating and bulimia nervosa. In this book Frank Bruni describes his helplessness as a man with an eating disorder. Although he realized that he had a problem, it took him years to get help, due to self-stigma and shame. Frank eventually sought help from a therapist, the process of which he describes, and moves forward toward living a life free of binge eating.

(2) "Hiding Under the Table" [46] is authored by Dennis Henning who suffered from BED, BN and AN. This book is written from a recovered perspective and focuses on the barriers experienced in trying to access treatment. Dennis provides an account of his misery as a man who had eating disorder. He desperately tried seeking treatment but often found his gender denied him access. After recovering from his eating issues Dennis pursued his goal to create public awareness about eating disorders. He is also co-founder for the Lifestyle Institute for Eating Disorders.

(3) "Weightless" [47] is an autobiography written by Gary A. Grahl that presents a sufferer's perspective of BED. In this account Greg moves through the process of illness and recovery. Presently, he is involved in creating awareness through his blog JustStopEatingSoMuch.com, which focuses on weight loss and food addiction.

(4) Michael Krasnow authored the autobiography "My Life as a Male Anorexic" [48] from a suffering perspective. He suffered from severe AN and wrote with the intention to help other young people, as well as to assist health professionals to better understand and provide help to sufferers. His account is almost exclusively focused on his experiences in treatment. Michael died three days after writing the final epilogue of this book.

(5) "My Thinning Years" [49] was written by Jon Derek Croteau. In this book he presents an account of how his denial of his own homosexuality led to the development of AN, BN, and other obsessional behavior.

(6) Gary Grahl wrote "The Skinny Boy" [50] and now is a professional counselor in Wisconsin and also a resource person for ANAD (National Association of Anorexia Nervosa and Associated Disorders) in Illinois. The narrative of Skinny Boy is about a young man suffering from AN. In his book Gary described in detail the daily struggles of living with AN and experiences of treatment that he had in the inpatient psychiatric unit of a hospital.

Three of the autobiographies were about men with a history of AN, of which two (The Skinny Boy & My Life as a Male Anorexic) provided details of experiences within eating disorder specific inpatient treatment settings. The other autobiography (My Thinning Years) discussed experiences of outpatient Cognitive Behavioral Therapy. BED was reported in two of the books, where one author discussed outpatient therapy sessions (Weightless) and the other (The Good Eater) did not describe the type of treatment experienced, excepting that it included self-help strategies such as "changing mindset" and exercise. Only one (Hiding Under the Table) author identified himself as suffering from BN and he describes his experiences seeking and receiving treatment from an inpatient rehabilitation center for eating disorders. All of the autobiographies described eating problems that first emerged during childhood. Two of the six authors identified themselves as homosexual. All autobiographies included rich detail about the authors' experiences of suffering from an eating disorder, and all but one included details about the authors' journey to recovery from their eating disorders. Treatment experiences were described in detail in 4 books, where text about treatment appeared on at least 15% of pages. This included two books (The Skinny Boy and My Life as a Male Anorexic), which were almost entirely about the treatment experienced by the authors. The remaining two books focused more about the reasons and situations that led to the eating disorder and discussion of treatment appeared on around 5% of all pages.

The analysis of data resulted in two broad themes. (1) Negative experiences of treatment and (2) Positive experiences of treatment, under which emerged several sub-themes.

Table 1. A brief summary of each of the autobiographies analysed in the study.

Book	Author	Country (Year)	ED Diagnosis	Self-Perceived Status at Writing	Sexual Orientation	Occupation	Age of ED Onset; Duration
Born Round [45]	Frank Bruni	US (2010)	Binge Eating, Bulimia Nervosa	Recovered	Homosexual	Restaurant critic	5 years; 30 years
Hiding Under the Table [46]	Dennis Henning	US (2004)	Binge Eating, Bulimia Nervosa, Anorexia Nervosa	Recovered	Heterosexual	Salesperson	9 years; 30 years
Weightless [47]	Gregg McBride	US (2014)	Binge Eating Disorder	Recovered	Heterosexual	Writer & Producer†	8 years; 23 years
My Life as a Male Anorexic [48]	Michael Krasnow	US (1996)	Anorexia Nervosa	Not Recovered (Later deceased)	Heterosexual	Library staff	15 years; 13 years
My Thinning Years [49]	Jon Derek Croteau	US (2014)	Anorexia Nervosa, Bulimia Nervosa	Recovered	Homosexual	Consultant, Writer & Speaker †	14 years; 18 years
Skinny Boy [50]	Gary A Grahl	US (2007)	Anorexia Nervosa	Recovered	Heterosexual	Professional ED Counsellor †	15 years; 5 years

NB: ED = eating disorder. † Occupation following eating disorder recovery.

6.2. *Negative Experiences of Treatment*

The authors provided many reasons for a negative experience. These included the behavior of the treating staff, negative thoughts and preconceptions of the men themselves, the time constraint of treatment sessions and also a lack of expertise of the health professionals.

(1) Unhelpful Interactions with Health Professionals

Judgmental. Firstly, the perceptions of authors about health professionals being invasive emerged as an important issue, though it was not the case every time. The authors identified that it was quite challenging for them to visit a health professional due to what was perceived as a stigmatized and judgmental stance against the patient. For example, one author mentioned that whenever he visited the doctor he felt as if he was being judged, which heightened his self-consciousness about his weight.

> "I had finally gotten around to selecting and paying a visit to a doctor. I'd neglected it before because I always avoided doctors, whose poking and prodding and above all weighing of me amounted to a judgment I didn't want rendered. Doctors made you stand naked or half naked in front of them." [45] (p. 203)

In the quote above, the author refers to feeling "naked" in front of the doctor, which may be interpreted both literally as well as metaphorically as being exposed. The "prodding" and "poking" referred to also suggests that rather than feeling accepted and understood by the health professional during such exposure, the author felt threatened and critically examined. The attitude of a therapist as being judgmental about the men's past also emerged as a common issue. As described in the account below, the author felt that his own healthy intentions toward therapy and recovery were being thwarted by the judgmental nature of the therapist:

> "I entered an eating disorder clinic. The therapist told me I had to really work on things and share in groups and to take my medications. I felt nervous but open. I rebelled against some groups and a yoga class, so the doctor came to visit me one day. He was very judgmental about my past and what I had done to survive." [46] (p. 65)

Unfriendly Attitude of the Therapist. A few authors described an "unfriendly" attitude of therapists toward them, which was thought to sometimes emanate from an antipathy against males. This type of attitude in a clinical setting plays a particularly important role because the treatment provided, as well as the patient's response to treatment, are influenced by the preconceptions of the therapist, as well as those of the patient.

> "There are people and therapists who want to help others, but who cannot even help themselves. There was this therapist who had issues with men that are not resolved and she became a therapist to help women who suffered like her. It is sad because they still harbor anger toward men and while treating men they are not able to really separate their anger." [46] (p. 83)

Another example of unfriendly and stern behavior is exemplified in this quote by another author, below. This author felt that his attempts to build rapport with his therapist were unsuccessful, which negatively affected the therapeutic relationship.

> "I also didn't like that he never laughed at my jokes and that he always had a stoic expression on his face whenever I explained some of the circumstances of my upbringing. Where was this guy's compassion? Didn't he knows I was a victim and unable to help myself? That none of this was my fault?" [47] (p. 163)

(2) Thoughts and Behaviors Impeding Treatment

Apart from the attitude and behavior of health professionals, the mindset of the person in treatment is very crucial for a positive outcome. The analysis of data found that sometimes it was the preformed notions of patients that negatively affected treatment outcomes, such that they were slow to engage in therapy.

Low expectations of therapists. Authors sometimes described unhelpful negative beliefs about therapy and therapists that influenced their attempts to seek and engage in treatment. The following excerpt from an autobiography indicates the self-assertive thinking of an author along with denigration of the health professionals.

> "I went into rehab knowing—and I mean knowing—that I knew it all and that the professionals there did not know jack shit." [46] (p. 177)

Similarly, an unsparing disclosure by one of the authors demonstrated the extent of the negative perceptions of treatment providers that may occur. The author in the following excerpt claims that psychiatric help is of no use.

> "Psychiatrists and psychiatric hospitals are pointless, if not detrimental." [48] (p. 52)

Such beliefs are likely formed on the basis of prior experience, however clearly place individuals in a position "against" rather than "in alliance" with the treatment team even before treatment commences.

High expectations of therapists. In contrast to the low expectations of the competencies of health providers, sometimes it was the patients' overly high expectations of health professionals, and the health professionals' subsequent inability to fulfill such expectations, that led to negative treatment experiences. An author, who was severely ill with AN in particular used the term "miracle workers" for therapists/doctors and reported that while initially he thought highly of doctors, over time, as he did not recover, they were viewed less favorably.

> "To us doctors were miracle workers. We had the incorrect belief that when you go to a doctor with your problem, he can solve it with a snap of his fingers." [48] (p. 11)

This alternating idealizing and demeaning of health professionals may be symptomatic of an unhealthy attachment or interpersonal style, which serves to create strain and distance in the therapeutic relationship, and thus hinder recovery.

Self-sabotaging. The authors of the autobiographies wrote that they felt that they were being judged within treatment centers, and were not well understood by others, including staff and other patients. This often resulted in unhelpful or self-sabotaging behavior in an attempt to have their need for acceptance met. In one instance an author recalled how he intentionally lied to a therapist in order to gain acceptance from him:

> "Jeff asked me to tell the truth during our first meeting and I thought that even though I was in a rehab and they were there to help me, he would think that I was a freak, a loser, unworthy of love, a pathetic excuse for a human being. I thought I had to lie to him to be accepted, so I lied." [46] (p. 167)

(3) Therapist Limitations

In continuation to the first theme of author's perception about the treatment providers' behavior, their knowledge regarding eating disorders and their expertise in the field as perceived by the men in this study emerged as a significant issue. All the authors unanimously acknowledged the expertise of therapists as an important factor in determining their treatment outcomes.

Lack of expertise in treating eating disorders. Perceived incompetency of therapists emerged as an important and critical issue in the study. After a person becomes sure that he is suffering from a health problem, the primary concern becomes the need for it to be resolved. In the case of an eating disorder this is not always simple, as exemplified in the following quote in which an author reported the inadequacy and unavailability of accurate treatment in men:

> "Some places tell me that they have a program for men, but the truth is they have no idea how to work with men, nor do they understand the differences between men and women who had eating disorders." [46] (p. 80)

The same author further added that the claims made by treatment centers that they were capable of treating eating disorders in men were false and there is a notable scarcity of centers that know how to treat a man with eating disorder.

> "Until this stay I had seen eight different professionals who tried to help me and at the same time only two knew how to work with someone who suffered from an eating disorder." [46] (p. 67)

Contradictory to his expectations that treatment providers would understand eating disorder issues, one author reported feeling misunderstood by the staff. Perceptions that eating disorders occur in women only may explain such disregard of the male author's symptoms.

> "The doctor and nurses made me feel as if I was crazy. None of them asked why I'd dropped so much weight." [49] (p. 172)

The experience of rehabilitation for men varied. One of the authors described his rehabilitation stay as a "real eye-opener" because of the conduct displayed by the staff members.

> "The one thing that was really an eye opener was to me in my last stay in rehab is that the people treating me were no healthier than I was." [46] (p. 67)

Ignorance of eating disorders in men. Furthermore, another author declared the therapist as ignorant and unaware of the occurrence of eating disorders in men. Interestingly, this author, who was severely underweight at the time, discussed how even though he was displaying excessive distress about fatness, the health professionals did not assess him for an eating disorder. To this author, such an experience spoke to the dismissal of the fact that eating disorders exist in men:

> "I was freaking out about how much fat was in the intravenous fluids they were giving me, but ironically, it never occurred to anyone to ask whether I had any kind of eating issues. It probably never occurred to them that a male could be anorexic. Even though I told the doctor I was running twelve miles or more a day on a bowl of cereal or a bagel and a handful of fat burners, he never asked about an eating disorder." [49] (p. 172)

Money-mindedness. Half of the men mentioned the money-mindedness of therapists. They quoted many instances where they felt their individual needs were neglected because the therapist prioritized monetary gains. This finding was similar, irrespective of the place of treatment (e.g., residential care, inpatient setting, or counseling session). The following excerpt clearly stated the frustration and misery of an author in this regard:

> "He was getting paid around sixty dollars per hour and we were staring at each other. That's all. No talking. I frequently told my parents that I wanted to stop seeing Dr P. He did not help and was a complete waste of time. I could be wrong but I believe he was more interested in money than anything else (either that or he was totally incompetent)." [48] (p. 24)

Ineffective Communication. Staff members have a critical role in the treatment setting of a clinic or hospital. According to the majority of authors the staff members were expected to be more authoritative, as opposed to authoritarian, in order to bring a subtle and long-lasting change in their behavior. For example in the following quote the author wished to have a tangible plan for recovery.

> "I needed something more concrete, something that was going to hold me accountable and responsible for my behaviors and actions." [46] (p. 170)

(4) Feeling Ostracized as a Man

By staff members. The role of staff members in the treatment setting was duly acknowledged. Being a man with an eating disorder is itself very challenging. A few men in treatment reported feeling unwanted in the treatment setting by the staff members due to their male gender.

> "Some of the staff had a problem with a male in the group and they did not have a problem letting me know." [46] (p. 67)

By other patients. Some men in treatment described feeling misunderstood and targeted by the prejudiced behavior of female patients towards men. For example, one author stated that women in the group could not accommodate his presence and wanted him to leave because they had some personal issues with men in their lives:

> "The meetings I first went to were all women and young girls - maybe a man once in a while. In these meetings, I was looked at as an outsider. In one OA (Overeaters Anonymous) meeting, a woman went as far as to ask me to leave because they had issues with men in their lives and a man in group was hard for them to deal with." [46] (p. 170)

(5) Treatment Side Effects

Two out of six authors wrote that antidepressants and electroconvulsive therapy were deleterious to their health. In particular, authors discussed unwanted side effects and/or ineffectiveness of medication:

> "Dr C prescribed antidepressant medication. Some were stopped because of side effects, such as drowsiness, light-headedness, fidgetiness (the most bothersome - like the jitters), and uncontrollable shaking. Others were stopped because they had no effect one way or the other." [48] (p. 11)

> "Prozac hadn't given me the speedy buzz it gave some people. It had given me the opposite: a gauzy lethargy." [45] (p. 200)

One author who described his treatment with electroconvulsive therapy, reported concern regarding memory loss that occurred following therapy:

> "One of the possible side effects of ECT is memory loss and this was the most prevalent result of my treatment." [48] (p. 11)

6.3. Positive Experiences of Treatment

The autobiographies focused very seldom on positive, as opposed to negative, treatment experiences. However in contrast to negative experiences, which were at times a result of the author's own thoughts and behaviors, it is interesting to note that the factors that were considered as positive in treatment were usually external, such as the behavior of staff members in hospital, therapists, or other patients in the treatment center.

(1) Therapist

Non-judgmental empathic behavior. Three of the six authors described non-judgmental behavior of therapists as an important positive experience in treatment. For example, one of the men felt encouraged to continue his therapy sessions because of the uncritical attitude of the therapist. In fact, he admitted that he actually liked being in her company.

> "She was the first therapist who took the time to help me and not judge me. I liked seeing her and listening to her." [46] (p. 92)

When the authors of the autobiographies perceived that the health professional was being empathic, this was important to them in regarding the treatment as positive. This is opposed to the negative treatment experience themes discussed above where the therapist was perceived as being judgmental or unfriendly. Thus, an understanding nature, non-judgmental behavior, and a caring and gentle attitude were therapist qualities that were discussed by authors as contributing to the success of their treatment. The following quote reflects on how a therapist who had a gentle nature was appreciated.

> "He had a careful, gentle way of helping me, as if he were carefully removing a bandage that had covered a massive wound for years. He didn't tear it off; he pulled back the adhesive slowly but steadily." [49] (pp. 228–229)

Expertise. The therapist had a very important role in defining the treatment outcome. Trust in the treatment aligned with the perceived expertise of the health professional, as exemplified in the following quote:

> "Once I started to work with the idea that the therapists knew more than I did at the same time, and I began to trust their input in my life, I began to trust myself and how I really felt." [46] (p. 86)

Interestingly, this theme appears to be in contrast to the negative treatment experience theme where authors described how their preconceptions of the treatment providers' incompetence at times sabotaged their ability to engage in therapy. Other authors acknowledged the expertise of therapists in helping them to address their symptoms.

> "I learned from Jeff R. and Jeff S. how to look at situations and handle them from a positive and realistic point of view, rather than turning to food, sex or the other dysfunctional behaviors I turned to as treatment for my emotional pain." [46] (p. 167)

Effective communication style. The adage that "one rule applies to all" defies for eating disordered patients, as is evident from the varied views presented by the authors regarding the style of communication they preferred from their treatment providers. Whereas some authors described a desire for a "tough" approach from their therapist, others clearly desired a more gentle approach. This demonstrates the need for therapists to assess the communication and relationship needs of their clients in informing their own interaction style.

Under the "non-judgmental" theme above, an example is provided of an author who appreciated a gentle and slow approach from his therapist: "*carefully removing a bandage*". On the other hand, for several of the authors, an authoritative nature of the doctor was considered as a welcoming effort to men in treatment. Perhaps this approach instilled confidence in the men, or gave them the permission to relinquish control over their eating to an authoritative figure. The metaphor of the bandage is used again here.

> "I have to admit that it was some of the best (and toughest) therapy I'd ever received. I'm not knocking whatever kind of therapy may work for someone else. But for me, this quick, tough love, rip-off-the-bandage-fast approach was really powerful." [47] (p. 168)

> "Dr X was making a major difference in my life. After he had earned my trust, he challenged me and never let me off easy. I liked that he pushed me." [49] (p. 263)

(2) Effect of Others in Hospital

Staff members. The role of staff members as being friendly and considerate had an important influence in forming the treatment experience as positive. One of the men in this study stated that being able to accept help from staff proved beneficial to him.

> "I have learned to let people into my life and trust them to help me, rather than to try to do everything alone and fail." [46] (p. 188)

Other patients. In addition to this, the supportive nature of group members emerged as a positive aspect of treatment.

> "We listen. We share pain and heartache. We ask questions. We empathize without feeling sorry for each other. We find the support to heal and gather strength to go on." [50] (p. 95)

(3) Treatment forms

There was lack of consensus in men with regards to the most effective form of treatment provided for an eating disorder.

Group therapy vs. individual therapy. In a hospital, the usual form of treatment includes medicine, counseling sessions, group therapy and behavioral therapy. In most of the instances being a part of group therapy was considered as an effective measure by the authors while in treatment. This could be attributed to the fact that talking about their eating disorder openly in group with other members with similar issues provided a sense of normalization and empathy. The following extract clearly outlines the perceived benefits of group therapy:

> "Sitting there in groups and slowly discussing my issues with a mind open for feedback made it easier to confront my fears, shame, guilt, anger, low, low, low self-esteem, self-hatred, and lack of self-respect. I no longer believed I had to hide and numb my pain." [46] (p. 175)

In contrast to this, other authors reported that they felt more supported in individual therapy. For example, in the following excerpt the author clearly stated that he felt safe and secure in therapy sessions where he does not have to acknowledge the presence of others as in group therapy:

> "I preferred the quiet safety and the anonymity of the one-on-one therapy." [49] (p. 213)

This clearly indicates that understanding the individual needs of men is central to tailoring an effective treatment regime.

Cognitive Behavioral Therapy. The effectiveness of treatment provided was frequently the primary concern of these men when discussing treatment experiences. In the majority of cases, cognitive behavioral therapy was followed and this approach was perceived as helpful.

> "After months of gaining my trust and respect through listening to my story, and understanding my past to help me move forward, she introduced me to cognitive behavioral therapy. This approach and other tools she gave me were meant to help me notice the behaviors I was engaging in and stop them." [49] (p. 214)

(4) Hospital Environment

The general atmosphere of the hospital environment was also mentioned as important. Although at times isolating, as reflected by one of the men, this characteristic of hospitalization was appreciated. This may in part be due to a desire to maintain control of the eating disorder, which may be threatened by the interference of others, as expressed here:

> "This hospital thing will fit my lifestyle quite nicely since I've recently become allergic to people. Social interaction makes me break out in a terrible rash called guilt; I simply can't seem to please enough people, no matter how hard I try." [50] (p. 9)

Maintaining a restrictive-type eating disorder requires significant self-control and determination, which is taxing for an individual. Quite a few men mentioned that being hospitalized provided temporary relief from this self-imposed control, which could be relinquished to staff.

"My feelings about the hospital were similar to those I had when I was taken out of the school. Deep down I think that I wanted to be hospitalized. It was a relief. Again it was a control issue." [48] (p. 14)

7. Discussion

The present study examined the treatment experiences of men who had or have had an eating disorder and engaged in any form of treatment. The analysis found that the factors that most commonly contributed to a negative experience were judgmental behavior of professionals and their perceived lack of expertise. The findings regarding the judgmental behavior of health professionals are commensurate with those reported in previous studies by women [28,29]. Additional themes also emerged however, such as the ulterior motives of therapists, like money-mindedness. Though financial cost of treatment had been discussed earlier [51–54], the putative "mercenary" attitudes of therapists has not been cited previously. Unexpectedly, a few of the men reported an antipathy of female practitioners towards them in treatment. This biased treatment was made sense of by the authors who assumed that some female practitioners had unresolved conflicts with men in their own lives and projected these towards the males they encountered in their treatment centers. All the negative experiences encountered by males thwarted their further engagement in therapy, as has been reported by women in other studies [55]. In contrast, an empathizing nature, non-judgmental behavior, good understanding and expertise with eating disorders in men, and a trustworthy relationship with the health professional formulated a positive experience of treatment. This finding is in consensus with studies in women [28].

Interestingly, the study found that sometimes men's own thoughts and behaviors impacted on treatment experiences. For example, having very high expectations of the therapist as a "miracle worker" led to disappointment when treatment was not progressing. Also, one author reported intentionally misleading therapists at times, to the detriment of their own outcomes. This self-sabotaging behavior may have occurred due to a fear of criticism, or a fear of losing the perceived positive aspects of an eating disorder, indicative of a lack of readiness to change [55]. Also, it was interesting that sometimes different approaches were preferred, for example some preferred a female therapist while others had no issues with the gender of the therapist. This highlights the importance of individualized or person-centered care [24] and increased availability of male providers.

In treatment, the role of group members and staff was recognized as important by the men in the present study and consistent with men reporting feelings of isolation in prior studies [14]. The study identified that men in the present study felt misunderstood and unwanted by staff members [26,27]. Some authors endorsed the desire for healthcare staff to be authoritative (expressing confidence in their expertise) but to also provide an equal distribution of power and to be empathic and friendly. Feminization of the disorder in society by referring it as women's disease or a "gay problem" [18] and also the stigma attached to men with eating disorders discouraged the male authors in this study to seek help [24,30]. Also, the sexuality of the authors was not a major theme as only 2 of 6 was identified as homosexual.

The study supports the limited literature that treatment approaches should consider men also and not only women [12]. However, it should be acknowledged that there are efforts being made to improve the situation and to provide educational material (e.g., videos) to clinicians. Examples include ways to ask questions to men about their eating patterns and exercise as described by Hildebrandt and Craigen [56].

In this study, there was a gender disparity in the number of treatment centers available to the men and there appeared to be a deficit in male-only treatment facilities. The men in treatment had varied opinions about the form of therapy. However, the majority of them promoted group therapy because of the supportive environment experienced within the group, as stated by Weltzin et al., [20]. In contrast to group therapy, there were few that reported positive experiences within individual therapy. Regarding the environment of the hospital, there was no consensus, as some pointed to the "stillness" of hospital as scary, whereas others preferred the isolation of the unit as a way to escape societal pressures. For these latter authors, the ability to relinquish control to hospital staff members in regards to diet and exercise schedules was experienced as a temporary relief from the pressures of the eating disorder.

8. Strengths and Limitations

Strengths of the study include autobiographical accounts of the men with eating disorders about their treatment experiences and broad inclusion criteria of all forms of eating disorders. Further strengths include that a systematic search was employed to identify autobiographies; two investigators read the autobiographies and coded themes, increasing the validity of the emergent themes; and the coding of themes by the authors continued until saturation was achieved. However, this study also has some limitations including: the very small sample size that consisted of a highly specific group of men who (1) decided to write an autobiography about their experiences and (2) found a publisher for it; selection of autobiographies to one language (English); and defined dates (years 1995–2015). It is possible that relevant autobiographies in other languages and/or from different (non-Western) cultures, or other time periods were missed. In addition the study did not include men younger than 18 years of age, so it was not possible to discuss how this age group reflect on their treatment experiences. On the other hand, all authors included in this study wrote about their childhood and adolescent experiences of eating disorder symptoms. In addition, while two authors who identified as homosexual were included in this study, it is possible that the treatment experiences of men with varied sexual identities differ and it would be relevant to include more men with homosexual or transgender identities in future studies. Autobiographies are also limited in that there are unknown motivations for writing (including income from royalties) although research [42] suggests several altruistic motivations for men who write about an eating disorder such as AN. Thus, it would be also important to follow this research with larger samples and with face-to-face interviews that would support the validity of these preliminary findings. Finally, while all authors wrote about treatment experience in the US, people's experiences may differ in other countries where health care services are government-funded, and where doctors are salaried (e.g., there may be less perceived "money mindedness" of the doctors).

9. Conclusions

This is the first study that used autobiographical accounts of men with eating disorders to understand their treatment experiences. The study identified that the behaviors and attitudes of both treatment providers and male patients may influence the outcome of treatment defining it as a positive or negative experience. Furthermore, the study provides a platform for designing further research and consideration of treatment strategies with a primary focus on attending to patients' perspectives. In particular, the findings highlight the importance of specialized expertise and a non-judgmental understanding in healthcare providers caring for men with eating disorders. Pre-treatment strategies aimed at educating patients as to expectations of treatment, and practitioner training interventions may be helpful to address barriers to positive treatment experiences.

Acknowledgments: Financial support was provided to PT from a Western Sydney University doctoral scholarship.

Author Contributions: P.H. designed the study. Data collection, analysis and interpretation was done by P.T. and D.M. P.T. drafted the article that is critically revised by D.M. and P.H. All the authors (P.T., D.M. and P.H.) gave their approval to publish this article.

References

1. American Psychiatric Association. *Diagnostic and Statistical Manual of Mental Disorders (DSM-5®)*; American Psychiatric Pub: Arlington, VA, USA, 2013.
2. Raevuori, A.; Keski-Rahkonen, A.; Hoek, H.W. A review of eating disorders in males. *Curr. Opin. Psychiatry* **2014**, 27, 426–430. [CrossRef] [PubMed]

3. Bulik, C.M.; Sullivan, P.F.; Tozzi, F.; Furberg, H.; Lichtenstein, P.; Pedersen, N.L. Prevalence, heritability, and prospective risk factors for anorexia nervosa. *Arch. Gen. Psychiatry* **2006**, *63*, 305–312. [CrossRef] [PubMed]
4. Keski-Rahkonen, A.; Hoek, H.W.; Susser, E.S.; Linna, M.S.; Sihvola, E.; Raevuori, A.; Bulik, C.M.; Kaprio, J.; Rissanen, A. Epidemiology and course of anorexia nervosa in the community. *Am. J. Psychiatry* **2007**, *164*, 1259–1265. [CrossRef] [PubMed]
5. Carlat, D.J.; Camargo, C.A., Jr.; Herzog, D.B. Eating disorders in males: A report on 135 patients. *Am. J. Psychiatry* **1997**, *154*, 1127. [PubMed]
6. Hall, A.; Delahunt, J.W.; Ellis, P.M. Anorexia nervosa in the male: Clinical features and follow-up of nine patients. *J. Psychiatr. Res.* **1985**, *19*, 315–321. [CrossRef]
7. Crisp, A.H.; Burns, T.; Bhat, A.V. Primary anorexia nervosa in the male and female: A comparison of clinical features and prognosis. *Psychol. Psychother. Theory Res. Pract.* **1986**, *59*, 123–132. [CrossRef]
8. Hudson, J.I.; Hiripi, E.; Pope, H.G.; Kessler, R.C. The prevalence and correlates of eating disorders in the National Comorbidity Survey Replication. *Biol. Psychiatry* **2007**, *61*, 348–358. [CrossRef] [PubMed]
9. Taylor, J.Y.; Caldwell, C.H.; Baser, R.E.; Faison, N.; Jackson, J.S. Prevalence of eating disorders among Blacks in the National Survey of American Life. *Int. J. Eat. Disord.* **2007**, *40*, S10–S14. [CrossRef] [PubMed]
10. Striegel, R.H.; Bedrosian, R.; Wang, C.; Schwartz, S. Why men should be included in research on binge eating: results from a comparison of psychosocial impairment in men and women. *Int. J. Eat. Disord.* **2012**, *45*, 233–240. [CrossRef] [PubMed]
11. Mitchison, D.; Hay, P.; Slewa-Younan, S.; Mond, J. The changing demographic profile of eating disorder behaviors in the community. *BMC Public Health* **2014**, *14*, 943. [CrossRef] [PubMed]
12. National Collaborating Centre for Mental Health. *Eating Disorders: Core Interventions in the Treatment and Management of Anorexia Nervosa, Bulimia Nervosa and Related Eating Disorders*; British Psychological Society: Leicester, UK, 2004.
13. Woodside, D.B.; Kaplan, A.S. Day hospital treatment in males with eating disorders—Response and comparison to females. *J. Psychosom. Res.* **1994**, *38*, 471–475. [CrossRef]
14. Andersen, A.E.; Holman, J.E. Males with eating disorders: Challenges for treatment and research. *Psychopharmacol. Bull.* **1997**, *33*, 391. [CrossRef] [PubMed]
15. Weltzin, T.E.; Weisensel, N.; Franczyk, D.; Burnett, K.; Klitz, C.; Bean, P. Eating disorders in men: Update. *J. Men's Health Gend.* **2005**, *2*, 186–193. [CrossRef]
16. Fernández-Aranda, F.; Krug, I.; Jiménez-Murcia, S.; Granero, R.; Núñez, A.; Penelo, E.; Solano, R.; Treasure, J. Male eating disorders and therapy: A controlled pilot study with one year follow-up. *J. Behav. Ther. Exp. Psychiatry* **2009**, *40*, 479–486. [CrossRef] [PubMed]
17. Greenberg, S.T.; Schoen, E.G. Males and eating disorders: Gender-based therapy for eating disorder recovery. *Prof. Psychol. Res. Pract.* **2008**, *39*, 464. [CrossRef]
18. Olivardia, R.; Pope, H.G., Jr.; Borowiecki, J.J., III; Cohane, G.H. Biceps and Body Image: The Relationship Between Muscularity and Self-Esteem, Depression, and Eating Disorder Symptoms. *Psychol. Men Masc.* **2004**, *5*, 112. [CrossRef]
19. Ming, T.S.; Lin Miao Shan, P.; Kuek Shu Cen, A.; Lian, L.E.; Boon Swee Kim, E. Men do get it: Eating disorders in males from an asian perspective. *ASEAN J. Psychiatry* **2014**, *15*, 72–82.
20. Weltzin, T.E.; Cornella-Carlson, T.; Fitzpatrick, M.E.; Kennington, B.; Bean, P.; Jefferies, C. Treatment issues and outcomes for males with eating disorders. *Eat. Disord.* **2012**, *20*, 444–459. [CrossRef] [PubMed]
21. Thapliyal, P.; Hay, P.J. Treatment experiences of males with an eating disorder: A systematic review of qualitative studies. *Transl. Dev. Psychiatry* **2014**, 2. [CrossRef]
22. De Beer, Z.; Wren, B. Eating Disorders in Males. In *Eating and its Disorders*; Fox, J.R.E., Goss, K.P., Eds.; John Wiley & Sons, Ltd.: Chichester, UK, 2012.
23. Dearden, A.; Mulgrew, K.E. Service provision for Men with eating issues in Australia: An analysis of Organisations', Practitioners', and Men's experiences. *Aust. Soc. Work* **2013**, *66*, 590–606. [CrossRef]
24. Robinson, K.J.; Mountford, V.A.; Sperlinger, D.J. Being men with eating disorders: Perspectives of male eating disorder service-users. *J. Health Psychol.* **2013**, *18*, 176–186. [CrossRef] [PubMed]
25. Drummond, M.J. Men, body image, and eating disorders. *Int. J. Men's Health.* **2002**, *1*, 89. [CrossRef]
26. Drummond, M. Life as a male 'anorexic'. *Aust. J. Prim. Health* **1999**, *5*, 80–89. [CrossRef]
27. Copperman, J. *Eating Disorders in the United Kingdom: Review of the Provision of Health Care Services for Men with Eating Disorders*; Eating Disorders Association Norwich: Norwich, UK, 2000.

28. Evans, E.J.; Hay, P.J.; Mond, J.; Paxton, S.J.; Quirk, F.; Rodgers, B.; Jhajj, A.K.; Sawoniewska, M.A. Barriers to help-seeking in young women with eating disorders: A qualitative exploration in a longitudinal community survey. *Eat. Disord.* **2011**, *19*, 270–285. [CrossRef] [PubMed]
29. Rich, E. Anorexic dis (connection): Managing anorexia as an illness and an identity. *Sociol. Health Illn.* **2006**, *28*, 284–305. [CrossRef] [PubMed]
30. Griffiths, S.; Mond, J.M.; Murray, S.B.; Touyz, S. The prevalence and adverse associations of stigmatization in people with eating disorders. *Int. J. Eat. Disord.* **2015**, *48*, 767–774. [CrossRef] [PubMed]
31. Marchel, C.; Owens, S. Qualitative research in psychology: Could William James get a job? *Hist. Psychol.* **2007**, *10*, 301. [CrossRef] [PubMed]
32. Espindola, C.R.; Blay, S.L. Anorexia nervosa's meaning to patients: A qualitative synthesis. *Psychopathology* **2009**, *42*, 69–80. [CrossRef] [PubMed]
33. Bezance, J.; Holliday, J. Adolescents with anorexia nervosa have their say: A review of qualitative studies on treatment and recovery from anorexia nervosa. *Eur. Eat. Disord. Rev.* **2013**, *21*, 352–360. [CrossRef] [PubMed]
34. Lamb, J.; Bower, P.; Rogers, A.; Dowrick, C.; Gask, L. Access to mental health in primary care: A qualitative meta-synthesis of evidence from the experience of people from 'hard to reach' groups. *Health* **2012**, *16*, 76–104. [CrossRef] [PubMed]
35. Tierney, S. The individual within a condition: A qualitative study of young people's reflections on being treated for anorexia nervosa. *J. Am. Psychiatr. Nurses Assoc.* **2008**, *13*, 368–375. [CrossRef] [PubMed]
36. Nakamura, H. Overcoming bulimia nervosa: A qualitative study of recovery in Japan. *Proceedings* **2012**, *17*, 101–109.
37. Reid, M.; Burr, J.; Williams, S.; Hammersley, R. Eating disorders patients' views on their disorders and on an outpatient service: A qualitative study. *J. Health Psychol.* **2008**, *13*, 956–960. [CrossRef] [PubMed]
38. Hay, P.J.; Cho, K. A qualitative exploration of influences on the process of recovery from personal written accounts of people with anorexia nervosa. *Women Health* **2013**, *53*, 730–740. [CrossRef] [PubMed]
39. Malson, H.; Finn, D.; Treasure, J.; Clarke, S.; Anderson, G. Constructing 'The Eating Disordered Patient' 1: A discourse analysis of accounts of treatment experiences. *J. Community Appl. Soc. Psychol.* **2004**, *14*, 473–489. [CrossRef]
40. Plummer, K. *Documents of Life 2: An Invitation to A Critical Humanism*; Sage: Newcastle upon Tyne, UK, 2001; Volume 2.
41. Bogdan, R.C.; Biklen, S.K. *Qualitative Research for Education*; Allyn and Bacon: Boston, MA, USA, 1992.
42. Aronson, J.K. Autopathography: The patient's tale. *Br. Med. J.* **2000**, *321*, 1599. [CrossRef]
43. Ritchie, J.; Spencer, L.; Bryman, A.; Burgess, R. *Analysing Qualitative Data*; Routledge: London, UK, 1994.
44. Pope, C.; Ziebland, S.; Mays, N. Analysing qualitative data. *Br. Med. J.* **2000**, *320*, 114. [CrossRef]
45. Bruni, F. *Born Round: The Story of Family Food and a Ferocious Appetite*; Penguin Book: New York, NY, USA, 2009.
46. Henning, D.; Woods, P. *Hiding Under the Table*; Americana Publishing Inc.: Albuquerque, NM, USA, 2004.
47. McBride, G. *Weightless: My Life as a Fat Man and How I Escaped*; Central Recovery Press: Las Vegas, NV, USA, 2014.
48. Krasnow, M. *My Life as a Male Anorexic*; Harrington Park Press: New York, NY, USA, 1996.
49. Croteau, J.D. *My Thinning Years: Starving the Gay Within*; Hazelden Publishing: Center City, MN, USA, 2014.
50. Grahl, G.A. *The Skinny Boy: A Young Man's Battle and Triumph over Anorexia*; American Legacy Media: Clearfield, UT, USA, 2007.
51. Becker, A.E.; Franko, D.L.; Nussbaum, K.; Herzog, D.B. Secondary prevention for eating disorders: The impact of education, screening, and referral in a college-based screening program. *Int. J. Eat. Disord.* **2004**, *36*, 157–162. [CrossRef] [PubMed]
52. Hepworth, N.; Paxton, S.J. Pathways to help-seeking in bulimia nervosa and binge eating problems: A concept mapping approach. *Int. J. Eat. Disord.* **2007**, *40*, 493–504. [CrossRef] [PubMed]
53. Escobar-Koch, T.; Banker, J.D.; Crow, S.; Cullis, J.; Ringwood, S.; Smith, G.; van Furth, E.; Westin, K.; Schmidt, U. Service users' views of eating disorder services: An international comparison. *Int. J. Eat. Disord.* **2010**, *43*, 549–559. [CrossRef] [PubMed]
54. National Eating Disorder Association, 2015. Available online: http://www.nationaleatingdisorders.org/ (accessed on 13 September 2016).

55. Leavey, G.; Vallianatou, C.; Johnson-Sabine, E.; Rae, S.; Gunputh, V. Psychosocial barriers to engagement with an eating disorder service: A qualitative analysis of failure to attend. *Eat. Disord.* **2011**, *19*, 425–440. [CrossRef] [PubMed]
56. Hildebrandt, T.; Craigen, K. Eating-Related Pathology in Men and Boys. In *Handbook of Assessment and Treatment of Eating Disorders*; Walsh, B.T., Attia, E., Glasofer, D.R., Sysko, R., Eds.; American Psychiatric Publishing, Inc.: Arlington, VA, USA, 2015; Chapter 6, pp. 105–118.

4

Perceived Family Functioning in Relation to Energy Intake in Adolescent Girls with Loss of Control Eating

Manuela Jaramillo [1,2], Natasha L. Burke [3], Lauren B. Shomaker [4], Sheila M. Brady [1], Merel Kozlosky [5], Jack A. Yanovski [1] and Marian Tanofsky-Kraff [1,2,*]

1 Section on Growth and Obesity, *Eunice Kennedy Shriver* National Institute of Child Health and Human Development (NICHD), National Institutes of Health (NIH), DHHS, 10 Center Drive, Bethesda, MD 20892-1103, USA; Manuela.Jaramillo@nih.gov (M.J.); BradyS@mail.nih.gov (S.M.B.); jy15i@nih.gov (J.A.Y.)
2 Department of Medical and Clinical Psychology, Uniformed Services University of the Health Sciences (USUHS), 4301 Jones Bridge Road, Bethesda, MD 20814, USA
3 Department of Psychology, Fordham University, 411 East Fordham Road, Bronx, NY 10458, USA; NBurke12@fordham.edu
4 Department of Human Development and Family Studies, Colorado State University, 303 Behavioral Sciences Building, 1570 Campus Delivery, Fort Collins, CO 80523, USA, Lauren.Shomaker@colostate.edu
5 Nutrition Department, Clinical Center, NIH, DHHS, 10 Center Drive, Bethesda, MD 20892, USA; KozloskyM@cc.nih.gov
* Correspondence: Marian.Tanofsky-Kraff@usuhs.edu

Abstract: Family functioning is hypothesized to influence the development, maintenance, and treatment of obesity and eating disorders. However, there are limited data examining family functioning in relation to energy intake in the laboratory among youth at high-risk for eating disorders and excess weight gain. Therefore, we examined the relationship between perceived family functioning and energy intake during a laboratory test meal designed to model a binge episode. We performed hierarchical multiple regression analyses among 108 adolescent girls in an excess weight gain prevention trial. Participants were at high-risk for eating disorders and excess weight gain due to reports of loss of control eating (LOC) and high body mass index (BMI). Participants completed the Family Adaptability and Cohesion Scale III to assess family adaptability and cohesion. Following an overnight fast, girls consumed lunch from a laboratory test meal. Poorer family adaptability, but not cohesion, was associated with lower percentage of total energy intake from protein and greater percentage of total energy intake from carbohydrates. Neither adaptability nor cohesion were significantly associated with total intake. We conclude that among girls with LOC eating and high BMI, poor reported family adaptability is associated with greater consumption of obesity-promoting macronutrients during binge episodes. Directionality and temporality of this association between unhealthy consumption and family rigidity requires further study.

Keywords: loss of control eating; obesity; BMI; adolescent; females; family functioning; energy intake

---

1. Introduction

Given the high prevalence of obesity among adolescents [1] and the relatively few effective treatment options for this age group [2], elucidating psychological factors that promote excess weight gain is warranted for the development of novel approaches. Loss of control eating (LOC), the subjective feeling that one cannot stop or control what or how much one consumes [3], may be one such factor. With approximately 33% of children with overweight or obesity engaging in LOC eating [4], LOC eating has been shown to be a robust predictor of excess weight and fat gain [5–7], exacerbate some components of the metabolic syndrome [8], and predict the development of partial or full-syndrome binge eating disorder [9,10]. Data have shown that, in general (for example, outside of the laboratory environment), youth with LOC eating consume more highly palatable, energy dense foods than youth without LOC eating [11–13], which may provide a mechanism for observed prospective outcomes.

The interpersonal model of binge eating disorder proposes that the link between difficulties in social functioning and LOC eating is largely mediated by negative affect resulting from relationship problems [14]. This model has been applied to adolescent girls with LOC eating [15]. While the theory focuses on any type of salient relationship, data suggest that among adolescent girls with LOC eating, family members may be most relevant to the interpersonal model [16]. Indeed, family dysfunction has been suggested to play a crucial role in child and adolescent overweight and obesity [17–19] and disordered eating [20–22].

Prior studies have operationalized family functioning as a person's perceived level of adaptability (i.e., ability of a family system to change its power structure, role relationships, and relationship rules in response to situational and developmental stress) and cohesion (i.e., emotional bonding that family members have toward one another) within their own family [23]. Research has shown that higher and/or balanced levels of perceived adaptability and/or cohesion can both relate to and predict healthy eating behaviors. Generally, it has been found that girls with diagnosed eating disorders (compared to girls without diagnosed eating disorders) report less functional levels of adaptability and/or cohesion [21,24]. For example, studies have shown that adolescents with binge-eating disorder perceive lower familial adaptability than adolescents without binge-eating disorder [25], report higher cohesion and flexibility compared to adolescent girls with anorexia nervosa or bulimia nervosa [26], and report more negative perceived maternal criticism than a control group [27]. Among non-clinical samples of adolescents with overweight, higher reports of overeating relate to lower perceived familial cohesion and adaptability [28], and mothers of adolescents with overweight also report higher psychopathology than mothers of adolescents without overweight [29].

Perceived family functioning has also been shown to relate to energy intake patterns [30,31]. For example, a cross-sectional study of youth and adults with diabetes assessing the relationships among family meal frequency, perceived familial cohesion, and reported intake found that cohesion mediated the relationship between family meal frequency and individuals' intake as measured through a food frequency questionnaire [32]. Specifically, higher levels of perceived familial cohesion were linked to a greater reported intake of several food items considered healthful, whereas lower levels of perceived familial cohesion were associated with a greater consumption of palatable and high-caloric density items like fried eggs, burgers, and chips. Similar findings were observed in a longitudinal study assessing the relationship between family cohesion and self-reported food intake in adolescents using a food diary. Perceived cohesion was positively related to healthier reported eating behaviors, such as breakfast consumption, and was negatively related to soda intake [31].

One limitation to the existing literature is the use of self-reported intake, which can be under (or over) reported [33,34], particularly among individuals with overweight and obesity [35,36] or those reporting LOC eating [37]. However, no study has examined total or macronutrient intake in relation to family functioning during actual meals, which may be more informative for understanding, and potentially preventing, obesity development. Lastly, there are no data specifically examining the family functioning and test meal intake of adolescent girls with LOC at high-risk for excess weight gain and eating disorders. We therefore related objectively measured intake at a meal designed to model a binge episode to reported familial functioning among high-risk adolescent girls. Given data showing that youth reporting LOC eating episodes tend to consume more energy from carbohydrate and fat and less energy from protein compared to youth not reporting LOC eating episodes [11,38], girls with overweight have greater overall energy consumption [13,39] and youth with LOC tend to have greater liking of foods in a test meal [40]. We hypothesized that lower levels of adaptability and cohesion would relate to greater total energy consumption, a greater percentage of energy consumed from fat and carbohydrates, and a lower percentage of energy consumed from protein.

2. Method

2.1. Participants

108 adolescent girls aged 12–17 years old and at high-risk for eating disorders and excess weight gain participated in a clinical study for the prevention of LOC eating (ClinicalTrials.gov ID#: NCT00680979). All data for the current analyses were collected at baseline prior to the initiation of any treatment. As previously described [41], inclusion criteria involved being between the 75th and 97th percentile for body mass index (BMI; kg/m^2) and having undergone at least one LOC episode in the last month. Exclusion criteria included any major medical or psychiatric diagnoses (other than binge eating disorder), regular use of medications that affect weight or appetite, current involvement in psychotherapy or a weight loss program, or weight loss in last 2 months exceeding >3% of body weight. A total of 185 participants were screened of whom 117 were eligible for the study. 108 participants completed the necessary measures for the current analysis. Signed informed consent and assent were obtained from parents and adolescents respectively. This protocol was approved by the Institutional Review Boards at the Eunice Kennedy Shriver National Institute of Child Health and Human Development and the Uniformed Services University of the Health Sciences.

2.2. Procedure

Demographic variables (e.g., age and race/ethnicity) were assessed by parent report and questionnaires and interviews were assessed by adolescent report. BMI, adiposity, and energy intake were assessed at the National Institutes of Health Clinical Research Center following an overnight fast initiated the night before at 10 p.m.

BMI and adiposity: BMI was calculated from height and weight. Weight was measured to the nearest tenth of a kilogram with a calibrated digital scale (Scale-Tronix, Wheaton, IL, USA). Height was measured in triplicate to the nearest millimeter with a calibrated electronic stadiometer (Holtain Ltd., Crymych, Wales, UK) and the average of the three heights was used. Fat mass (kg) was measured by dual energy X-ray absorptiometry (DXA) using a Hologic QDR-4500A or Discovery instrument (Bedford, MA, USA) as previously described [41].

LOC eating: The presence of LOC eating over the past month was assessed by the overeating section of the Eating Disorder Examination, Version 14 OD/C.2 (EDE; [42]). The Eating Disorder Examination is a semi-structured diagnostic clinical interview used to assess disordered attitudes and behaviors related to eating, body shape, and weight. This instrument has been shown to be reliable and valid in pediatric samples [43,44].

Family functioning: Family functioning was defined as an adolescent's perceived level of adaptability and cohesion within their own family [23]. Perceived familial adaptability and cohesion were assessed with the Family Adaptability and Cohesion Scale III (FACES III), a 20-item self-report instrument that measures perceived levels of familial adaptability (e.g., "Parent(s) and children discuss punishment together") and cohesion (e.g., "Family members like to spend free time with each other"). The FACES has been used frequently in the literature to assess family function and is based on the hypothesis that functional family systems have more balanced levels of adaptability and cohesion than do dysfunctional family systems. Items were rated on a 5-point Likert scale (i.e., almost never, once in a while, sometimes, frequently, almost always) and scales were derived by summing items. The possible subscale score ranges for adaptability and cohesion were 10–50, with higher scores indicating greater (more positive) adaptability or cohesion. The FACES III has exhibited good test–retest reliability for both subscales (adaptability Cronbach's alpha = 0.80 at the 5-week interval; cohesion Cronbach's alpha = 0.83 at the 5-week interval) and strong discriminant validity given a low correlation between adaptability and cohesion ($r = 0.03$) [23]. Cronbach's alpha for the current study was 0.75 for adaptability and 0.87 for cohesion. Considering that the data for the current study was collected between 2008 and 2011, the FACES version used is not the most current as of 2011. However, if adaptability and cohesion are analyzed as continuous variables (as was done in the current study) and not categorical variables, the FACES III is a valid and interpretable measure [23].

Energy intake: At 11:00 a.m., participants were presented with a 9835 kcal buffet test meal with individual items representing a wide assortment of foods that varied in macronutrient composition (12% protein, 51% carbohydrate, and 37% fat across all foods). Adolescents entered the room containing the buffet and were provided with the tape-recorded instruction stating, "let yourself go and eat as much as you want." Participants were then left alone in the room until they indicated that they were finished eating. Total consumption of each food item was assessed by weighing the food items before and after presentation to each participant. This paradigm has effectively distinguished adolescents with LOC eating from those without reported LOC eating [11]. Some of the test meal data collected at baseline have been published in previous reports [45–48].

Pre-meal hunger: A single item-assessment was used to measure pre-meal hunger. The item asked, "how hungry do you feel right now?" and individuals responded on a 1 (Not at all) to 100 (Extremely) sliding scale.

Depressive symptoms: A single item-assessment was used to measure pre-meal depressive symptoms from the Brunel Mood Scale [49]. The item asked participants to select their current level of depression on a 1 (Not at all) to 5 (Extremely) Likert scale.

Post-meal subjective evaluation of LOC eating: A single item-assessment was used to measure post-meal subjective evaluation of LOC eating. The item asked, "how much is the eating you just completed like a meal when you feel 'loss of control'?" on a 1 (Extremely) to 5 (Not at all) Likert scale.

2.3. Statistical Analyses

Analyses were performed using SPSS version 25. Hierarchical multiple regression analyses were conducted with perceived adaptability and cohesion as independent variables and macronutrients (protein, carbohydrates, and fat as a percentage of total energy consumption) and total energy intake as dependent variables. R squared values indicate the proportion of variance in the dependent variable that is explained by the model. Height, body fat (%), lean body mass (kg), age, race, depressive symptoms, pre-meal hunger, and total energy intake (kcal) were considered as covariates in the models predicting percentage of macronutrients. Age, race, depressive symptoms, and pre-meal hunger did not contribute to any model and were removed from analyses. Height was highly correlated with lean body mass ($r = 0.77$) and was not included in analyses to meet multicollinearity assumptions. Macronutrient intake percentages were arcsine square root transformed to achieve normality. All other assumptions for model testing were met. Significance was set at $\alpha = 0.05$, two-tailed. We also conducted a series of follow up analyses for participants with overweight or obesity (BMI percentile ≥ 85).

3. Results

Participants were 108 adolescent girls (M $\pm$ SD 14.49 $\pm$ 1.66 years) who had above-average weight with a mean BMIz of 1.54 (SD = 0.33). Racial breakdown was as follows: 58.3% White, 25.0% Black, 9.3% Multiple Races, 2.8% Asian, 0.9% American Indian or Alaskan Native, and 3.7% Other or unknown. 9.3% of the sample identified as Latina or Hispanic. (See Table 1).

Table 1. Descriptive characteristics of participants.

	N = 108
Age, year *	14.5 (1.7)
BMIz *	1.54 (0.33)
Race/Ethnicity, %	
White	58.3
Black	25.0
Asian	2.8
American Indian	0.9
Hispanic	9.3
More than one race	9.3
Other/Unknown	3.7
FACES Score *	
Adaptability	31.6 (6.2)
Cohesion	26.2 (8.1)
LOC Eating Episodes	
Episodes 1 month pre-test meal *	4.69 (6.2)
Proportion of youth reporting at least 4 episodes per month in 3 months pre-test meal	14.8%
Test Meal *	
Total kcals consumed	1,177.3 (453.7)
Kcal from protein %	12.9 (3.2)
Kcal from carbohydrates %	50.9 (8.2)
Kcal from fat %	36.2 (7.0)
Pre-meal hunger (Scale 1–100)	62.7 (18.6)
Pre-meal depressive symptoms (Scale 1–5)	0.44 (1.02)
Post-meal subjective evaluation of LOC eating (Scale 1–5)	3.94 (1.1)

* = Mean (SD).

Total and Macronutrient Intake

Total energy intake: The first step of the model (base model) included covariates and the second step (full model) added the predictors of family adaptability and cohesion. Neither the base ($F(2, 105) = 0.63$, $p = 0.534$) nor full ($F(4, 103) = 0.69$, $p = 0.598$) models significantly predicted total energy intake. The full model accounted for only 2.6% of the variance in total energy intake. Adaptability ($\beta = -0.04$, $p = 0.683$) and cohesion ($\beta = 0.13$, $p = 0.222$) were not significant contributors to the full model.

Protein: Covariates (first step) explained 5.4% of the variance in percentage protein consumed but the base model was not significant overall, $F(3, 104) = 1.98$, $p = 0.12$. Adding adaptability and cohesion to the model improved model fit and accounted for an additional 6% of the variance in percentage of protein consumed ($\Delta R^2 = 0.06$, $p = 0.038$) and the full model was significant, $F(5, 102) = 2.59$, $p = 0.030$. Percentage of body fat was a significant predictor of percentage of protein consumed ($\beta = 0.24$, $p = 0.016$) as was family adaptability ($\beta = 0.26$, $p = 0.015$), but not family cohesion ($\beta = -0.18$, $p = 0.081$) (see Table 2). Specifically, lower percentage of body fat and worse family adaptability were both significantly related to less percentage of protein consumed.

Carbohydrates: The first step of the model explained 7.2% of the variance in percentage of carbohydrates consumed and the base model was significant, $F(3, 104) = 2.70$, $p = 0.049$. Adding adaptability and cohesion to the model improved model fit and accounted for an additional 5% of the variance in percentage of carbohydrates consumed ($\Delta R^2 = 0.053$, $p = 0.049$) and the full model was significant, $F(5, 102) = 2.93$, $p = 0.016$. Total energy consumed was a significant predictor of percentage of carbohydrates consumed ($\beta = -0.24$, $p = 0.011$) as was family adaptability ($\beta = -0.26$, $p = 0.015$), but not family cohesion ($\beta = 0.12$, $p = 0.232$). Specifically, less total energy consumed and worse family adaptability were related to higher percentage of carbohydrates consumed, even when accounting for all other variables in the model.

Table 2. Hierarchical regression for total intake and macronutrients.

		Outcome Variables															
		Total Intake				Protein				Carbohydrates				Fat			
Model	Predictor Variables	β	t	*p*	ΔR²	β	t	*p*	ΔR²	β	t	*p*	ΔR²	β	t	*p*	ΔR²
1	Constant		13.0	0.00 *	0.01		3.82	0.00 *	0.05		7.87	0.00 *	0.07		1.47	0.15	0.11 †
	Total lean fat	0.06	0.61	0.54		−0.03	−0.31	0.76		−0.06	−0.62	0.54		0.08	0.82	0.42	
	Total % fat	−0.08	−0.79	0.43		0.21	2.18	0.03 *		−0.15	−1.55	0.12		0.07	0.74	0.46	
	Total intake (kcals)					−0.05	−0.53	0.60		−0.23	−2.45	0.02 *		0.32	3.39	0.00 *	
2	Constant		11.77	0.00 *	0.01		3.34	0.00 *	0.06 †		8.32	0.00 *	0.05 †		1.02	0.31	0.03
	Total lean fat	0.007	0.69	0.50		−0.07	−0.69	0.49		−0.03	−0.27	0.79		0.05	0.55	0.59	
	Total % fat	−0.08	−0.81	0.42		0.24	2.45	0.02 *		−0.17	−1.81	0.07		0.09	0.92	0.36	
	Total intake (kcals)					−0.03	−0.35	0.73		−0.24	−2.60	0.01 *		0.32	3.46	0.00 *	
	Adaptability	−0.04	−0.41	0.68		0.26	2.47	0.02 *		−0.26	−2.49	0.02 *		0.20	1.90	0.06	
	Cohesion	0.13	1.23	0.22		−0.18	−1.76	0.08		0.12	1.20	0.23		−0.07	−0.70	0.49	

† = Model significant; * = $p < 0.05$; Note: Percentages of protein, carbohydrates, and fat intake were arcsine-square root transformed for analyses.

Fat: The first step of the model explained 10.8% of the variance in percentage of fat consumed and the base model was significant, $F(3, 104) = 4.20$, $p = 0.008$. Adding adaptability and cohesion to the model did not significantly improve model fit ($\Delta R^2 = 0.031$, $p = 0.169$). The full model was significant, $F(5, 102) = 3.28$, $p = 0.009$, but adaptability and cohesion were not significant predictors. Significance was driven by total energy consumed, ($\beta = 0.32$, $p = 0.001$), with more total energy consumed related to higher percentage of fat consumed (see Table 2).

Follow-up analyses: Follow-up analyses were conducted for girls with a BMI percentile indicating overweight status (above 85th percentile) and with girls reporting four or more LOC eating episodes in the past 28 days. Follow-up analyses were conducted to assess whether results in the sub-groups would differ from the full sample. A total of 101 girls in the study had a BMI percentile above the 85th percentile and 37 girls reported four or more LOC eating episodes. Neither those with overweight nor those reporting four or more LOC eating episodes differed from the entire sample for any outcome.

4. Discussion

In this analysis of perceived family functioning and objective energy intake, we found that adolescent girls with reported LOC eating who perceived their families as being less adaptable consumed a lower percentage of energy from protein and a higher percentage from carbohydrates. Perceived level of family cohesion did not significantly relate to test meal intake measures. We found that familial adaptability was associated with degree of carbohydrate and protein intake, but not with total energy or degree of fat intake. These results are generally consistent with data comparing youth with and without LOC eating, such that those with LOC eating consume more energy from carbohydrate and less from protein [11,50,51]. Given that all participants in our sample reported LOC eating, and that poorer adaptability was specifically linked to macronutrient intake that may promote excess weight [52–55], interpersonal functioning linked to less familial flexibility may provide a more fine-grained understanding of the interpersonal model. Indeed, adolescent girls with LOC eating [15,56] and adults with binge eating [57] often describe rigidity within families. Supporting this notion, low levels of familial adaptability have been shown to correspond with high levels of stress [58] and thus, it is possible that girls consume higher amounts of carbohydrate-rich "comfort" food to cope with the stress of a relatively inflexible family environment. Likewise, protein consumption has generally been associated with healthier body weight [59,60] and eating patterns [61–63] and may thus explain how poorer family adaptability was related to adolescents' lower protein intake. Of note, the relationship between family functioning and energy intake accounted for only a small proportion of variance. This could be due to family functioning being a global construct that may be persistent whereas energy intake in the laboratory is situational (e.g., may be affected by hunger, current mood, environment, etc.). As a result, future research including a more naturalistic measure of eating behavior outside of the laboratory, such as ecological momentary assessment, is warranted.

The lack of an association between family cohesion and intake was unexpected. Previous studies have found that higher cohesion correlates with healthier food intake [30–32,64]. It is possible that the nature of our sample and test meal design may explain differences in results. Previous studies were primarily conducted in children and adolescents who were not selected for disordered eating behaviors. Moreover, studies based on self-reported intake were focused on eating in general, as opposed to a meal designed to capture a binge episode. It is possible that we would have found a significant link with family cohesion had we assessed girls' intake during a "normal" test meal. Indeed, our prior research has demonstrated that girls with overweight and reported LOC eating can distinguish between "binge" and "normal" meals in the laboratory [11]. However, this notion requires testing. Furthermore, perceived cohesion has been linked to more meals eaten as a family [31] and thus, authors of prior studies suggest that the cohesion–healthy eating relationship might be interpreted within this family-eating context, which promotes healthy food consumption [65,66]. Therefore, another possible explanation for our findings is that given that youth with LOC eating tend to consume fewer regular meals compared to those without LOC eating [67], cohesion may be less relevant with regard to intake among adolescents who report LOC eating behaviors in the context of a meal modeled to capture a binge episode. Indeed, girls ate alone during the test meal. Further, data based on self-reports tends to find that binge episodes often take place when others are not present [39,68,69].

Strengths of this investigation include the objective measure of energy intake, use of DXA to assess body composition, and the diverse sample of participants of various ethnic groups and races. Limitations of the study include that the FACES is a self-report measure, which may be vulnerable to subjective bias. Also, the cohort contained only adolescent girls of above-average weight with LOC eating, potentially limiting the generalizability of the findings. As we did not include control samples of girls with or without overweight and without LOC eating, future research should address this gap. Lastly, given the cross-sectional nature of the results, no conclusions on temporality between perceived family functioning and intake can be made.

In conclusion, we found that adolescent girls with LOC who perceived their families as being relatively less adaptable consumed significantly more carbohydrates and less protein from a test meal that modeled a LOC episode. The findings of this study underscore the importance of addressing family functioning in the clinical setting and potentially including family members in interventions involving the modification of adolescent girls' eating behaviors. Future prospective research is required to elucidate whether familial functioning plays a role in the development of adverse outcomes and intervention response.

Author Contributions: Conceptualization, M.J. and M.T.K.; designing of study, M.T.K. and J.A.Y.; data collection, M.T.K., L.B.S., S.M.B., M.K., and J.A.Y.; data analysis, M.J., N.L.B., and M.T.K.; writing-original draft preparation, M.J., M.T.K., and N.L.B.; writing-review and editing, all authors.

References

1. Hales, C.M.; Fryar, C.D.; Carroll, M.D.; Freedman, D.S.; Ogden, C.L. Trends in obesity and severe obesity prevalence in us youth and adults by sex and age, 2007-2008 to 2015-2016. *JAMA* **2018**, *319*, 1723–1725. [CrossRef] [PubMed]
2. Ryder, J.R.; Fox, C.K.; Kelly, A.S. Treatment options for severe obesity in the pediatric population: Current limitations and future opportunities. *Obesity* **2018**, *26*, 951–960. [CrossRef] [PubMed]
3. American Psychiatric Association. *Diagnostic and Statistical Manual of Mental Disorders*, 5th ed.; American Psychiatric Association: Washington DC, USA, 2013.
4. Morgan, C.M.; Yanovski, S.Z.; Nguyen, T.T.; McDuffie, J.; Sebring, N.G.; Jorge, M.R.; Keil, M.; Yanovski, J.A. Loss of control over eating, adiposity, and psychopathology in overweight children. *Int. J. Eat. Disord.* **2002**, *31*, 430–441. [CrossRef] [PubMed]
5. Tanofsky-Kraff, M.; Cohen, M.L.; Yanovski, S.Z.; Cox, C.; Theim, K.R.; Keil, M.; Reynolds, J.C.; Yanovski, J.A. A prospective study of psychological predictors of body fat gain among children at high risk for adult obesity. *Pediatrics* **2006**, *117*, 1203–1209. [CrossRef] [PubMed]
6. Tanofsky-Kraff, M.; Yanovski, S.Z.; Schvey, N.A.; Olsen, C.H.; Gustafson, J.; Yanovski, J.A. A prospective study of loss of control eating for body weight gain in children at high risk for adult obesity. *Int. J. Eat. Disord.* **2009**, *42*, 26–30. [CrossRef] [PubMed]
7. Sonneville, K.R.; Horton, N.J.; Micali, N.; Crosby, R.D.; Swanson, S.A.; Solmi, F.; Field, A.E. Longitudinal associations between binge eating and overeating and adverse outcomes among adolescents and young adults: Does loss of control matter? *JAMA Pedatr.* **2013**, *167*, 149–155. [CrossRef] [PubMed]
8. Tanofsky-Kraff, M.; Shomaker, L.B.; Stern, E.A.; Miller, R.; Sebring, N.; DellaValle, D.; Yanovski, S.Z.; Hubbard, V.S.; Yanovski, J.A. Children's binge eating and development of metabolic syndrome. *Int. J. Obes.* **2012**, *36*, 956. [CrossRef]

9. Tanofsky-Kraff, M.; Shomaker, L.B.; Olsen, C.; Roza, C.A.; Wolkoff, L.E.; Columbo, K.M.; Raciti, G.; Zocca, J.M.; Wilfley, D.E.; Yanovski, S.Z.; Yanovski, J.A. A prospective study of pediatric loss of control eating and psychological outcomes. *J. Abnorm. Psychol.* **2011**, *120*, 108–118. [CrossRef]
10. Hilbert, A.; Hartmann, A.S.; Czaja, J.; Schoebi, D. Natural course of preadolescent loss of control eating. *J. Abnorm. Psychol.* **2013**, *122*, 684. [CrossRef]
11. Tanofsky-Kraff, M.; McDuffie, J.R.; Yanovski, S.Z.; Kozlosky, M.; Schvey, N.A.; Shomaker, L.B.; Salaita, C.; Yanovski, J.A. Laboratory assessment of the food intake of children and adolescents with loss of control eating. *Am. J. Clin. Nutr.* **2009**, *89*, 738–745. [CrossRef]
12. Mirch, M.C.; McDuffie, J.R.; Yanovski, S.Z.; Schollnberger, M.; Tanofsky-Kraff, M.; Theim, K.R.; Krakoff, J.; Yanovski, J.A. Effects of binge eating on satiation, satiety, and energy intake of overweight children. *Am. J. Clin. Nutr.* **2006**, *84*, 732–738. [CrossRef] [PubMed]
13. Theim, K.R.; Tanofsky-Kraff, M.; Salaita, C.G.; Haynos, A.F.; Mirch, M.C.; Ranzenhofer, L.M.; Yanovski, S.Z.; Wilfley, D.E.; Yanovski, J.A. Children's descriptions of the foods consumed during loss of control eating episodes. *Eat. Behav.* **2007**, *8*, 258–265. [CrossRef] [PubMed]
14. Wilfley, D.E.; Welch, R.R.; Stein, R.I.; Spurrell, E.B.; Cohen, L.R.; Saelens, B.E.; Dounchis, J.Z.; Frank, M.A.; Wiseman, C.V.; Matt, G.E. A randomized comparison of group cognitive-behavioral therapy and group interpersonal psychotherapy for the treatment of overweight individuals with binge-eating disorder. *Arch. Gen. Psychiatry* **2002**, *59*, 713–721. [CrossRef] [PubMed]
15. Tanofsky-Kraff, M.; Wilfley, D.E.; Young, J.F.; Mufson, L.; Yanovski, S.Z.; Glasofer, D.R.; Salaita, C.G. Preventing excessive weight gain in adolescents: Interpersonal psychotherapy for binge eating. *Obesity* **2007**, *15*, 1345–1355. [CrossRef] [PubMed]
16. Berger, S.S.; Elliott, C.; Ranzenhofer, L.M.; Shomaker, L.B.; Hannallah, L.; Field, S.E.; Young, J.F.; Sbrocco, T.; Wilfley, D.E.; Yanovski, J.A. Interpersonal problem areas and alexithymia in adolescent girls with loss of control eating. *Compr. Psychiatry* **2014**, *55*, 170–178. [CrossRef] [PubMed]
17. Halliday, J.A.; Palma, C.L.; Mellor, D.; Green, J.; Renzaho, A.M. The relationship between family functioning and child and adolescent overweight and obesity: A systematic review. *Int. J. Obes. (Lond).* **2014**, *38*, 480–493. [CrossRef] [PubMed]
18. Vincent, M.A.; McCabe, M.P. Gender differences among adolescents in family, and peer influences on body dissatisfaction, weight loss, and binge eating behaviors. *J. Youth Adolesc.* **2000**, *29*, 205–221. [CrossRef]
19. Tanofsky-Kraff, M.; Haynos, A.F.; Kotler, L.A.; Yanovski, S.Z.; Yanovski, J.A. Laboratory-based studies of eating among children and adolescents. *Curr. Nutr. Food Sci.* **2007**, *3*, 55–74. [CrossRef]
20. Waller, G.; Slade, P.; Calam, R. Family adaptability and cohesion: Relation to eating attitudes and disorders. *Int. J. Eat. Disord.* **1990**, *9*, 225–228. [CrossRef]
21. Vidović, V.; Jureša, V.; Begovac, I.; Mahnik, M.; Tocilj, G. Perceived family cohesion, adaptability and communication in eating disorders. *Eur. Eat. Disord. Rev.* **2005**, *13*, 19–28. [CrossRef]
22. Lundholm, J.K.; Waters, J.E. Dysfunctional family systems: Relationship to disordered eating behaviors among university women. *J. Subst. Abuse.* **1991**, *3*, 97–106. [CrossRef]
23. Olson, D.; Portner, J.; Lavee, Y. *Family Adaptability and Cohesion Evaluation Scale (faces iii)*, 1st ed.; Life Innovations: Minneapolis, MN, USA, 1985; pp. 1–17.
24. Wisotsky, W.; Dancyger, I.; Fornari, V.; Katz, J.; Wisotsky, W.L.; Swencionis, C. The relationship between eating pathology and perceived family functioning in eating disorder patients in a day treatment program. *Eat. Disord.* **2003**, *11*, 89–99. [CrossRef] [PubMed]
25. Tetzlaff, A.; Schmidt, R.; Brauhardt, A.; Hilbert, A. Family functioning in adolescents with binge-eating disorder. *Eur. Eat. Disord. Rev.* **2016**, *24*, 430–433. [CrossRef] [PubMed]
26. Cerniglia, L.; Cimino, S.; Tafà, M.; Marzilli, E.; Ballarotto, G.; Bracaglia, F. Family profiles in eating disorders. Family functioning and psychopathology. *Psychol. Res. Behav. Manag.* **2017**, *10*, 305–312. [CrossRef] [PubMed]
27. Schmidt, R.; Tetzlaff, A.; Hilbert, A. Perceived expressed emotion in adolescents with binge-eating disorder. *J. Abnorm. Child Psychol.* **2015**, *43*, 1369–1377. [CrossRef] [PubMed]
28. Cromley, T.; Neumark-Sztainer, D.; Story, M.; Boutelle, K.N. Parent and family associations with weight-related behaviors and cognitions among overweight adolescents. *J. Adolesc. Health* **2010**, *47*, 263–269. [CrossRef] [PubMed]

29. Blanco, M.; Sepulveda, A.R.; Lacruz, T.; Parks, M.; Real, B.; Martin-Peinador, Y.; Román, F.J. Examining maternal psychopathology, family functioning and coping skills in childhood obesity: A case–control study. *Eur. Eat. Disord. Rev.* **2017**, *25*, 359–365. [CrossRef]
30. Bourdeaudhuij, I.D.; Oost, P.V. Personal and family determinants of dietary behaviour in adolescents and their parents. *Psychol. Health* **2000**, *15*, 751–770. [CrossRef]
31. Franko, D.L.; Thompson, D.; Bauserman, R.; Affenito, S.G.; Striegel-Moore, R.H. What's love got to do with it? Family cohesion and healthy eating behaviors in adolescent girls. *Int. J. Eat. Disord.* **2008**, *41*, 360–367. [CrossRef]
32. Ruhee, D.; Mahomoodally, F. Relationship between family meal frequency and individual dietary intake among diabetic patients. *J. Diabetes Metab. Disord.* **2015**, *14*, 66. [CrossRef]
33. Livingstone, M.B.E.; Robson, P.; Wallace, J. Issues in dietary intake assessment of children and adolescents. *Br. J. Nutr.* **2004**, *92*, S213–S222. [CrossRef] [PubMed]
34. Gersovitz, M.; Madden, J.P.; Smiciklas-Wright, H. Validity of the 24-hr. Dietary recall and seven-day record for group comparisons. *J. Am. Diet. Assoc.* **1978**, *73*, 48–55. [PubMed]
35. Mendez, M.A.; Wynter, S.; Wilks, R.; Forrester, T. Under-and overreporting of energy is related to obesity, lifestyle factors and food group intakes in jamaican adults. *Public Health Nutr.* **2004**, *7*, 9–19. [CrossRef] [PubMed]
36. Johansson, L.; Solvoll, K.; Bjørneboe, G.-E.; Drevon, C.A. Under-and overreporting of energy intake related to weight status and lifestyle in a nationwide sample. *Am. J. Clin. Nutr.* **1998**, *68*, 266–274. [CrossRef] [PubMed]
37. Wolkoff, L.E.; Tanofsky-Kraff, M.; Shomaker, L.B.; Kozlosky, M.; Columbo, K.M.; Elliott, C.A.; Ranzenhofer, L.M.; Osborn, R.L.; Yanovski, S.Z.; Yanovski, J.A. Self-reported vs. Actual energy intake in youth with and without loss of control eating. *Eat. Behav.* **2011**, *12*, 15–20. [CrossRef] [PubMed]
38. Goldschmidt, A.B.; Tanofsky-Kraff, M.; Wilfley, D.E. A laboratory-based study of mood and binge eating behavior in overweight children. *Eat. Behav.* **2011**, *12*, 37–43. [CrossRef]
39. Tanofsky-Kraff, M.; Goossens, L.; Eddy, K.T.; Ringham, R.; Goldschmidt, A.; Yanovski, S.Z.; Braet, C.; Marcus, M.D.; Wilfley, D.E.; Olsen, C. A multisite investigation of binge eating behaviors in children and adolescents. *J. Consult. Clin. Psychol.* **2007**, *75*, 901. [CrossRef]
40. Kurz, S.; Schoebi, D.; Dremmel, D.; Kiess, W.; Munsch, S.; Hilbert, A. Satiety regulation in children with loss of control eating and attention-deficit/hyperactivity disorder: A test meal study. *Appetite* **2017**, *116*, 90–98. [CrossRef]
41. Tanofsky-Kraff, M.; Shomaker, L.B.; Wilfley, D.E.; Young, J.F.; Sbrocco, T.; Stephens, M.; Ranzenhofer, L.M.; Elliott, C.; Brady, S.; Radin, R.M.; et al. Targeted prevention of excess weight gain and eating disorders in high-risk adolescent girls: A randomized controlled trial. *Am. J. Clin. Nutr.* **2014**, *100*, 1010–1018. [CrossRef]
42. Fairburn, C.G.; Wilson, G.T.; Schleimer, K. *Binge Eating: Nature, Assessment, and Treatment*, 12th ed.; Guilford Press: New York, NY, USA, 1993; pp. 317–360.
43. Tanofsky-Kraff, M.; Shomaker, L.B.; Wilfley, D.E.; Young, J.F.; Sbrocco, T.; Stephens, M.; Brady, S.M.; Galescu, O.; Demidowich, A.; Olsen, C.H. Excess weight gain prevention in adolescents: Three-year outcome following a randomized controlled trial. *J. Consult. Clin. Psychol.* **2017**, *85*, 218. [CrossRef]
44. Tanofsky-Kraff, M.; Yanovski, S.Z.; Wilfley, D.E.; Marmarosh, C.; Morgan, C.M.; Yanovski, J.A. Eating-disordered behaviors, body fat, and psychopathology in overweight and normal-weight children. *J. Consult. Clin. Psychol.* **2004**, *72*, 53. [CrossRef] [PubMed]
45. Shank, L.M.; Crosby, R.D.; Grammer, A.C.; Shomaker, L.B.; Vannucci, A.; Burke, N.L.; Stojek, M.; Brady, S.M.; Kozlosky, M.; Reynolds, J.C. Examination of the interpersonal model of loss of control eating in the laboratory. *Compr. Psychiatry.* **2017**, *76*, 36–44. [CrossRef] [PubMed]
46. Vannucci, A.; Shomaker, L.B.; Field, S.E.; Sbrocco, T.; Stephens, M.; Kozlosky, M.; Reynolds, J.C.; Yanovski, J.A.; Tanofsky-Kraff, M. History of weight control attempts among adolescent girls with loss of control eating. *Health Psychol.* **2014**, *33*, 419. [CrossRef] [PubMed]
47. Glasofer, D.R.; Haaga, D.A.; Hannallah, L.; Field, S.E.; Kozlosky, M.; Reynolds, J.; Yanovski, J.A.; Tanofsky-Kraff, M. Self-efficacy beliefs and eating behavior in adolescent girls at-risk for excess weight gain and binge eating disorder. *Int. J. Eat. Disord.* **2013**, *46*, 663–668. [CrossRef] [PubMed]
48. Ranzenhofer, L.M.; Hannallah, L.; Field, S.E.; Shomaker, L.B.; Stephens, M.; Sbrocco, T.; Kozlosky, M.; Reynolds, J.; Yanovski, J.A.; Tanofsky-Kraff, M. Pre-meal affective state and laboratory test meal intake in adolescent girls with loss of control eating. *Appetite* **2013**, *68*, 30–37. [CrossRef] [PubMed]

49. Terry, P.C.; Lane, A.M.; Lane, H.J.; Keohane, L. Development and validation of a mood measure for adolescents. *J. Sports Sci.* **1999**, *17*, 861–872. [CrossRef] [PubMed]
50. Hilbert, A.; Tuschen-Caffier, B.; Czaja, J. Eating behavior and familial interactions of children with loss of control eating: A laboratory test meal study. *Am. J. Clin. Nutr.* **2010**, *91*, 510–518. [CrossRef]
51. Yanovski, S.Z.; Leet, M.; Yanovski, J.A.; Flood, M.N.; Gold, P.W.; Kissileff, H.R.; Walsh, B.T. Food selection and intake of obese women with binge-eating disorder. *Am. J. Clin. Nutr.* **1992**, *56*, 975–980. [CrossRef]
52. McCrory, M.A.; Fuss, P.J.; McCallum, J.E.; Yao, M.; Vinken, A.G.; Hays, N.P.; Roberts, S.B. Dietary variety within food groups: Association with energy intake and body fatness in men and women. *Am. J. Clin. Nutr.* **1999**, *69*, 440–447. [CrossRef]
53. Paddon-Jones, D.; Westman, E.; Mattes, R.D.; Wolfe, R.R.; Astrup, A.; Westerterp-Plantenga, M. Protein, weight management, and satiety. *Am. J. Clin. Nutr.* **2008**, *87*, 1558–1561. [CrossRef]
54. Schoeller, D.A.; Buchholz, A.C. Energetics of obesity and weight control: Does diet composition matter? *J. Am. Diet. Assoc.* **2005**, *105*, 24–28. [CrossRef]
55. Westerterp-Plantenga, M.S. The significance of protein in food intake and body weight regulation. *Curr. Opin. Clin. Nutr. Metab. Care* **2003**, *6*, 635–638. [CrossRef] [PubMed]
56. Berger, S.S.; Elliott, C.; Ranzenhofer, L.M.; Shomaker, L.B.; Hannallah, L.; Field, S.E.; Young, J.F.; Sbrocco, T.; Wilfley, D.E.; Yanovski, J.A.; Tanofsky-Kraff, M. Interpersonal problem areas and alexithymia in adolescent girls with loss of control eating. *Compr. Psychiatry* **2014**, *55*, 170–178. [CrossRef] [PubMed]
57. Wilfley, D.E. *Interpersonal Psychotherapy for Group*, 1st ed.; Basic Books: New York, NY, USA, 2000.
58. Glenn, S.; Cunningham, C.; Poole, H.; Reeves, D.; Weindling, M. Maternal parenting stress and its correlates in families with a young child with cerebral palsy. *Child Care Health Dev.* **2009**, *35*, 71–78. [CrossRef] [PubMed]
59. Anderson, G.H.; Moore, S.E. Dietary proteins in the regulation of food intake and body weight in humans. *J. Nutr.* **2004**, *134*, 974–979. [CrossRef] [PubMed]
60. Noakes, M.; Keogh, J.B.; Foster, P.R.; Clifton, P.M. Effect of an energy-restricted, high-protein, low-fat diet relative to a conventional high-carbohydrate, low-fat diet on weight loss, body composition, nutritional status, and markers of cardiovascular health in obese women. *Am. J. Clin. Nutr.* **2005**, *81*, 1298–1306. [CrossRef] [PubMed]
61. Xie, B.; Gilliland, F.D.; Li, Y.-F.; Rockett, H.R. Effects of ethnicity, family income, and education on dietary intake among adolescents. *Prev. Med.* **2003**, *36*, 30–40. [CrossRef]
62. Kerver, J.M.; Yang, E.J.; Obayashi, S.; Bianchi, L.; Song, W.O. Meal and snack patterns are associated with dietary intake of energy and nutrients in us adults. *J. Am. Diet. Assoc.* **2006**, *106*, 46–53. [CrossRef]
63. Neumark-Sztainer, D.; Hannan, P.J.; Story, M.; Croll, J.; Perry, C. Family meal patterns: Associations with sociodemographic characteristics and improved dietary intake among adolescents. *J. Am. Diet. Assoc.* **2003**, *103*, 317–322. [CrossRef]
64. Kintner, M.; Boss, P.G.; Johnson, N. The relationship between dysfunctional family environments and family member food intake. *J. Marriage Fam.* **1981**, 633–641. [CrossRef]
65. Videon, T.M.; Manning, C.K. Influences on adolescent eating patterns: The importance of family meals. *J. Adolesc. Health* **2003**, *32*, 365–373. [CrossRef]
66. Hammons, A.J.; Fiese, B.H. Is frequency of shared family meals related to the nutritional health of children and adolescents? *Pediatrics* **2010**. [CrossRef] [PubMed]
67. Matheson, B.E.; Camacho, C.; Peterson, C.B.; Rhee, K.E.; Rydell, S.A.; Zucker, N.L.; Boutelle, K.N. The relationship between parent feeding styles and general parenting with loss of control eating in treatment-seeking overweight and obese children. *Int. J. Eat. Disord.* **2015**, *48*, 1047–1055. [CrossRef] [PubMed]
68. Goldschmidt, A.B.; Crosby, R.D.; Cao, L.; Engel, S.G.; Durkin, N.; Beach, H.M.; Berg, K.C.; Wonderlich, S.A.; Crow, S.J.; Peterson, C.B. Ecological momentary assessment of eating episodes in obese adults. *Psychosom. Med.* **2014**, *76*, 747. [CrossRef] [PubMed]
69. Hilbert, A.; Rief, W.; Tuschen-Caffier, B.; de Zwaan, M.; Czaja, J. Loss of control eating and psychological maintenance in children: An ecological momentary assessment study. *Behav. Res. Ther.* **2009**, *47*, 26–33. [CrossRef] [PubMed]

5

The Role of Regular Eating and Self-Monitoring in the Treatment of Bulimia Nervosa: A Pilot Study of an Online Guided Self-Help CBT Program

Sarah Barakat [1,*], Sarah Maguire [2], Lois Surgenor [3], Brooke Donnelly [4], Blagica Miceska [2], Kirsty Fromholtz [2], Janice Russell [5], Phillipa Hay [6] and Stephen Touyz [1]

1 School of Psychology, University of Sydney, Sydney, NSW 2006, Australia; stephen.touyz@sydney.edu.au
2 Centre for Eating and Dieting Disorders, Boden Institute, University of Sydney, Sydney, NSW 2006, Australia; servicedevelopmentofficer@gmail.com (S.M.); bm405@uowmail.edu.au (B.M.); kfromholtz@gmail.com (K.F.)
3 Department of Psychological Medicine, University of Otago at Christchurch, Christchurch 8140, New Zealand; lois.surgenor@otago.ac.nz
4 Sydney Local Health District, Sydney, NSW 2006, Australia; brooke.donnelly@sswahs.nsw.gov.au
5 School of Medicine, University of Sydney, Sydney, NSW 2006, Australia; janice.russell@sydney.edu.au
6 Translational Health Research Institute, School of Medicine, Western Sydney University, Sydney, NSW 2751, Australia; p.hay@westernsydney.edu.au
* Correspondence: sbar1821@uni.sydney.edu.au

Abstract: *Background*: Despite cognitive behavioural therapy (CBT) being regarded as the first-line treatment option for bulimia nervosa (BN), barriers such as its time-consuming and expensive nature limit patient access. In order to broaden treatment availability and affordability, the efficacy and convenience of CBT could be improved through the use of online treatments and selective emphasis on its most 'potent' components of which behavioural techniques form the focus. *Method:* Twenty-six individuals with BN were enrolled in an online CBT-based self-help programme and 17 completed four weeks of regular eating and food-monitoring using the online Food Diary tool. Participants were contacted for a weekly check-in phone call and had their bulimic symptom severity assessed at five time points (baseline and weeks 1–4). *Results*: There was a significant decrease in the frequency of self-reported objective binge episodes, associated loss of control and objective binge days reported between pre- and post-treatment measures. Significant improvements were also observed in most subscales of the Eating Disorder Examination-Questionnaire. *Conclusion*: This study provides encouraging preliminary evidence of the potential of behavioural techniques of online CBT in the treatment of BN. Online therapy with this focus is potentially a viable and practical form of treatment delivery in this illness group. These preliminary findings support the need for larger studies using control groups.

Keywords: bulimia nervosa; online treatment; self-monitoring; regular eating; cognitive behavioural therapy; objective binge episodes; purging

---

1. Introduction

Therapist-led cognitive behavioural therapy (CBT) currently forms the most empirically validated treatment for bulimia nervosa (BN), and accordingly is widely recommended as the first line treatment for adults with BN [1,2]. However, the empirical support which this "gold-standard" treatment enjoys is challenged by the statistic that on average only 23.2% of eating disorder (ED) sufferers actually access treatment [3], with this figure substantially lower in some urban and rural regions with no specialist ED services [4]. Importantly, the quality of CBT delivered in the community is inconsistent. Tobin, Banker, Weisberg and Bowers [5] report that only 6% of clinicians adhere to an evidence-based manualised version of CBT for eating disorders (EDs), concluding that therapist 'drift' from CBT is the norm rather than the exception [6]. Moreover, CBT for BN is a specialist treatment, which for a routine delivery costs US$6000.00 per individual case [7], with the Australian healthcare system rebating less than half of the CBT sessions for a routine case treated by a psychologist [4].

Modification of CBT-BN structure and delivery is vital to ensure treatment is accessible [8]. Broadening the format of CBT delivery beyond the current therapist-led structure to an online, self-help program will offset the shortage of ED specialist clinicians. Additionally, overcoming the lengthy nature of CBT-BN can be achieved through investigation of the most powerful therapeutic components of CBT-BN, of which behavioural techniques are a promising candidate [9].

1.1. *Treatment Delivery Formats to Increase Access*

In order to address barriers to accessing treatment, a number of alternative treatment formats have evolved. These are briefly reviewed.

1.1.1. Guided Self-Help

Various forms of guided self-help for BN have been available for several decades now, allowing a body of research to have evolved assessing its effectiveness. People who receive professional therapeutic support throughout their self-help treatment program display superior treatment outcomes to those independently engaging in self-help, producing equivalent outcomes to therapist led CBT for one-third of BN patients [10]. Accordingly, the addition of monthly thirty-minute guidance sessions for patients' observing Fairburn's *Overcoming Binge Eating* self-help manual [11] raised symptomatic improvement from 25% for those receiving no guidance, to 36% for telephone guidance and 50% for face-to-face guidance [12]. Supervision requirements for self-help treatment options are one-fifth of that required for a complete CBT course [13], advocating for a "stepped-care" approach which allows for the appropriate allocation of therapeutic skills according to one's clinical severity [14,15].

1.1.2. Online Self-Help

The successful application of CBT's primary principles into recent technological advancements has been demonstrated across a range of formats including online programs [16–21], email correspondence [22,23], text messaging [24] and CD-ROM programs [25]. Pretorius et al. [19] recently evaluated a web-based CBT intervention consisting of eight 30–40 min interactive online sessions for a sample of 101 patients diagnosed with BN or eating disorder not otherwise specified (EDNOS) with bulimic features. In addition to weekly email support, completion of the eTherapy program resulted in a significant improvement in the frequency of objective binge episodes (OBEs), purge episodes and global Eating Disorder Examination (EDE) [26] maintained at the six-month follow up. Additional support for eTherapy has been provided by a study of 75 BN or EDNOS patients of whom 25.8% displayed abstinence from bulimic behaviours following engagement in an eight-session online CBT-based program [21]. These findings are comparable to the 20% and 30% post-treatment abstinence from bulimic behaviours observed following the use of manual-based CBT self-help books and face-to-face CBT treatment, respectively [10,14].

Self-monitoring via a technological device upholds numerous benefits to traditional pen and paper methods, including in-built reminders to prompt higher completion, more ecologically valid data, real-time monitoring and personalised, immediate feedback on one's entries [27,28]. The recent popularity of a smartphone application for ED self-monitoring, known as 'Recovery Record', has seen 108,000 downloads across a two-year period, of which the majority of users logged their daily meals on the application for a thirty-day period [28]. However, Walsh and colleagues [27] found that while people with EDs viewed the idea of online monitoring favourably, they did not experience any benefit in practising the technique themselves.

1.2. Behavioural Components of CBT

Despite the extensive number of clinical trials assessing CBT as an entire treatment package, little empirical evidence exists on the effectiveness of CBT's individual therapeutic techniques [29]. Component analyses of CBT treatment for depression and anxiety demonstrate that therapy consisting purely of behavioural techniques produces equivalent outcomes to therapy involving both behavioural and cognitive techniques [30]. Moreover, in a comparative treatment trial for BN, CBT produced a greater shift in patients' distorted attitudes regarding shape, weight and extreme dieting as compared to a simplified behavioural version of CBT, yet was equivalent in all other treatment outcomes [31]. Key behavioural components of CBT for BN are briefly reviewed below.

1.2.1. Self-Monitoring

Self-monitoring is one of the first behavioural tasks introduced in CBT whereby patients record a target behaviour and any associated antecedents as they occur within their natural context [32]. Self-monitoring allows the clinician and patient to jointly evaluate problematic behavioural patterns, work to reduce them and can spark reactive effects due to the inherently reinforcing or punishing nature of self-records [32].

In CBT-BN, daily self-monitoring is introduced in the first session and requires patients to record their food and drink intake, including binge or compensatory behaviours, time, meal type and associated feelings at each meal [33]. A number of experts credit self-monitoring as the most powerful therapeutic intervention in the treatment of BN [9,34]. In support of this, investigations of the temporal effectiveness of CBT reveal the largest reduction in key bulimic behaviours occurs within the first four to six weeks of treatment, while self-monitoring and regular eating are being introduced, and is the best predictor of short and long term treatment outcomes for BN patients [35–39].

Latner and Wilson [9] conducted one of the very few studies examining the effect of self-monitoring in BN treatment. Following six to seven days of food-monitoring, 30 individuals diagnosed with either BN or binge eating disorder (BED) reported a significant decrease in OBEs. It has also been found that in addition to a reduction in OBEs, self-monitoring produces a simultaneous increase in subjective binge episodes (SBEs). Such a response was termed 'binge drift', with Hildebrandt and Latner [34] claiming that although food monitoring allows for greater awareness of one's eating behaviours, it may not target the destructive thoughts and negative affect, characteristic of the loss of control (LOC) experienced during binges. Other studies have examined the efficacy of self-monitoring alone in small or non-clinical samples, also suggesting its effectiveness [40,41].

1.2.2. Regular Eating: The Three-Hour Rule

Paired with food monitoring is another behavioural activity known as the three-hour rule whereby patients are instructed to consume three planned meals and two or three planned snacks daily to ensure food deprivation does not exceed three to four hours [42,43]. Regular eating interrupts the heavy dietary restriction practiced by individuals with BN, reducing vulnerability to psychological and physical triggers for a binge [44].

Despite emphasis on regular eating as a fundamental component of CBT for BN [45], there has been limited empirical investigation into its effectiveness as a singular component. Shah, Passi, Bryson and Agras [46] reported the consumption of three meals and one snack daily resulted in the highest abstinence from binge eating and purging in a sample of 158 BN patients receiving either CBT or interpersonal psychotherapy (IPT). Additionally, high adherence to regular eating has also been shown to lower weekly binge frequency in a sample of 38 university students presenting with regular binge eating [44].

The current study endeavours to expand upon the preliminary research examining self-monitoring and regular eating to investigate their joint effectiveness in a modified CBT treatment program. In an attempt to enhance the efficacy of online CBT and consequently improve treatment outcomes for people with BN, the current study explores the therapeutic effectiveness of food monitoring and the "three-hour rule" via an online, low-intensity CBT program known as Binge Eating eTherapy (BEeT), recently developed by the Centre for Eating and Dieting Disorders (CEDD) at the University of Sydney.

Firstly, it was hypothesised that following Stage 1 low-intensity CBT (online self-monitoring and "three-hour rule" training), participants will display a significant reduction in OBEs, LOC and compensatory behaviours. Secondly, in line with prior findings of 'binge drift', we hypothesise an increase in SBE pre-post treatment measures.

BN possesses the highest psychiatric comorbidity of the ED's [47], with up to 94.5% of sufferers meeting criteria for at least one DSM-IV disorder axis I diagnosis [48] and evidence suggests this comorbidity can be linked to more severe BN psychopathology [49,50] and symptom persistence [51]. For this reason, consideration of these factors was also considered pertinent in the current study. Specifically, we expected that a preliminary exploratory analysis of participants with comorbid mood disorders and/or severe bulimic behaviours in this cohort will display lower treatment compliance and poorer therapeutic outcomes.

2. Materials and Methods

2.1. Participants

Participants were recruited from the general Australian community using online advertisements on health websites, social media announcements, referrals from health professionals and paper advertisements placed on the grounds of the University of Sydney. The study was approved by the Sydney Local Health District Ethics Review Committee, Royal Prince Alfred Hospital Zone (Ethics Approval Number: X14-0302).

Of the 69 individuals who expressed interest, 26 females entered the study (See Figure 1). Participants were eligible for this study if they were aged between 16 to 65 years of age and met a full DSM-5 [52] diagnostic criteria for BN (purging or non-purging type). Participants below 18 years of age were required to provide parental consent. As assessed by the Eating Disorder Examination Questionnaire (EDE-Q) [53], participants must have engaged in OBEs and inappropriate compensatory behaviours (inclusive of vomiting, excessive laxative or diuretic use, extreme exercise or severe dietary restriction) at least once per week in the preceding 28 days from when the questionnaire was taken. The presence of such behaviours across the preceding three months was confirmed by a senior clinical psychologist with experience in treating ED patients who discussed symptom presentation with the patient in a thorough phone interview. As part of the interview, participants' self-evaluation due to shape and weight, as assessed on the EDE-Q, was also confirmed.

Exclusion criteria included a body mass index (BMI) below 18.5 and current participation in a CBT psychological treatment specifically for their eating disorder. Individuals engaging in general psychological or pharmacological treatment were not excluded from the study, neither were participants with a comorbid psychiatric disorder. If a safety plan and regular monitoring of risk could not be established for participants with self-harm and suicide behaviours, they were excluded from the study. Monitoring of risk included follow-up phone calls if participants' displayed thoughts of self-harm or suicide in their weekly questionnaires or Food Diary entries. In this phone call, the severity of these thoughts was clarified and regular contact of the participant with an informed health professional was confirmed. Previous or acute active suicidality or self-harm behaviours did not obviate inclusion.

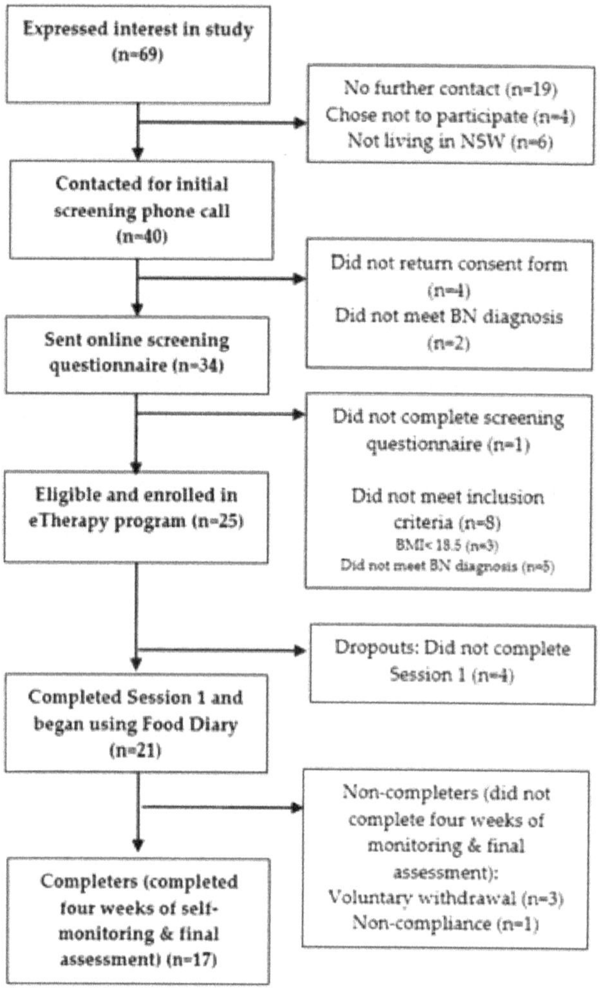

Figure 1. Flowchart of study participants.

2.2. Materials

2.2.1. Binge Eating eTherapy Program (BEeT)

The BEeT program consists of ten, one-hour interactive, multi-media sessions employing low-intensity CBT delivered by a pre-recorded therapist. Session 1 addresses the regular eating according to the "three-hour rule" and self-monitoring of eating using the online Food Diary. Access to the Food Diary tool was provided upon completion of Session 1 of the online program. Specifically, participants were educated on the impact of severe dietary restriction and how "delayed eating" is linked to urges to binge. Participants were encouraged to offset this by structuring their eating around three planned meals and two to three planned snacks daily.

The Food Diary tool is based upon the self-monitoring procedure for recording of eating behaviours as specified in most eating disorder therapies, including all existing CBT programs for BN [42,43,54,55]. Participants were to log a separate diary entry for each meal recording the following details: meal type, type and quantity of food and beverage consumed, the time at which intake occurred, whether the meal was considered to be a binge or over-eating, any urge to binge, type and quantity or length of any compensatory behaviours and associated events or feeling. On participants' entry of their dinner record in the diary, end of day on-screen feedback is provided on the "three-hour rule" and on the presence of binges across that day. Importantly, the feedback encouraged participants to continue practising the behavioural activities.

2.2.2. SMS Reminders

A daily SMS is sent to participants' mobile phones at approximately 9 a.m. as a reminder to record their meals using the Food Diary tool throughout the day. An additional evening SMS is sent at approximately 6 p.m. to participants who had not completed a Food Diary entry for the preceding two days to prompt reengagement.

2.3. *Psychometric Measures*

All the psychometric measures listed below formed part of the pre- and post-treatment maxi eScreens. The mini eScreen weekly assessments consisted of a shortened version of the EDE-Q, the Kessler Psychological Distress Scale (K10) and the self-harm and suicidality risk assessment. All psychometric measures were self-report assessments administered online. There exists a high correspondence between the psychometric measures delivered using online and written formats [56].

2.3.1. Eating Disorder Examination Questionnaire (EDE-Q)

The 16th edition of the EDE-Q [53] is a 30-item self-report version of the interview-delivered EDE [26]. The EDE-Q examines the behavioural features of one's ED, including the frequency and days of OBEs and SBEs as well as the frequency of purging, laxative use and excessive exercise over the preceding 28 days. The EDE-Q also contains four subscales (Shape Concern, Weight Concern, Eating Restraint, and Eating Concern) assessing the cognitive and emotional aspects of the ED, which utilise a seven-point Likert scale ranging from scores of 0 to 6, with higher scores indicative of more severe symptomology.

The EDE-Q was used to validate a diagnosis of BN and determine the severity of patients' bulimic behaviours, with frequency of binging and compensatory behaviours constituting the primary outcome measures. The EDE-Q upholds good reliability (Cronbach's $\alpha = 0.90$) [57].

2.3.2. Kessler Psychological Distress Scale (K10)

The K10 [58] is a screening tool used to monitor psychological distress experienced by patients and comprises of ten questions, each consisting of five response options, which assess the degree of negative emotionality experienced across the past 28 days (pre- and post-treatment questionnaires) or 7 days (weekly questionnaires). The K10 has good reliability (Cronbach's $\alpha = 0.93$) [58].

2.3.3. Eating Disorder Quality of Life Questionnaire (EDQOL)

The EDQOL [59] consists of 25-items examining the quality of life experienced by individuals suffering with an ED. Four subscales assess the impairment upon four primary domains including Psychological, Physical/Cognitive, Work/School and Financial domains. The EDQOL has good reliability (Cronbach's $\alpha = 0.94$) [59].

2.3.4. Three-Factor Eating Questionnaire (TFEQ)

The TFEQ [60] consists of three subscales assessing dietary restraint, disinhibition or loss of control over eating and hunger perception. The self-report assessment consists of 36 items with a yes/no response option, 14 items using a 1–4 response scale and a single vertical rating item.

2.3.5. General Information and Demographics

This series of questions concerns the general demographic information including age, gender, occupation, cultural background/ethnicity and setting of residence.

2.3.6. General Mental Health

This series of questions gathers information regarding participants' current primary and secondary mental health concerns, such as eating/weight issues, anxiety, stress, depression or substance/alcohol issues, whether or not these mental health concerns are being treated and by which mental health service, such as psychiatrist, psychologist, mental health nurse, social worker, counsellor, medical doctor or self-help book, and the type of treatment they are accessing, such as CBT, general counselling, hypnosis, antipsychotics or antidepressants.

2.3.7. Self-Harm and Suicidality Risk Assessment

This assessment reviews the history of participants' suicidal and self-harming thoughts and actions. It explores whether participants have had thoughts of suicide, attempted suicide or tried to injure or harm themselves in the previous 12 months or 28 days prior to completing the assessment.

2.4. Procedure

A brief telephone assessment screened participants for suitability; those eligible completed written informed consent and were then administered a comprehensive online assessment. Participants were instructed to complete Session 1 of the program and upon completion to immediately begin recording subsequent meals and episodes of binging and/or compensation in the online Food Diary for the following 28 days (See Figure 2).

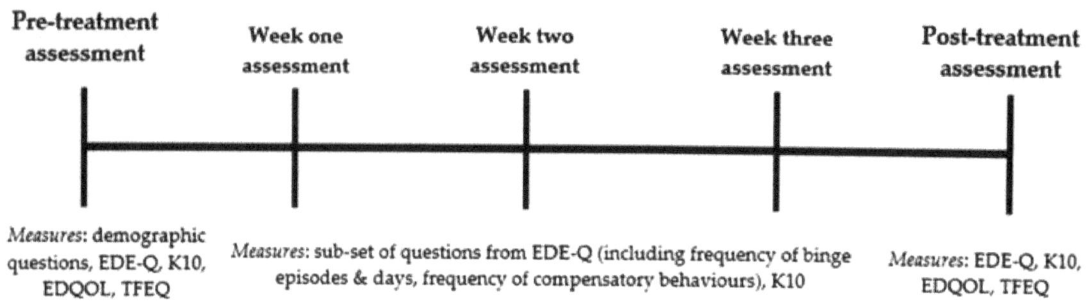

Figure 2. Schematic of the timing and sequence of assessments and included measures. Note: Week one, week two and week three assessments were identical. EDE-Q = Eating Disorder Examination-Questionnaire; K10 = Kessler Psychological Distress Scale; EDQOL = Eating Disorder Quality of Life Scale; TFEQ = Three Factor Eating Questionnaire.

On the 7th, 14th and 21st day following their first Food Diary entry, participants completed a mini eScreen questionnaire and received a 15- to 20-min check-in phone call from a research assistant trained by the CI (clinical psychologist). Each phone call was guided by a standardised set of questions and feedback developed by a clinical psychologist (S.M.) with over 15 years of experience using CBT for BN. Obstacles hindering participants' ability to adopt the Food Diary and three-hour rule were discussed, with a member of the treatment team presenting solutions in accordance with key CBT techniques of psychoeducation and positive reinforcement. Participants were sent an email the day prior to the scheduled phone call prompting completion of the mini eScreen questionnaire, followed by reminder text message on the day of the phone call.

On the 28th day of using the Food Diary, participants completed the final comprehensive online assessment (maxi eScreen) and received a final check-in phone call. Participants then gained access to remaining components of the BEeT program to engage in a pure self-help format independent of the study protocol.

2.5. Statistical Analysis

The data were cleaned and inspected for normality and baseline features of participants were examined. The statistical analysis was conducted in several stages, focusing on compliance then symptom outcome variance. First, attrition and compliance of participants with the treatment program was examined using the variables of mean number of days a Food Diary entry was made and the average number of daily Food Diary entries.

Secondly, linear regression analysis was used to test the statistical significance of differences between the pre- and post-treatment dependent variables of OBE frequency, OBE days, SBE days, LOC frequency, purge frequency, laxative frequency, exercise frequency, EDE-Q subscale scores, global EDE-Q score, global EDQOL score and global TFEQ score. Comparisons between groups were based upon a two-tailed Bonferroni-corrected α of 0.0036 (0.05/14). Linear regression analyses and pairwise comparisons were used to assess changes in OBE frequency, OBE days, purge frequency, laxative frequency, SBE frequency, dietary restriction and the number of days of Food Diary entries between the week one, two and three measures.

Finally, in order to determine if differences in participants' clinical and demographic features at baseline were associated with their treatment compliance, bulimic symptom severity and bulimic symptom improvement, these three outcome variables were converted into binary variables.

Treatment compliance variables (treatment completion, days of Food Diary entries, number of Food Diary entries) and treatment outcome variables (pre- to post-treatment change in binge frequency, purge frequency, laxative frequency, excessive exercise frequency, dietary restraint score) were converted into three binary distributions with the reference point (or cut-off) specified at 50%, 75% and 90% of the original variable value. Three distributions were created as a precautionary measure in the absence of any prior convention from previous BN treatment studies regarding the conversion of continuous dependent variables into binary variables.

A series of paired t-tests were used to examine differences between the binary variable levels in terms of the continuous variables of age and K10 score. Similarly, a Fisher's exact test examined differences between binary variable levels in terms of the categorical predictor variables of secondary mental health concerns, active/past suicidality and active/past self-harm. Analyses were conducted using the SPSS for Mac OS X version 22.0.

3. Results

3.1. Participant Characteristics

The mean age of the 25 female participants enrolled in the eTherapy program was 30.24 years (range 16–47 years, *SD* = 9.37) and the mean BMI was 25.1 (range 18.8–50.7, *SD* = 6.88). Only one participant was below 18 years of age. The sample included participants with normal weight BN and overweight BN. All participants met the DSM-5 criteria for BN at baseline [52]. Five participants (20.0%) satisfied the DSM-5 criteria for BN, non-purging type [52], the remainder met the purging type category. A high proportion of participants reported comorbid anxiety (32.0%) or depression (40.0%) as a secondary mental health concern. No participants were excluded on the basis of their self-harm or suicidality assessment. Nineteen participants (76.0%) reported engaging in another form of treatment at baseline. The most commonly reported treating professional was a psychologist or psychiatrist (56.0%), followed by GP (24.0%) and dietitian (12.0%). The sociodemographic variables of participants as reported at baseline are displayed in Table 1.

3.2. Attrition and Compliance

Of the 25 participants enrolled in the online program, four participants (16.0%) did not complete Session 1 and therefore did not access the Food Diary tool (dropouts). Four participants (16.0%) failed to complete the four weeks of monitoring and the final assessment (non-completers) and 17 participants (68.0%) engaged in the four-weeks of treatment and completed the final assessment (completers). The non-completers engaged in the Food Diary tool for an average of 18.8 days (*SD* = 2.06), that is approximately 2.5 weeks, prior to disengaging from the treatment program.

On average, the 17 completers logged at least one entry in the online Food Diary for 87.1% of the possible 28 days (range: 16–28 days, *M* = 24.4, *SD* = 4.76). The most common number of daily Food

Diary entries made by all participants was five per day. There was a significant difference in the mean number of days of self-monitoring (indexed by at least one Food Diary entry) between the four weeks of treatment, Wald χ^2 (3, N = 17) = 15.03, p = 0.002. Specifically, there was a significant decrease in the mean number of days monitored between week one (M = 6.7, SD = 0.86) and week two (M = 6.1, SD = 1.52, p = 0.042); week three (M = 6.06, SD = 1.89) and week four (M = 5.47, SD = 2.04, p = 0.05) and week one and week four (p = 0.002). Generally, the mean number of days monitored decreased each week, although at the end of treatment (week four) the average was still approximately 5.5 days of the 7. Participants' (n = 17) regularly monitored their food intake (indexed by five or more Food Diary entries) for an average of 21.2% of the possible 28 days (range: 0–28 days, M = 5.9 days, SD = 8.00).

Table 1. Baseline characteristics of participants (n = 25).

Participant Feature	Frequency (%)
Employed	60
Student	24
White/Caucasian	84
Asian	12
Metropolitan residence	64
Regional residence *	24
Rural residence	12
Comorbid anxiety	32
Comorbid depression	40
Comorbid substance/alcohol issues	16
Receiving concurrent treatment	76
Frequent alcohol consumption (4 or more times per week)	36
Past suicidality	60
Active suicidality (within previous 28 days)	20
Past self-harm	48
Active self-harm (within previous 28 days)	12

* NSW Health categorises regional residence as outside a major metropolitan city (e.g., Sydney) but not a rural location. Examples of regional locations include Wyong and Wagga Wagga.

Due to scheduling constraints, 13.2% of weekly phone calls were not completed at the exact seven-day mark. On average, these phone calls occurred 2.0 days (range: 1–8 days, SD = 2.35) later than the scheduled date and five phone calls did not take place. Moreover, 26.4% of the weekly questionnaires were not completed on time at the 7-day mark and were delayed by an average of 2.83 days (range: 1–11 days, SD = 2.81).

3.3. Treatment Outcomes

Table 2 provides the means and standard deviations for all dependent variables at each assessment period, as well as regression analysis results. Participants (n = 17) displayed a significant pre-post treatment decrease in the mean frequency of objective binge episodes, Wald χ^2 (1, N = 17) = 21.62, $p < 0.00$, mean number of days participants' experienced OBEs, Wald χ^2 (1, N = 17) = 12.99, $p < 0.001$ and frequency of perceived loss of control experienced during OBEs, Wald χ^2 (1, N = 17) = 12.47, $p < 0.001$. Pairwise comparisons revealed a significant increase in the mean number of objective binge days experienced in week one (M = 2.7, SD = 2.03) to week two (M = 3.5, SD = 2.07), p = 0.006.

There was no significant change in the number of days participants experienced subjective binge episodes between pre- and post-treatment measures, Wald χ^2 (1, N = 17) = 0.704, p = 0.401.

Using the Bonferroni correction, the decrease in the pre-post treatment frequency of purging episodes was no longer significant, Wald χ^2 (1, N = 13) = 4.30, p = 0.038. No significant differences were found in other compensatory behaviours of laxative use and excessive exercise.

There was a significant decrease from baseline to post-treatment in the mean global score on the EDE-Q, Wald χ^2 (1, N = 17) = 12.86, $p < 0.001$, as well as the mean scores on three EDE-Q subscales including dietary restraint, Wald χ^2 (1, N = 17) = 10.75, p = 0.001, eating concern, Wald χ^2 (1, N = 17) = 10.18, p = 0.001 and shape concern, Wald χ^2 (1, N = 17) = 9.92, p = 0.002.

The results of the Wilcoxon signed rank test (non-parametric sensitivity analysis) supported the respective statistical significance and non-significance of the preceding regression analyses examining the difference in bulimic symptomology between pre- and post-treatment measures.

Table 2. Treatment outcomes for Eating Disorder Examination-Questionnaire (EDE-Q), Eating Disorder Quality of Life Scale (EDQOL) and Three Factor Eating Questionnaire (TFEQ) Scores (n = 17).

Outcome	Pre-Treatment Means (*SD*)	Post-Treatment Means (*SD*)	p Value	Test Statistic Wald χ^2 (df = 1)
EDE-Q				
Objective binge frequency	23.7 (16.63)	14.9 (12.55)	$p < 0.001$ *	21.62
Objective binge days	17.9 (6.17)	10.8 (9.31)	$p < 0.001$ *	12.99
Loss of control frequency	21.0 (12.01)	14.1 (13.87)	$p < 0.001$ *	12.47
Subjective binge days (n = 16)	9.7 (9.60)	7.4 (6.26)	$p = 0.401$	0.70
Purge frequency (n = 13)	20.4 (20.45)	14.4 (18.85)	$p = 0.038$	4.30
Laxative use frequency (n = 7)	11.9 (11.45)	9.3 (10.61)	$p = 0.071$	3.25
Excessive exercise frequency (n = 11)	9.5 (10.58)	6.5 (8.42)	$p = 0.123$	2.38
Dietary restraint	4.1 (1.14)	2.9 (1.84)	$p = 0.001$ *	10.75
Eating concern	4.1 (1.11)	3.0 (1.41)	$p = 0.001$ *	10.18
Shape concern	5.3 (0.72)	4.5 (1.25)	$p = 0.002$ *	9.92
Weight concern	5.0 (0.60)	4.4 (1.48)	$p = 0.076$	3.14
Global score	4.6 (0.55)	3.7 (1.31)	$p < 0.001$ *	12.86
Other Outcomes				
EDQOL global score	1.9 (0.71)	1.8 (0.865)	$p = 0.564$	0.33
TFEQ global score	34.5 (4.91)	34.7 (4.61)	$p = 0.888$	0.02

* Statistically significant ($p < 0.0036$). Comparisons based upon Bonferroni-corrected α of 0.0036 (0.05/14). Note: EDE-Q = Eating Disorder Examination-Questionnaire; EDQOL = Eating Disorder Quality of Life Scale; TFEQ = Three Factor Eating Questionnaire.

3.4. *Predictors of Outcome and Dropout*

The Fisher's Exact Test revealed a significant association between the participants' level of bulimic severity and their degree of improvement in binge frequency, p = 0.002. Participants who displayed a 50% or greater reduction in binge frequency all were classed as less severe in bulimic presentation (defined by an average of 1–7 compensatory behaviours per week). In contrast, the majority (77.8%) of participants who displayed less than 50% reduction in binge frequency were classified as more severe in bulimic presentation.

Bulimic symptom severity was also associated with dietary restraint, p = 0.050. A statistical trend emerged whereby a larger number of participants who displayed a 50% or greater reduction in dietary restraint scores, had low bulimic severity (87.5%) as compared to high bulimic severity (12.5%). Conversely, more participants with high bulimic severity (66.7%) displayed less than 50% reduction in restraint scores as compared to those with low bulimic severity (33.3%).

Overall, treatment compliance and degree of improvement in compensatory behaviours were not significantly associated with participants' age, secondary mental health concern, K10 score, active/past suicidality, active/past self-harm and bulimic symptom severity.

4. Discussion

The findings of this study provide preliminary support for the food monitoring and regular eating techniques of CBT delivered online. Four weeks of guided, online stage 1 CBT resulted in a significant decrease in the frequency of OBEs, number of OBE days and frequency of associated LOC from baseline to post-treatment measures. There was also a significant decrease in both global EDE-Q scores and the EDE-Q subscales of dietary restraint, eating concern and shape concern. No change was observed in frequency of SBEs and compensatory behaviours including purging, laxative use and excessive exercise.

4.1. Attrition and Compliance

The current study has a considerably lower dropout rate (16%) than other online CBT studies (35% to 82%) [20]. Treatment compliance remained high with the Food Diary being entered at least once for an average of 87.1% of the possible 28 days. The food-monitoring compliance reported by previous studies is varied, ranging from 100% compliance for six to seven days of self-monitoring [9,34] to 46% compliance for 56 days of self-monitoring [41] The compliance achieved by the present study fits within the range reported by others and suggests that 28 days of food-monitoring may be an appropriate compromise between harnessing the technique's therapeutic potential and maintaining motivation to engage. Furthermore, many participants reported that the repetitive and tiresome nature of food monitoring was largely offset by the motivating nature of the weekly phone calls, with such anecdotal feedback suggesting an important role for therapeutic contact treatment compliance. However, due to the absence of appropriate control groups, the role of regular therapeutic contact and digital access to the Food Diary in producing heightened treatment compliance is yet to be elucidated.

Inaccuracies in the logging of meals in the Food Diary prevented accurate evaluation of participants' compliance with the "three-hour rule". The absence of such valuable information is due to the inaccurate recording of meal time or meal type, with most participants not adjusting the default settings of 7:00 a.m. and Breakfast when entering in the Food Diary. Consequently, an analysis of this data was not conducted. We recommend future studies adopt more stringently formatted systems to ensure accurate timing of meals is recorded [44].

4.2. Treatment Outcomes

The brief four week intervention achieved key symptom improvement comparable to the treatment outcomes of considerably longer online CBT self-help programs lasting for two to four months on average [16–19,21,61]. The preliminary results here contradict a recent review reporting that people with EDs do not find self-monitoring beneficial in practice [27] and rather supports the potential for concise, online self-monitoring programs. It is possible, however, that the observed improvements may possess short-term therapeutic effect, necessitating self-monitoring be examined over an extended time period which may cause the task to become burdensome.

The absence of a significant reduction across compensatory behaviours, despite an observed improvement in binging measures, may be due to several features of the current study. These include the short intervention period of four weeks and the small subset of participants having reported engaging in purging (n = 13), laxative use (n = 7) and excessive exercise (n = 11) as compensatory behaviours. Alternatively, given that the primary objective of food monitoring and the "three-hour rule" is to establish a regular eating pattern [42], it would appear logical for earlier change to be observed in binge frequency prior to compensatory behaviours. The paucity of evidence regarding the therapeutic effect of regular eating upon compensatory behaviours [46] necessitates future replication using larger sample sizes to confirm such suggestions. Additionally, considering early treatment response is known to predict short and long term BN treatment outcomes [38,39], the significant improvement observed in OBEs, LOC and dietary restraint following the use of only two behavioural techniques from Fairburn's 20-week program [42] may be indicative of future improvement.

Although participants' displayed an overall reduction in the number of OBE days from pre- to post-treatment measures, there was an unexpected increase in OBE days from week one (2.65 days) to week two (3.53 days). Given that the week two questionnaire was completed at the mid-point of treatment, perhaps the observed trend represents participants' initial motivation for recovery becoming later overpowered by the strength and habitual nature of their disordered eating behaviours. Alternatively, having people with BN closely review their egodystonic symptoms in the form of a Food Diary may prompt a decrease in mood and increase the likelihood of binges to regulate the distress and shame surrounding their eating behaviours [62]. More simply, participants may have developed heightened awareness regarding their behaviours in the second week of monitoring or perhaps documented their binges more truthfully once they became more comfortable with the treatment process. Further research is required to clarify whether an initial rise in OBE days is a typical BN treatment response or an anomaly of the current study.

Contrary to Hypothesis 2, no significant change was found in the number of days participants' recorded experiencing SBEs, and this challenges Hildebrandt and Latner's [34] 'binge drift' observation. The theoretical justification for 'binge drift' as the inability of self-monitoring to adjust dysfunctional cognitions [34] is also challenged by the observed decrease in the EDE-Q measures of attitudinal eating disorder psychopathology. Self-help CBT programs consisting of a longer two month treatment program have been unable to achieve such attitudinal change, similarly claiming that additional treatment time and greater focus upon cognitive elements are required [63,64]. Thus, the attitudinal improvement brought about by a considerably shorter behaviourally-based program alludes to suggestions that cognitive adjustments can be prompted by engaging in behavioural activities [30]. For example, persistence in implementing the "three-hour rule" allows for first-hand experience of the benefits of regular eating and provokes correction of certain fears or maladaptive cognitions regarding their shape. In a similar manner to the component analyses of CBT for depression [65], the ability of behavioural techniques to harness improvement in cognitive measures must be validated through direct comparison of the cognitive and behavioural components of CBT-BN.

4.3. Predictors of Treatment Compliance and Outcome

Participants with a more severe clinical presentation of BN displayed a smaller improvement in both OBE frequency and dietary restraint as compared to participants with less severe BN symptomology. Differential treatment responses as a function of one's clinical severity is mirrored in similar studies of guided self-help treatment [13,15] and fits within the "stepped-care" structure of treatment allocation [14]. Online stage 1 CBT appears to approach the therapeutic effectiveness of face-to-face treatment for a sub-set of less severe BN patients, whilst overcoming the barriers of cost, accessibility and duration of a treatment format, which may be unnecessarily excessive for their condition [8]. However, given the small sample size, it is possible that the statistical trend observed between dietary restraint and bulimic severity may represent a Type 2 error and requires replication in larger samples.

In contrast with existing literature on CBT treatment for BN [49,66,67], in this sample treatment compliance and bulimic symptom improvement was not significantly associated with baseline measures of depression or the presence of comorbid mood or anxiety disorders. The absence of such association may be due to the heavy concentration of behavioural techniques within the current study. Behavioural activities provide a practical and "hands-on" approach to treatment that is likely to enhance self-efficacy and offset the hopelessness brought upon by depressive traits and the bulimic symptoms [65,68,69]. Specifically, self-monitoring allows for direct observation of one's efforts to adhere to the "three-hour rule" and provides objective evidence of their attempts. Taken together with the encouragement provided by a therapeutic assistant, behavioural activities provide direct, observable change in depressed participants which may shift their external locus of control [66] and offset poor treatment compliance. Such justification is supported by recent suggestions regarding the importance of motivation as a predictor of BN treatment success [70] and should be included as a baseline measure in future studies. Additionally, the equivalent treatment compliance and therapeutic effectiveness across participants aged between 16 to 47 years, once more broadens the scope of candidates suitable for this treatment.

4.4. Strengths, Limitations and Future Research

The current study provides a novel contribution to the literature on BN treatment by offering preliminary pilot study evidence for the clinical effectiveness of an online, stage 1 CBT program.

The BEeT program employed in the study is a highly structured and sophisticated program, professionally developed by team of ED specialists and constructed based upon relevant empirical research on CBT-BN. Additionally, therapeutic guidance was provided by a non-expert trained in how to deliver the behavioural components of CBT treatment, offering promise as a method that could be used broadly by non-experts. The present study improves upon methodological limitations in the existing literature [71] having recruited a pure clinical sample of BN patients. Additionally, all communication took place via email and the telephone, maintaining the largely anonymous nature of online treatment and increasing the accessibility for patients who are busy with work, study or carer commitments as face-to-face interviews were not required.

Due to the relatively small sample size, these findings must be considered tentative until an adequately powered study is conducted. The absence of a waitlist control condition also limits the conclusions regarding the causal role of the treatment program and necessitates other robust research designs be conducted. A randomised controlled trial will also allow for comparison of online, stage 1 CBT against conventional CBT programs, with the presence of control arms providing further clarity regarding the role of therapeutic guidance techniques, such as reminder text messages and weekly phone calls, in provoking the greatest change in one's behaviours.

Given that 56% of participants reported receiving additional treatment, other than CBT, for their ED, it is possible that improvement observed may be partly attributed to their concurrent treatment program. However, seeing as all participants were engaged in their additional treatment prior to entering the current study, it appears that the self-monitoring and regular eating techniques enforced may have been instrumental in bringing about change.

Future research should control for concurrent treatment to isolate the effects of behavioural techniques and strengthen claims regarding its therapeutic effectiveness. Furthermore, considering previous research [72] suggests that the reactive effects of self-monitoring are limited to the time period for which the individual actively engages in self-monitoring, future studies should include a follow-up.

5. Conclusions

The present study provides preliminary evidence for the clinical effectiveness of brief behavioural self-monitoring and regular eating training (BEeT) delivered online which, if replicated in a larger sample, may result in the development of shorter, yet equally effective, forms of treatment. Concise programs would make treatment accessible for a much broader range of people with BN for whom their work or study commitments and financial constraints make it extremely difficult for them to engage in three months of one-hour weekly therapy sessions [14]. Additionally, the digital format of treatment delivery overcomes the barriers of accessibility and cost inherent in the treatment of EDs and which are of particular concern for rural and regional residents. The current findings provide the justification for a randomised controlled trial to elucidate the clinical benefits of emphasising behavioural techniques which form part of typical CBT-BN delivery by online modalities.

Acknowledgments: The development of the Binge Eating eTherapy program was funded by NSW Health.

Author Contributions: Sarah Barakat, Sarah Maguire, Phillipa Hay and Stephen Touyz conceived and designed the experiments; Sarah Barakat and Sarah Maguire performed the experiments; Sarah Barakat analyzed the data; Sarah Barakat, Sarah Maguire, Lois Surgenor, Brooke Donnelly, Blagica Miceska, Kirsty Fromholtz, Janice Russell, Phillipa Hay and Stephen Touyz contributed reagents/materials/analysis tools; Sarah Barakat wrote the paper.

References

1. Hay, P.; Chinn, D.; Forbes, D.; Madden, S.; Newton, R.; Sugenor, L.; Touyz, S.; Ward, W. Royal Australian and New Zealand College of Psychiatrists clinical practice guidelines for the treatment of eating disorders. *Aust. N. Z. J. Psychiatry* **2014**, *48*, 977–1008. [CrossRef] [PubMed]

2. National Collaborating Centre for Mental Health. *Eating Disorders: Core Interventions in the Treatment and Management of Anorexia Nervosa, Bulimia Nervosa and Related Eating Disorders*; NICE guideline (CG9); British Psychological Society: Leicester, UK; Royal College of Psychiatrists: London, UK, 2004.
3. Hart, L.M.; Granillo, M.T.; Jorm, A.F.; Paxton, S.J. Unmet need for treatment in the eating disorders: A systematic review of eating disorder specific treatment seeking among community cases. *Clin. Psychol. Rev.* **2011**, *31*, 727–735. [CrossRef] [PubMed]
4. National Eating Disorders Collaboration (NEDC). *Eating Disorders Prevention, Treatment and Management: An Evidence Review*; Commissioned by the Commonwealth Department of Health and Aging; National Eating Disorders Collaboration: Canberra, Australia, 2010.
5. Tobin, D.L.; Banker, J.D.; Weisberg, L.; Bowers, W. I know what you did last summer (and it was not CBT): A factor analytic model of international psychotherapeutic practice in the eating disorders. *Int. J. Eat. Disord.* **2007**, *40*, 754–757. [CrossRef] [PubMed]
6. Waller, G. Evidence-based treatment and therapist drift. *Behav. Res. Ther.* **2009**, *47*, 119–127. [CrossRef] [PubMed]
7. Stuhldreher, N.; Konnopka, A.; Wild, B.; Herzog, W.; Zipfel, S.; Löwe, B.; König, H.H. Cost-of-illness studies and cost-effectiveness analyses in eating disorders: A systematic review. *Int. J. Eat. Disord.* **2012**, *45*, 476–491. [CrossRef] [PubMed]
8. Williams, C. New technologies in self-help: Another effective way to get better? *Eur. Eat. Disord. Rev.* **2003**, *11*, 170–182. [CrossRef]
9. Latner, J.D.; Wilson, G.T. Self-monitoring and the assessment of binge eating. *Behav. Ther.* **2002**, *33*, 465–477. [CrossRef]
10. Hay, P.; Bacaltchuk, J.; Stefano, S. Psychotherapy for bulimia nervosa and binging. *Cochrane Database Syst. Rev.* **2004**, *1*, 1–73.
11. Fairburn, C.G. *Overcoming Binge Eating*, 1st ed.; Guilford Press: New York, NY, USA, 1995.
12. Palmer, R.L.; Birchall, H.; McGrain, L.; Sullivan, V. Self-help for bulimic disorders: A randomised controlled trial comparing minimal guidance with face-to-face or telephone guidance. *Br. J. Psychiatry* **2002**, *181*, 230–235. [CrossRef] [PubMed]
13. Thiels, C.; Schmidt, U.; Troop, N.; Treasure, J.; Garthe, R. Binge frequency predicts outcome in guided self-care treatment of bulimia nervosa. *Eur. Eat. Disord. Rev.* **2000**, *8*, 272–278. [CrossRef]
14. Treasure, J.; Schmidt, U.; Troop, N.; Tiller, J.; Todd, G.; Turnbull, S. Sequential treatment for bulimia nervosa incorporating a self-care manual. *Br. J. Psychiatry* **1996**, *168*, 94–98. [CrossRef] [PubMed]
15. Agras, W.S.; Crow, S.J.; Halmi, K.A.; Mitchell, J.E.; Wilson, G.T.; Kraemer, H.C. Outcome predictors for the cognitive behavior treatment of bulimia nervosa: Data from a multisite study. *Am. J. Psychiatry* **2000**, *157*, 1302–1308. [CrossRef] [PubMed]
16. Carrard, I.; Rouget, P.; Fernández-Aranda, F.; Volkart, A.C.; Damoiseau, M.; Lam, T. Evaluation and deployment of evidence based patient self-management support program for bulimia nervosa. *Int. J. Med. Inform.* **2006**, *75*, 101–109. [CrossRef] [PubMed]
17. Fernández-Aranda, F.; Núñez, A.; Martínez, C.; Krug, I.; Cappozzo, M.; Carrard, I.; Rouget, P.; Jiménez-Murcia, S.; Granero, R.; Penelo, E.; et al. Internet-based cognitive-behavioral therapy for bulimia nervosa: A controlled study. *Cyberpsychol. Behav.* **2009**, *12*, 37–41. [CrossRef] [PubMed]
18. Mitchell, J.E.; Crosby, R.D.; Wonderlich, S.A.; Crow, S.; Lancaster, K.; Simonich, H.; Swan-Kremeier, L.; Lysne, C.; Myers, T.C. A randomized trial comparing the efficacy of cognitive–behavioral therapy for bulimia nervosa delivered via telemedicine versus face-to-face. *Behav. Res. Ther.* **2008**, *46*, 581–592. [CrossRef] [PubMed]
19. Pretorius, N.; Arcelus, J.; Beecham, J.; Dawson, H.; Doherty, F.; Eisler, I.; Gallagher, C.; Gowers, S.; Isaacs, G.; Johnson-Sabine, E.; et al. Cognitive-behavioural therapy for adolescents with bulimic symptomatology: The acceptability and effectiveness of internet-based delivery. *Behav. Res. Ther.* **2009**, *47*, 729–736. [CrossRef] [PubMed]
20. Ruwaard, J.; Lange, A.; Broeksteeg, J.; Renteria-Agirre, A.; Schrieken, B.; Dolan, C.V.; Emmelkamp, P. Online cognitive–behavioural treatment of bulimic symptoms: A randomized controlled trial. *Clin. Psychol. Psychother.* **2013**, *20*, 308–318. [CrossRef] [PubMed]

21. Sánchez-Ortiz, V.C.; Munro, C.; Stahl, D.; House, J.; Startup, H.; Treasure, J.; Williams, C.; Schmidt, U. A randomized controlled trial of internet-based cognitive-behavioural therapy for bulimia nervosa or related disorders in a student population. *Psychol. Med.* **2011**, *41*, 407–417. [CrossRef] [PubMed]
22. Ljotsson, B.; Lundin, C.; Mitsell, K.; Carlbring, P.; Ramklint, M.; Ghaderi, A. Remote treatment of bulimia nervosa and binge eating disorder: A randomized trial of Internet-assisted cognitive behavioural therapy. *Behav. Res. Ther.* **2007**, *45*, 649–661. [CrossRef] [PubMed]
23. Robinson, P.H.; Serfaty, M.A. The use of e-mail in the identification of bulimia nervosa and its treatment. *Eur. Eat. Disord. Rev.* **2001**, *9*, 182–193. [CrossRef]
24. Bauer, S.; Okon, E.; Meermann, R.; Kordy, H. Technology-enhanced maintenance of treatment gains in eating disorders: Efficacy of an intervention delivered via text messaging. *J. Consult. Clin. Psychol.* **2012**, *80*, 700–706. [CrossRef] [PubMed]
25. Schmidt, U.; Andiappan, M.; Grover, M.; Robinson, S.; Perkins, S.; Dugmore, O.; Treasure, J.; Landau, S.; Eisler, I.; Williams, C. Randomised controlled trial of CD–ROM-based cognitive–behavioural self-care for bulimia nervosa. *Br. J. Psychiatry* **2008**, *193*, 493–500. [CrossRef] [PubMed]
26. Fairburn, C.G.; Cooper, Z. The Eating Disorder Examination (12th ed.). In *Binge Eating: Nature, Assessment and Treatment*; Fairburn, C.G., Wilson, G.T., Eds.; Guilford Press: New York, NY, USA, 1993; pp. 317–360.
27. Walsh, S.; Golden, E.; Priebe, S. Systematic review of patients' participation in and experiences of technology-based monitoring of mental health symptoms in the community. *Br. Med. J. Open* **2016**, *6*, e008362. [CrossRef] [PubMed]
28. Tregarthen, J.P.; Lock, J.; Darcy, A.M. Development of a smartphone application for eating disorder self-monitoring. *Int. J. Eat. Disord.* **2015**, *48*, 972–982. [CrossRef] [PubMed]
29. Geller, J.; Srikameswaran, S. What effective therapies have in common. *Adv. Eat. Disord. Theor. Res. Pract.* **2015**, *3*, 191–197. [CrossRef]
30. Longmore, R.J.; Worrell, M. Do we need to challenge thoughts in cognitive behavior therapy? *Clin. Psychol. Rev.* **2007**, *27*, 173–187. [CrossRef] [PubMed]
31. Fairburn, C.G.; Jones, R.; Peveler, R.C.; Carr, S.J.; Solomon, R.A.; O'Connor, M.E.; Burton, J.; Hope, R.A. Three psychological treatments for bulimia nervosa: A comparative trial. *Arch. Gen. Psychiatry* **1991**, *48*, 463–469. [CrossRef] [PubMed]
32. Korotitsch, W.J.; Nelson-Gray, R.O. An overview of self-monitoring research in assessment and treatment. *Psychol. Assess.* **1999**, *11*, 415–425. [CrossRef]
33. Wilson, G.T.; Vitousek, K.M. Self-monitoring in the assessment of eating disorders. *Psychol. Assess.* **1999**, *11*, 480–489. [CrossRef]
34. Hildebrandt, T.; Latner, J. Effect of self-monitoring on binge eating: Treatment response or 'binge drift'? *Eur. Eat. Disord. Rev.* **2006**, *14*, 17–22. [CrossRef]
35. Fairburn, C.G.; Agras, W.S.; Walsh, B.T.; Wilson, G.T.; Stice, E. Prediction of outcome in bulimia nervosa by early change in treatment. *Am. J. Psychiatry* **2004**, *161*, 2322–2324. [CrossRef] [PubMed]
36. Le Grange, D.; Doyle, P.; Crosby, R.D.; Chen, E. Early response to treatment in adolescent bulimia nervosa. *Int. J. Eat. Disord.* **2008**, *41*, 755–757. [CrossRef] [PubMed]
37. Raykos, B.C.; Watson, H.J.; Fursland, A.; Byrne, S.M.; Nathan, P. Prognostic value of rapid response to enhanced cognitive behavioral therapy in a routine clinic sample of eating disorder outpatients. *Int. J. Eat. Disord.* **2013**, *46*, 764–770. [CrossRef] [PubMed]
38. Thompson-Brenner, H.; Shingleton, R.M.; Sauer-Zavala, S.; Richards, L.K.; Pratt, E.M. Multiple measures of rapid response as predictors of remission in cognitive behavior therapy for bulimia nervosa. *Behav. Res. Ther.* **2015**, *64*, 9–14. [CrossRef] [PubMed]
39. Vall, E.; Wade, T.D. Predictors of treatment outcome in individuals with eating disorders: A systematic review and meta-analysis. *Int. J. Eat. Disord.* **2015**, *48*, 946–971. [CrossRef] [PubMed]
40. Cash, T.F.; Hrabosky, J.I. The effects of psychoeducation and self-monitoring in a cognitive-behavioral program for body-image improvement. *Eat. Disord.* **2003**, *11*, 255–270. [CrossRef] [PubMed]
41. Nichols, S.; Gusella, J. Food for thought: Will adolescent girls with eating disorders self-monitor in a CBT group. *Can. Child Psychiatry Rev.* **2003**, *12*, 37–39.
42. Fairburn, C.G. *Cognitive Behavior Therapy and Eating Disorders*; Guilford Press: New York, NY, USA, 2008.
43. Cooper, M.; Todd, G.; Wells, A. *Treating Bulimia Nervosa and Binge Eating: An Integrated Metacognitive and Cognitive Therapy Manual*; Routledge, Taylor & Francis Group: London, UK, 2009.

44. Zendegui, E.A.; West, J.A.; Zandberg, L.J. Binge eating frequency and regular eating adherence: The role of eating pattern in cognitive behavioral guided self-help. *Eat. Behav.* **2014**, *15*, 241–243. [CrossRef] [PubMed]
45. Telch, C.F.; Agras, S.W. The effects of short-term food deprivation on caloric intake in eating-disordered subjects. *Appetite* **1996**, *26*, 221–234. [CrossRef] [PubMed]
46. Shah, N.; Passi, V.; Bryson, S.; Agras, W.S. Patterns of eating and abstinence in women treated for bulimia nervosa. *Int. J. Eat. Disord.* **2005**, *38*, 330–334. [CrossRef] [PubMed]
47. Swanson, S.A.; Crow, S.J.; Le Grange, D.; Swendsen, J.; Merikangas, K.R. Prevalence and correlates of eating disorders in adolescents: Results from the national comorbidity survey replication adolescent supplement. *Arch. Gen. Psychiatry* **2011**, *68*, 714–723. [CrossRef] [PubMed]
48. Hudson, J.I.; Hiripi, E.; Pope, H.G.; Kessler, R.C. The prevalence and correlates of eating disorders in the National Comorbidity Survey Replication. *Biol. Psychiatry* **2007**, *61*, 348–358. [CrossRef] [PubMed]
49. Grilo, C.M.; Masheb, R.M.; Wilson, G.T. Subtyping binge eating disorder. *J. Consult. Clin. Psychol.* **2001**, *69*, 1066–1072. [CrossRef] [PubMed]
50. Grilo, C.M.; White, M.A.; Masheb, R.M. DSM-IV psychiatric disorder comorbidity and its correlates in binge eating disorder. *Int. J. Eat. Disord.* **2009**, *42*, 228–234. [CrossRef] [PubMed]
51. Stice, E.; Bohon, C.; Marti, C.N.; Fischer, K. Subtyping women with bulimia nervosa along dietary and negative affect dimensions: Further evidence of reliability and validity. *J. Consult. Clin. Psychol.* **2008**, *76*, 1022–1033. [CrossRef] [PubMed]
52. American Psychiatric Association. *Diagnostic and Statistical Manual of Mental Disorders*, 5th ed.; American Psychiatric Publishing: Arlington, VA, USA, 2013.
53. Fairburn, C.G.; Beglin, S.J. Eating Disorder Examination Questionnaire (6.0). In *Cognitive Behavior Therapy and Eating Disorders*; Fairburn, C.G., Ed.; Guildford Press: New York, NY, USA, 2008; pp. 309–315.
54. Fairburn, C.G.; Marcus, M.D.; Wilson, G.T. Cognitive-Behavioral Therapy for Binge Eating and Bulimia Nervosa: A Comprehensive Treatment Manual. In *Binge Eating: Nature, Assessment and Treatment*; Fairburn, C.G., Wilson, G.T., Eds.; Guildford Press: New York, NY, USA, 1993; pp. 361–404.
55. Fairburn, C.G.; Cooper, Z.; Shafran, R. Cognitive behaviour therapy for eating disorders: A "transdiagnostic" theory and treatment. *Behav. Res. Ther.* **2003**, *41*, 509–528. [CrossRef]
56. Luce, K.H.; Winzelberg, A.J.; Das, S.; Osborne, M.I.; Bryson, S.W.; Taylor, C.B. Reliability of self-report: Paper versus online administration. *Comput. Hum. Behav.* **2007**, *23*, 1384–1389. [CrossRef]
57. Peterson, C.B.; Crosby, R.D.; Wonderlich, S.A.; Joiner, T.; Crow, S.J.; Mitchell, J.E.; Bardone-Cone, A.M.; Klein, M.; Le Grange, D. Psychometric properties of the eating disorder examination-questionnaire: Factor structure and internal consistency. *Int. J. Eat. Disord.* **2007**, *40*, 386–389. [CrossRef] [PubMed]
58. Kessler, R.C.; Andrews, G.; Colpe, L.J.; Hiripi, E.; Mroczek, D.K.; Normand, S.L.; Walters, E.E.; Zaslavsky, A.M. Short screening scales to monitor population prevalences and trends in non-specific psychological distress. *Psychol. Med.* **2002**, *32*, 959–976. [CrossRef] [PubMed]
59. Engel, S.G.; Wittrock, D.A.; Crosby, R.D.; Wonderlich, S.A.; Mitchell, J.E.; Kolotkin, R.L. Development and psychometric validation of an eating disorder-specific health-related quality of life instrument. *Int. J. Eat. Disord.* **2006**, *39*, 62–71. [CrossRef] [PubMed]
60. Stunkard, A.J.; Messick, S. The three-factor eating questionnaire to measure dietary restraint, disinhibition and hunger. *J. Psychosom. Res.* **1985**, *29*, 71–83. [CrossRef]
61. Banasiak, S.J.; Paxton, S.J.; Hay, P. Guided self-help for bulimia nervosa in primary care: A randomized controlled trial. *Psychol. Med.* **2005**, *35*, 1283–1294. [CrossRef] [PubMed]
62. Williamson, D.A.; Muller, S.L.; Reas, D.L.; Thaw, J.M. Cognitive bias in eating disorders: Implications for theory and treatment. *Behav. Modif.* **1999**, *23*, 556–577. [CrossRef] [PubMed]
63. Cooper, P.J.; Coker, S.; Fleming, C. An evaluation of the efficacy of supervised cognitive behavioral self-help for bulimia nervosa. *J. Psychosom. Res.* **1996**, *40*, 281–287. [CrossRef]
64. Perkins, S.S.; Murphy, R.R.; Schmidt, U.U.; Williams, C. Self-help and guided self-help for eating disorders. *Cochrane Database Syst. Rev.* **2006**, *4*, 1–3.
65. Ilardi, S.S.; Craighead, W.E. The role of nonspecific factors in cognitive-behavior therapy for depression. *Clin. Psychol. Sci. Pract.* **1994**, *1*, 138–155. [CrossRef]
66. Steel, Z.; Jones, J.; Adcock, S.; Clancy, R.; Bridgford-West, L.; Austin, J. Why the high rate of dropout from individualized cognitive-behavior therapy for bulimia nervosa? *Int. J. Eat. Disord.* **2000**, *28*, 209–214. [CrossRef]

67. Chen, E.Y.; Le Grange, D. Subtyping adolescents with bulimia nervosa. *Behav. Res. Ther.* **2007**, *45*, 2813–2820. [CrossRef] [PubMed]
68. Bandura, A. Self-efficacy: Toward a unifying theory of behavioral change. *Psychol. Rev.* **1977**, *84*, 191–215. [CrossRef] [PubMed]
69. Cooper, P.J.; Coker, S.; Fleming, C. Self-help for bulimia nervosa: A preliminary report. *Int. J. Eat. Disord.* **1994**, *16*, 401–404. [CrossRef]
70. Steele, A.L.; Bergin, J.; Wade, T.D. Self-efficacy as a robust predictor of outcome in guided self-help treatment for broadly defined bulimia nervosa. *Int. J. Eat. Disord.* **2011**, *44*, 389–396. [CrossRef] [PubMed]
71. Hay, P.J.; Claudino, A.M. Bulimia nervosa: Online interventions. *Br. Med. J. Clin. Evid.* **2015**, *3*, 1–16.
72. Nelson, R.O.; Boykin, R.A.; Hayes, S.C. Long-term effects of self-monitoring on reactivity and on accuracy. *Behav. Res. Ther.* **1982**, *20*, 357–363. [CrossRef]

6

Mother and Infant Body Mass Index, Breast Milk Leptin and their Serum Leptin Values

Francesco Savino [1,*,†], Allegra Sardo [1,†], Lorenza Rossi [1,†], Stefania Benetti [1,†], Andrea Savino [1,†] and Leandra Silvestro [2]

1 Department of Pediatrics, Regina Margherita Children' Hospital, Città della Salute e della Scienza di Torino, Piazza Polonia 94, Torino I-10126, Italy; allegra.sardo@gmail.com (A.S.); lory_rossi@hotmail.it (L.R.); stefy_benetti@virgilio.it (S.B.); andrea.savino817@edu.unito.it (A.S.)

2 Department of Public Health and Pediatric Sciences, University of Turin I-10126, Italy; leandra.silvestro@unito.it

* Correspondence: francesco.savino@unito.it

† These authors contributed equally to this work.

Abstract: Purpose: This study investigates correlations between mother and infant Body Mass Index (BMI), their serum leptin values and breast milk leptin concentration in early infancy. Subjects and Methods: We determined serum leptin values in 58 healthy infants and leptin values in their mothers' breast milk, using radioimmunoassay (RIA). Infant and maternal anthropometrics were measured. Results: Median leptin concentration was 3.9 ng/mL (interquartile range (IQR): 2.75) in infant serum, 4.27 ng/mL (IQR: 5.62) in maternal serum and 0.89 ng/mL (IQR: 1.32) in breast milk. Median maternal BMI and weight were 24 kg/m^2 (IQR: 4.41) and 64 kg (IQR: 15). Median infant BMI was 15.80 kg/cm^2 (IQR: 4.02), while average weight was 5.130 kg (IQR: 1.627). Infants serum leptin values positively correlated with infants' BMI (p = 0.001; r = 0.213) and breast milk leptin (p = 0.03; r = 0.285). Maternal serum leptin values positively correlated with maternal BMI (p = 0.000, r = 0.449) and breast milk leptin ones (p = 0.026; r = 0.322). Conclusion: Breast milk leptin and maternal BMI could influence infant serum leptin values. Further studies are needed to better elucidate the role of genetics and environment on infant leptin production and risk of obesity later in life.

Keywords: mothers; serum leptin; BMI; breast milk; infancy

1. Introduction

Leptin is a polypeptide hormone, made of 167 amino acids and discovered by Zhang *et al.* in 1994 thanks to studies on ob/ob gene in mice [1]. This hormone is the product of the ob gene, located on chromosome 7q31.3. It circulates in plasma free or bound to proteins and it exerts its action through the soluble-OB (s-OB) receptor [2]. The primary function of this hormone is to inhibit food intake and to promote energy expenditure by regulating neuronal activity in hypothalamic arcuate nuclei: leptin, in fact, activates anorectic Pro-opiomelanocortin/ Cocaine-and amphetamine-regulated-transcript (POMC/CART) neurons and hinders the activity of those which stimulate food intake Neuropeptide Y/Agouti-related protein (NPY/AgRP) [3].

There are increasing data that environmental factors in early life predict later health. The early adiposity rebound recorded in most obese subjects suggests that factors promoting body fat development operate in the first years of life [4]. It has been shown that higher serum leptin values correlate with lower body mass index (BMI) in childhood and with lower predisposition to develop metabolic disorders in adolescence and adulthood [5].

Schuster *et al.* suggest that milk leptin could provide a link between maternal body composition and infant growth and development and also plays a role in regulating infant appetite and food intake during early infancy [6].

Increased maternal body mass index is a well-established risk factor for later infant obesity [7–9] and prevalence of obesity women is increasing worldwide [10]. Evidence suggests that human milk may decrease the transmission of obesity from mothers to their children, for example exerting its effects on early growth of the infant microbiome, as recently proposed by Lemas *et al.* [11].

It is known that leptin is mainly produced by white adipose tissue; this is the reason why serum leptin values directly correlate with body fat stores. During fasting or weight loss, leptin levels decrease, while during overeating, they increase [12]. Leptin is also released by the hypothalamus, pituitary gland, skeletal muscle, stomach, liver, placenta and mammary gland [13,14].

Leptin is found in breast milk and, interestingly, it is not only related with infants' body fat mass, but also with that of their mothers [15]. It is produced by mammary epithelial cells and it is associated with fat globules. Studies conducted on mice have shown that this hormone is transferred from maternal blood to breast milk and that it is then transferred from milk to mice puppies' bloodstream. Interestingly, the presence of leptin receptors has been found on gastric and intestinal epithelial cells of both humans and rats, suggesting that leptin may play a role in the regulation of GI functions [16]. It could be assumed that leptin taken by children with breast milk can directly pass into their bloodstream through gut since leptin receptor isoform has been found in brush border, basolateral membrane, and cytoplasm of enterocytes [17].

The amount of different adipokines in human breast milk is supposed to affect energy intake of the infant. [18] It is not well determined whether only leptin plays a causal role in early life fat deposition prevention since recently it has been reported that also sOB receptor values could have a part in the regulation of infant energy intake and infant growth and development [19].

The aim of this study is to measure leptin in mother and infant serum and in breast milk in order to look for correlations between mother and infant BMI, their serum leptin values and breast milk leptin concentration in early infancy.

2. Materials and Methods

2.1. Subjects

2.1.1. Infants

We enrolled 58 AGA healthy term infants who were admitted to the Department of Pediatrics of the University of Turin, Regina Margherita Children's Hospital, between June 2013 and July 2015. The infants underwent blood tests during routine outpatient examinations. The study protocol was approved by the local Ethical Committee at Ospedale Mauriziano—Ospedale Infantile Regina Margherita (Ethical approval code: 4698, Protocol Version 1.0., 23 May 2013)—S. Anna Torino, and infants' parents gave their written consent.

Criteria for enrollment were as follows:

Age: children from 10 days of life to 6 months and 15 days of life;

Gestational age: from 38 to 40 weeks;

Birth characteristics: birth weight from 2500 g to 4500 g, APGAR equal or above 7 and absence of neonatal diseases;

Nutrition: infants were fed with breast milk and they had not been weaned;

Clinical condition: at the time of blood sampling, infants did not have acute diseases and were afebrile.

At the time of sampling, infants were exclusively breastfed and they had not received any complementary feeding.

2.1.2. Mothers

Fifty-eight caucasian mothers belonging to a rural or urban setting were enrolled with their children. Regarding delivery, 19 mothers underwent a Caesarian section, while 39 had a spontaneous delivery. Criteria for enrollment were as follows:

Mothers who delivered infants at 38 to 40 weeks' gestation;
Mothers who were planning to exclusively breastfeed;

Mothers who signed written informed consent. Eligibility criteria for mothers were no maternal medical complications, non-smoking mothers, normal response to a glucose tolerance test, no mastitis, no prescribed medication, no digestive disorders.

2.2. *BMI Measurement*

Anthropometric measures were collected by two trained medical doctors with high intra-observer and inter-observer reliability.

Infants were weighed with an electronic integrating scale (SECA, model 757, Vogel & Halke, Hamburg, Germany), were measured in length with a stat meter and BMI was calculated as the ratio of body weight (kg) to the square of length (m^2). Mothers were weighed with a scale (Wunder, Italy), measured in height with a stat meter (Holtain Limited, Crymych, Dyfed, UK) and BMI was calculated as above.

2.3. *Blood Sampling and Hormone Analysis*

For the evaluation of leptin in serum, infants underwent four hours fasting before blood testing usually at 8.00 in the morning. The sample was stored in a refrigerator for 60 min and was then put in the refrigerated centrifuge at 4 °C at 4000 revolutions/min for 10 min. The serum obtained was divided into 2 test tubes and was stored in a freezer at −30 °C. The same procedure was carried out for mothers.

Hormone analysis was conducted with a commercially available radioimmunoassay (RIA) kit (LEP R-40, Multispecie-Leptin-RIA-Sensitive, Mediagnost, Reutlingen, Germany) with a sensitivity of 0.04 ng/mL (0.01 ng/mL with the procedure for increased sensitivity). The intra-assay variation was less than 5%, and the inter-assay variation did not exceed 7.6%.

2.4. *Breast Milk Sampling and Hormone Analysis*

About 5 mL of foremilk samples were collected from the lactating women by hand expression between 07:00 and 09:00. All milk samples were collected in tubes containing protease inhibitors (Sigma-Aldrich Company Ltd., Dorset, England) and immediately frozen at −20 °C. Samples were thawed at 4–6 °C overnight and centrifuged at 2500 revolutions at 4 for 20 min to separate the fat milk. Like serum leptin, 2 mL of skimmed breast milk leptin was analyzed with a RIA kit (LEP R-40, Multispecie-Leptin-RIA-Sensitive, Mediagnost, Reutlingen, Germany) with a sensitivity of 0.04 ng/mL (0.01 ng/mL with the procedure for increased sensitivity).

2.5. *Statistical Analysis*

Statistical analyses were conducted using SPSS software (version 21.0, SPSS, Inc., Chicago, IL, USA). First, we performed univariate descriptive analysis. The normal distribution of the variables was tested by the Shapiro-Wilk test. Continuous variables were expressed as median and interquartile range (IQR). Data that were not normally distributed were analysed with the Mann-Whitney U test and the Kruskal-Wallis test. Correlations are expressed by the Spearman correlation coefficient. All tests were done with two tails, with a fixed significance alpha =5%.

3. Results

Median leptin concentration was 3.9 ng/mL (IQR: 2.75) in infant serum, 4.27 ng/mL (IQR: 5.62) in maternal serum and 0.89 ng/mL (IQR: 1.32) in breast milk (Tables 1 and 2). Statistical significance was set at $p < 0.05$ and correlations were assessed using Spearman's rho.

Table 1. Infant anthropometric parameters and serum leptin values (median + interquartile range (IQR)).

Parameters	Infants
	$n = 58$
Age (days)	61 (76.5)
Gestational Age (weeks)	39 (1.5)
Birth Weight (kg)	3.275 (0.622)
Birth Length (cm)	49.45 (2.2)
Birth Cranial Circumference (cm)	34.05 (1.5)
Weight (kg)	5.130 (1.269)
Height (cm)	55 (3.25)
Cranial Circumference (cm)	39 (3)
BMI (kg/m^2)	15.80 (2.47)
Serum Leptin (ng/mL)	3.9 (2.75)

Table 2. Maternal anthropometric parameters, serum leptin and Breast Milk (BM) leptin values (median + IQR).

Parameters	Mothers
	$n = 58$
Age (years)	28.5 (8)
Weight (kg)	64 (12.59)
Height (cm)	164 (0.064)
BMI (kg/m^2)	24 (4.52)
Serum Leptin (ng/mL)	4.27 (5.62)
Breast Milk Leptin (ng/mL)	0.89 (1.32)

We evaluated the impact of potential confounders on breast milk leptin values and maternal and infant serum leptin values. Particularly, we analyzed the effect of infant age and gender on leptin concentrations.

Regarding infant age, we divided our cohort into three age groups at enrollment. We obtained a median (IQR) leptin concentration of 2.87 (2.53) ng/mL in infant serum, 3.27 (5.38) ng/mL in maternal serum and 0.83 (1.17) ng/mL in breast milk in group 1 (<2 months; $n = 30$), of 4.54 (9.89) ng/mL in infant serum, 2.46 (1.49) ng/mL in maternal serum and 1.18 (1.29) ng/mL in breast milk in group 2 (<4 months; $n = 18$) and of 4.85 (7.51) ng/mL in infant serum, 3.21 (2.25) ng/mL in maternal serum and 0.87 (3.55) ng/mL in breast milk in group 3 (4–6 months; $n = 10$). No significant differences in breast milk and infant and serum leptin values were detected among the three groups ($p > 0.05$).

We divided patients by gender into two groups: as concernes males ($n = 26$), the median (IQR) leptin concentration was 2.83 (2.16) ng/mL in infant serum, 3.27 (5.13) ng/mL in maternal serum and 0.83 (1.32) ng/mL in breast milk; in females ($n = 32$), the median (IQR) leptin concentration was 4.79 (8.46) ng/mL in infant serum, 2.84 (2.14) ng/mL in maternal serum and 0.93 (2.59) ng/mL in breast milk. With reference to gender, we did not observe any statistical differences in breast milk leptin values and maternal and infant serum leptin values ($p > 0.05$).

3.1. *Infant Serum Leptin Values and Infant BMI*

Serum leptin values positively correlated with infants' weight ($p = 0.002$; $r = 0.2$) and BMI ($p = 0.001$; $r = 0.213$), as shown in Figure 1.

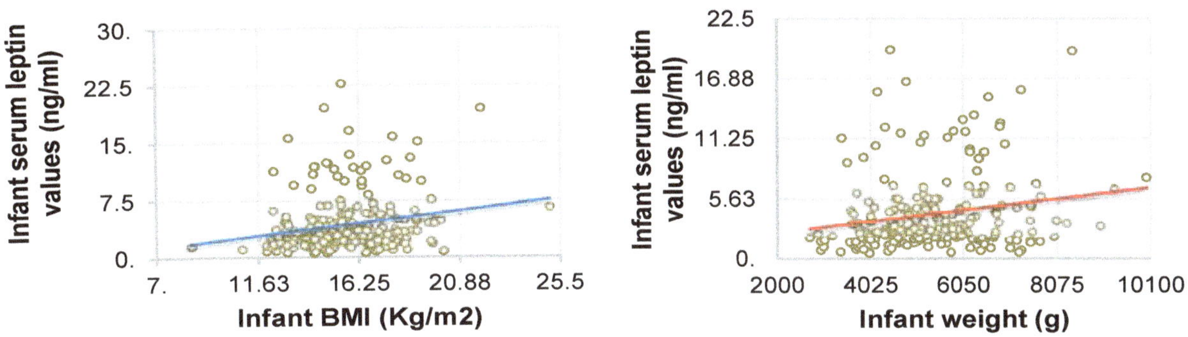

(a) (b)

Figure 1. Correlation between infant serum leptin values and infant Body Mass Index (BMI) and weight. (**a**) Association between serum leptin values and BMI; (**b**) Association between serum leptin values and weight.

The positive correlation between infant serum leptin values and both infant BMI and weight suggests that leptin concentrations are directly related to body fat stores. This hormone is primarily released by adipocytes in adipose white tissue [15]. This is the reason why infants with higher BMI have higher serum leptin values [20].

3.2. Maternal Serum Leptin Values, Maternal BMI and Breast Milk Leptin

Maternal BMI positively correlated with maternal serum leptin levels ($p = 0.000$; $r = 0.449$) and breast milk leptin ($p = 0.004$; $r = 0.368$) as illustrated in Figure 2. We found a significant correlation between breast milk leptin and maternal serum leptin values ($p = 0.026$; $r = 0.322$) as shown in Figure 3.

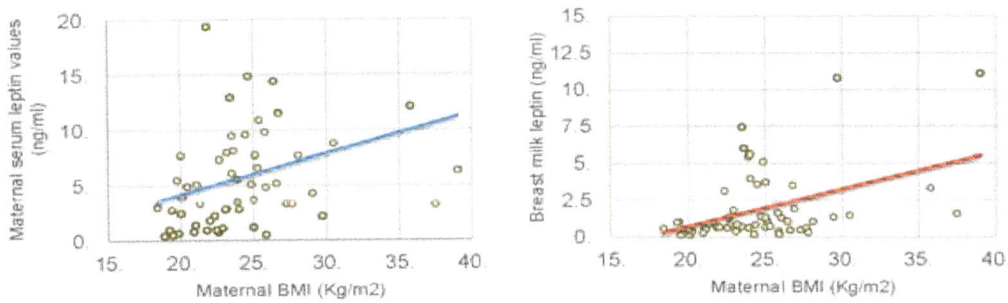

(a) (b)

Figure 2. Correlation between maternal BMI and maternal serum leptin and breast milk leptin. (**a**) Association between maternal BMI and maternal serum leptin values; (**b**) Association between maternal BMI and breast milk leptin.

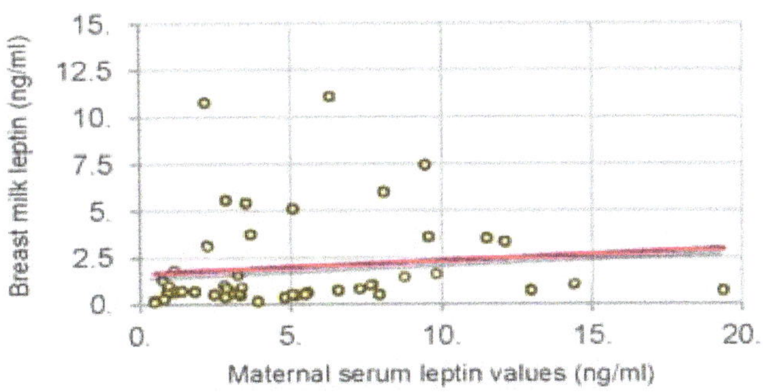

Figure 3. Correlation between maternal serum leptin and breast milk leptin.

We found a positive and significant correlation between BMI and serum leptin values. As shown for infants, mothers with higher BMI have higher serum leptin values, suggesting that leptin concentration is directly proportional to body fat mass percentage [20].

Regarding breast milk, it is interesting that a positive correlation exists between maternal BMI and leptin levels in breast milk [21]. It could be that not only breast milk leptin depends on the amount produced by mammary epithelial cells, but also on the amount released from maternal body fat stores.

A significant correlation was observed between maternal serum leptin values and breast milk leptin [22]. Also Weyermann *et al.* [23] observed that leptin concentration in breast milk correlated positively with leptin in maternal serum.

3.3. Infant Serum Leptin Values, Maternal Serum Leptin Values and Breast Milk Leptin

We did not find any significant correlation between maternal and infant serum leptin values ($p > 0.05$), suggesting that further studies are required to investigate the possible role of maternal leptin in the regulation of infant metabolism [24]. Regarding breast milk leptin and infant serum leptin values, we obtained a positive correlation, as illustrated in Figure 4 ($p = 0.03$; $r = 0.285$).

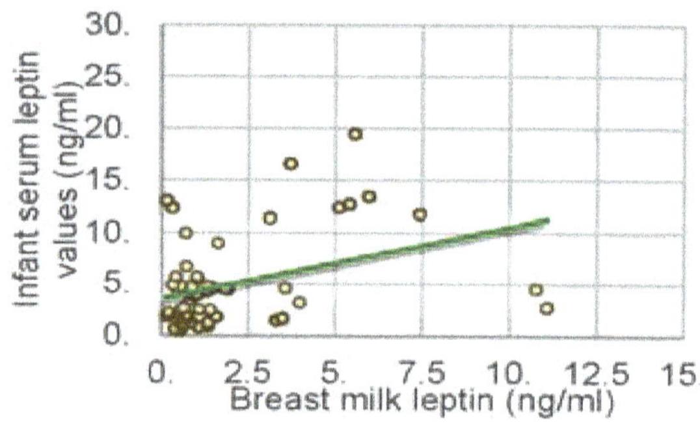

Figure 4. Correlation between breast milk leptin and infant serum leptin values.

The higher the breast milk leptin concentration is, the higher infant serum leptin values are. These findings suggest a possible association between breast milk components and infant adiposity [18].

4. Discussion

This study presents data of a positive correlation between breast milk leptin and infant serum leptin values. Furthermore, our study is strengthened by the fact that we found that breast milk leptin directly correlates with maternal serum leptin values. Actually, we did not obtain a significant association between maternal and infant serum leptin values. Regarding maternal and infant BMI, we showed that breast milk leptin and maternal serum leptin values directly correlate with materal BMI. In addition, we demonstrated a positive association between infant BMI and infant serum leptin values. We evaluated the possible impact of infant age and gender on infant and maternal serum leptin values and breast milk leptin concentrations. We did not obtain any significant differences in leptin values among the created groups.

4.1. Serum Leptin Values and BMI

Leptin is mainly produced by adipocytes; thus its levels are strictly associated to body fat mass percentage. During fasting, this hormone decreases; on the other hand, in overeating, its levels increase [25]. Both in infants and their mothers, we found that this hormone correlates with BMI and weight. Higher BMI correlates with higher serum leptin levels. It is known that people with an elevated BMI have high serum leptin levels not only because they have a larger amount of fat mass, but also because their adipocytes are bigger. What is more, Dusserre *et al.* showed that leptin values vary according to the type of adipose tissue that releases them: omental adipocytes express leptin mRNA less than subcutaneous adipocytes [26].

4.2. Breast Milk Leptin and Maternal Serum Leptin Values

Casabiell *et al.* showed that leptin is transferred from maternal bloodstream to breast milk in mice [16]. We found a positive correlation between breast milk leptin values and maternal serum leptin ones. It is thus possible that leptin in breast milk depends not only on the amount produced by mammary epithelial cells, but also on the amount in maternal bloodstream. It would be interesting to evaluate if maternal leptin values represent a predictor for infant obesity [27].

4.3. Breast Milk Leptin and Infant Serum Leptin Values

Leptin receptors have been found on gastrointestinal epithelial cells, suggesting that this hormone could be absorbed from infant mucosa and then transferred to infant bloodstream. The significant correlation that we found between breast milk leptin and infant serum leptin values could indicate that leptin in children is influenced by both infant fat stores and breast milk leptin. In previous studies, we demonstrated that formula fed infants have lower leptin levels than breast milk fed ones [28]. Data on the presence of leptin in infant formula are still controversial [29], however more investigations are needed to detect if hormones present in breast milk have a beneficial effect on obesity later in life [30,31].

4.4. Study Limitations

This study has several limitations. We could not assess the influence of leptin circadian variations since we do not have daily access to serum leptin samples, nor were we able to assess daily changes in breast milk leptin.

Moreover, we did not measure serum leptin at the same age time in all subjects enrolled.

However, baseline characteristics were similar among the infants in the study group.

Further, we were unable to measure fat mass at the same time of leptin sampling in mothers and infants.

Finally, since this study is observational it is important to interpret our correlations with caution.

Our findings are consistent with the possibility that breast milk leptin affects infant health later in life and opens new implications for research such as the role of breastfeeding and infant metabolic response.

Therefore, a follow-up of our patients, based on these results, will help us build a stronger overall evidence base and fill the gap in knowledge.

It is known that early nutrition plays an important role in the development of metabolic diseases in adolescence and adulthood. It has been shown that breastfed infants are at lower risk to become obese than formula-fed ones [32]. The positive correlation observed between maternal serum leptin concentration and maternal BMI is strictly linked to breast milk leptin values, suggesting that the amount of leptin in breast milk is influenced not only by mammary gland, but also by leptin released from maternal fat storages [33]. Interestingly, in a previous study, we demonstrated that infant serum leptin values are correlated to maternal BMI, thus showing that infants breast-fed by mothers with high BMI receive higher amounts of leptin [34]. Children with obese mothers seem to be at higher risk to become obese themselves [35]. The protective effect of breastfeeding against early childhood obesity may differ with race and ethnicity [36].

Many factors related to breastfeeding may influence childhood weight outcomes and obesity such as breastfeeding duration [37]; however, it should be considered that, ingesting high amounts of leptin, infants with obese mothers become leptin resistant and have alterations in appetite regulation [7,9,38]. In animal models it has been shown that obese phenotype can be transmitted by mothers to the following generations [39]. Since recently it has been observed that higher perinatal leptin is associated with lower adiposity at 3 years of life [40], leptin could be a key to understand the relationship between maternal BMI and infant growth and development. Intersting data showed that breast feeding affects infant's self-regulation of milk intake during late infancy [41].

5. Conclusions

Understanding the determinants of infant body mass index is relevant for the study of childhood obesity and the related risk of obesity in adulthood.

The existing data of the effects of breast milk leptin on infant growth and adiposity are controversial. Growing evidence suggests that human milk may reduce the transfer of obesity from mother to progenies and leptin is one of the possible factors involved.

In this study we investigated the possible correlations between maternal and infant serum leptin values, breast milk leptin concentrations and infant and maternal BMI. We demonstrated a positive correlation between infants' serum leptin concentrations and both maternal and infant BMI.

Regarding breast milk leptin values, we obtained a positive association not only with maternal BMI but also with maternal and infant serum leptin values.

There was no association between infant and maternal serum leptin concentrations.

Leptin is a peptide hormone produced by both adipocytes and mammary gland and it could be considered a marker that may signify excess fat accumulation.

Overall, our findings show that breast feeding and maternal BMI could influence infant serum leptin values. Further studies are needed to better elucidate the role of genetics on infant leptin production and risk of obesity later in life.

Acknowledgments: We are grateful to Sapienza, D. for perfoming hormone assays at the Laboratory analysis "Baldi and Riberi", Molinette—Città della Salute e della Scienza di Torino, Italy.

Author Contributions: F.S. conceived the study and designed the research, and wrote the manuscript. A.S. performed the experiments and wrote the manuscript. L.R. performed the experiments; analyzed the data. A.S. searched references and revised the manuscript. L.S. conceived the study and revised the manuscript. All authors read and approved the final manuscript.

References

1. Zhang, Y.; Proenca, R.; Maffei, M.; Barone, M.; Leopold, L.; Friedman, J.M. Positional cloning of the mouse obese gene and its human homologue. *Nature* **1994**, *372*, 425–432. [CrossRef] [PubMed]
2. Tartaglia, L.; Dembski, M.; Weng, X.; Deng, N.; Culpepper, J.; Devos, R.; Richards, G.J.; Campfield, L.A.; Clark, F.T.; Deeds, J.; *et al.* Identification and expression cloning of a leptin receptor. *Cell* **1995**, *83*, 1263–1271. [CrossRef]
3. Spanswick, D.; Smith, M.; Groppi, V.E.; Logan, S.; Ashford, M.L. Leptin inhibits hypothalamic neurons by activation of ATP-sensitive potassium channels. *Nature* **1997**, *390*, 521–525. [PubMed]
4. Rolland-Cachera, M.F.; Akrout, M.; Péneau, S. Nutrient intakes in early life and risk of obesity. *Int. J. Environ. Res. Public Health* **2012**, *13*, 564. [CrossRef] [PubMed]
5. Savino, F.; Liguori, S.; Benetti, S.; Sorrenti, M.; Fissore, M.F.; di Montezemolo, L.C. High serum leptin levels in infancy can potentially predict obesity in childhood, especially in formula-fed infants. *Acta Paediatr. Int. J. Paediatr.* **2013**. [CrossRef] [PubMed]
6. Miralles, O.; Sánchez, J.; Palou, A.; Picó, C. A physiological role of breast milk leptin in body weight control in developing infants. *Obesity* **2006**, *14*, 1371–1377. [CrossRef] [PubMed]
7. Andreas, N.; Hyde, M.; Gale, C.; Parkinson, J.; Jeffries, S.; Holmes, E.; Modi, N. Effect of maternal body mass index on hormones in breast milk: A systematic review. *PLoS ONE* **2014**. [CrossRef] [PubMed]
8. Bider-Canfield, Z.; Martinez, M.P.; Wang, X.; Yu, W.; Bautista, M.P.; Brookey, J.; Page, K.A.; Buchanan, T.A.; Xiang, A.H. Maternal obesity, gestational diabetes, breastfeeding and childhood overweight at age 2 years. *Pediatr. Obes.* **2016**. [CrossRef] [PubMed]
9. Gruszfeld, D.; Kułaga, Z.; Wierzbicka, A.; Rzehak, P.; Grote, V.; Martin, F.; Poncelet, P.; Closa-Monasterolo, R.; Escribano, J.; Verduci, E.; *et al.* Leptin and adiponectin serum levels from infancy to school age: Factors influencing tracking. *Child Obes.* **2016**, *12*, 179–187. [CrossRef] [PubMed]

10. NCD Risk Factor Collaboration (NCD-RisC). Trends in adult body-mass index in 200 countries from 1975 to 2014: A pooled analysis of 1698 population-based measurement studies with 19.2 million participants. *Lancet* **2016**, *387*, 1377–1396.
11. Lemas, D.J.; Young, B.E.; Baker, P.R., II; Tomczik, A.C.; Soderborg, T.K.; Hernandez, T.L. Alterations in human milk leptin and insulin are associated with early changes in the infant intestinal microbiome. *Am. J. Clin. Nutr.* **2016**, *103*, 1291–1300. [CrossRef] [PubMed]
12. Havel, P.; Townsend, R. High-fat meals reduce 24-h circulating leptin concentrations in women. *Diabetes* **1999**, *48*, 334–341. [CrossRef] [PubMed]
13. Hassink, S.; de Lancey, E.; Sheslow, D.V.; Smith-Kirwin, S.M.; O'Connor, D.M.; Considine, R.V.; Opentanova, I.; Dostal, K.; Spear, M.L.; Leef, K.; *et al.* Placental leptin: An important new growth factor in intrauterine and neonatal development? *Pediatrics* **1997**. [CrossRef]
14. Bado, A.; Levasseur, S.; Attoub, S.; Kermorgant, S.; Laigneau, J.P.; Bortoluzzi, M.N.; Moizo, L.; Lehy, T.; Guerre-Millo, M.; le Marchand-Brustel, Y.; *et al.* The stomach is a source of leptin. *Nature* **1998**, *394*, 790–793. [PubMed]
15. Houseknecht, K.; McGuire, M.; Portocarrero, C.P.; McGuire, M.A.; Beerman, K. Leptin is present in human milk and is related to maternal plasma leptin concentration and adiposity. *Biochem. Biophys. Res. Commun.* **1997**, *240*, 742–747. [CrossRef] [PubMed]
16. Casabiell, X.; Piñeiro, V.; Tomé María, A.; Peinó, R.; Diéguez, C.; Casanueva, F. Presence of leptin in colostrum and/or breast milk from lactating mothers: A potential role in the regulation of neonatal food intake. *J. Clin. Endocrinol. Metab.* **1997**, *82*, 4270–4273. [CrossRef] [PubMed]
17. Barrenetxe, J.; Villaro, C.; Guembe, L.; Pascual, I.; Muñoz-Navas, M.; Barber, A.; Lostao, M.P. Distribution of the long leptin receptor isoform in brush border, basolateral membrane, and cytoplasm of enterocytes. *Gut* **2002**, *50*, 797–802. [CrossRef] [PubMed]
18. Fields, D.A.; Schneider, C.R.; Pavela, G. A narrative review of the associations between six bioactive components in breast milk and infant adiposity. *Obesity* **2016**, *24*, 1213–1221. [CrossRef] [PubMed]
19. Zepf, F.D.; Rao, P.; Moore, J.; Stewart, R.; Ladino, Y.M.; Hartmann, B.T. Human breast milk and adipokines—A potential role for the soluble leptin receptor (sOb-R) in the regulation of infant energy intake and development. *Med. Hypothesis* **2016**, *86*, 53–55. [CrossRef] [PubMed]
20. Sinha, M.; Caro, J. Clinical aspects of leptin. *Vitam. Horm.* **1998**, *54*, 1–30. [PubMed]
21. Uysal, F.; Onal, E.; Aral, Y.Z.; Adam, B.; Dilmen, U.; Ardiçolu, Y. Breast milk leptin: Its relationship to maternal and infant adiposity. *Clin. Nutr.* **2002**, *21*, 157–160. [CrossRef] [PubMed]
22. Schuster, S.; Hechler, C.; Gebauer, C.; Kiess, W.; Kratzsch, J. Leptin in maternal serum and breast milk: Association with infants' body weight gain in a longitudinal study over 6 months of lactation. *Pediatr. Res.* **2011**, *70*, 633–637. [CrossRef] [PubMed]
23. Weyermann, M.; Beermann, C.; Brenner, H.; Rothenbacher, D. Adiponectin and leptin in maternal serum, cord blood, and breast milk. *Clin. Chem.* **2006**, *52*, 2095–2102. [CrossRef] [PubMed]
24. Castagno, E.; Liguori, S.A.; Viola, S.; Lupica, M.M.; Oggero, R.; Savino, F. Serum leptin levels in breastfed infants in the first six months of life, in their mothers and in breast milk. *Dig. Liver Dis.* **2009**, *41*, S226. [CrossRef]
25. Ahima, R.; Prabakaran, D.; Mantzoros, C.; Qu, D.; Lowell, B.; Maratos-Flier, E.; Flier, J.S. Role of leptin in the neuroendocrine response to fasting. *Nature* **1996**, *382*, 250–252. [CrossRef] [PubMed]
26. Dusserre, E.; Moulin, P.; Vidal, H. Differences in mRNA expression of the proteins secreted by the adipocytes in human subcutaneous and visceral adipose tissues. *Biochim. Biophys.* **2000**, *1500*, 88–96. [CrossRef]
27. Misra, V.; Straughen, J.; Trudeau, S. Maternal serum leptin during pregnancy and infant birth weight: The influence of maternal overweight and obesity. *Obesity* **2013**, *21*, 1064–1069. [CrossRef] [PubMed]
28. Savino, F.; Liguori, S.A.; Petrucci, E.; Lupica, M.M.; Fissore, M.F.; Oggero, R.; Silvestro, L. Evaluation of leptin in breast milk, lactating mothers and their infants. *Eur. J. Clin. Nutr.* **2010**, *64*, 972–977. [CrossRef] [PubMed]
29. Lage, M.; Baldelli, R.; Camiña, J.P.; Rodriguez-Garci, J.; Peñalva, A.; Dieguez, C.; Casanueva, F.F. Presence of bovine leptin in edible commercial milk and infant formula. *J. Endocrinol. Invest.* **2002**, *25*, 670–674. [CrossRef] [PubMed]

30. Savino, F.; Fissore, M.; Liguori, S.A.; Oggero, R. Can hormones contained in mothers' milk account for the beneficial effect of breast-feeding on obesity in children? *Clin. Endocrinol.* **2009**, *81*, 757–765. [CrossRef] [PubMed]
31. Savino, F.; Liguori, S.; Fissure, M.; Oggero, R. Breast milk hormones and their protective effect on obesity. *Int. J. Pediatr. Endocrinol.* **2009**. [CrossRef]
32. Oddy, W. Infant feeding and obesity risk in the child. *Breastfeed. Rev.* **2012**, *20*, 7–12. [PubMed]
33. Savino, F.; Sorrenti, M.; Bennetti, S.; Lupica, M.M.; Liguori, S.A.; Oggero, R. Resistin and leptin in breast milk and infants in early life. *Early Hum. Dev.* **2012**, *88*, 779–782. [CrossRef] [PubMed]
34. Savino, F.; Liguori, S.A.; Oggero, R.; Silvestro, L.; Miniero, R. Maternal BMI and serum leptin concentration of infants in the first year of life. *Acta Paediatr.* **2006**, *95*, 414–418. [CrossRef] [PubMed]
35. Parsons, T.; Power, C.; Manor, O. Fetal and early life growth and body mass index from birth to early adulthood in 1958 British cohort: Longitudinal study. *BMJ* **2001**, *323*, 1331–1335. [CrossRef] [PubMed]
36. Ehrenthal, D.B.; Wu, P.; Trabulsi, J. Differences in the protective effect of exclusive breastfeeding on child overweight and obesity by mother's race. *Matern. Child Health J.* **2016**. [CrossRef] [PubMed]
37. Modrek, S.; Basu, S.; Harding, M.; White, J.S.; Bartick, M.C.; Rodriguez, E.; Rosenberg, K.D. Does breastfeeding duration decrease child obesity? An instrumental variables analysis. *Pediatr. Obes.* **2016**. [CrossRef] [PubMed]
38. Doneray, H.; Orbak, Z.; Yildiz, L. The relationship between breast milk leptin and neonatal weight gain. *Acta Paediatr.* **2009**, *98*, 643–647. [CrossRef] [PubMed]
39. Wang, H.; Ji, J.; Yu, Y.; Wei, X.; Chai, S.; Liu, D.; Huang, D.; Li, Q.; Dong, Z.; Xiao, X. Neonatal overfeeding in female mice predisposes the development of obesity in their male offspring via altered central leptin signalling. *J. Neuroendocrinol.* **2015**, *27*, 600–608. [CrossRef] [PubMed]
40. Boeke, C.E.; Mantzoros, C.S.; Hughes, M.D.; Rifas-Shiman, S.L.; Villamor, E.; Zera, C.A.; Gillman, M.W. Differential associations of leptin with adiposity across early childhood. *Obesity* **2013**, *21*, 1430–1437. [CrossRef] [PubMed]
41. Li, R.; Fein, S.B.; Grummer-Strawn, L.M. Do infants fed from bottles lack self-regulation of milk intake compared with directly breastfed infants? *Pediatrics* **2010**, *125*, 1386–1393. [CrossRef] [PubMed]

7

Managing Risk of Non-Communicable Diseases in Women with Bulimia Nervosa or Binge Eating Disorders: A Randomized Trial with 12 Months Follow-Up

Therese Fostervold Mathisen [1,*], Jorunn Sundgot-Borgen [1], Jan H. Rosenvinge [2] and Solfrid Bratland-Sanda [3]

1 Department of Sports Medicine, Norwegian School of Sport Sciences; Sognsvegen 220, 0806 Oslo, Norway; jorunn.sundgot-borgen@nih.no
2 Department of Psychology, Faculty of Health Sciences, UiT- the Arctic University of Norway, N-9037 Tromsø, Norway; jan.rosenvinge@uit.no
3 Department of Sports and Physical Education and Outdoor Sciences, University of South-Eastern Norway, N-3800 Bø in Telemark, Norway; solfrid.bratland-sanda@usn.no
* Correspondence: t.f.mathisen@nih.no

Abstract: Persons with bulimia nervosa (BN) or binge eating disorder (BED) have an elevated risk of non-communicable diseases (NCDs). However, lowering this risk is rarely addressed in standard cognitive-behavioral treatment (CBT). We aimed to compare CBT with an intervention combining physical exercise and dietary therapy (PED-t), and hypothesized that the PED-t would do better than CBT in lowering the risk of NCD both initially and longitudinally. In this study, 164 women with bulimia nervosa or binge eating disorder were randomly assigned to 16-weeks of outpatient group therapy with either PED-t or CBT. Body composition (BC) was measured by dual-energy X-ray absorptiometry. Measures of physical fitness (VO_2peak and one repetition maximum (1RM) in squats, bench press, and seated row) were also recorded. All measurements were completed baseline, post-treatment, and at 6- and 12-month follow-ups, respectively. Our results showed that PED-t improved more than CBT on mean (99% CI) absolute Vo2peak; 57,2 (84.4, 198.8) mL ($g = 0.22$, $p < 0.001$) post-treatment. There were small to medium long-term differences in 1RM after PED-t compared to CBT. BC deteriorated in both groups during follow-up. Neither the PED-t nor the CBT lowered the risk for NCDs. Clearly, other approaches need to be considered to promote physical fitness and lower the risk of NCDs among individuals with BN and BED.

Keywords: physical fitness; visceral adipose tissue; obesity; eating disorders; nutrition; physical activity; exercise; bulimia; binge eating disorder

---

1. Introduction

Poor physical fitness is a major public health challenge, and it has been found to be prevalent among those suffering from bulimia nervosa (BN) or binge eating disorders (BED) [1,2]. Poor physical fitness may in return increase the risk of non-communicable diseases (NCDs) such as type 2 diabetes, obesity, and cardiovascular symptoms [3]: risk profiles previously identified in BN and BED [4–9].

It is well documented that lifestyle interventions focusing on diet and physical activity may reduce the risk of obesity and many NCDs [10]. However, in the treatment of BN, and notably, anorexia nervosa, there is a reluctance to focus on physical activity because of fear of triggering or exacerbating dieting, compulsive exercise, and other eating disorder symptoms (ED-symptoms) [11,12]. Further, with respect to BN, and BED in particular, a need to focus on physical activity due to a risk of obesity is hampered by the fact that many treatment guidelines recommend postponing such a focus until eating disorder symptoms have been successfully treated [12,13]. Another problem regarding the limited attention to somatic comorbidity during treatment of BN and BED is the poor specificity of body mass index (BMI) categories and the waist-circumference ratio to detect overweight problems. Thus, "masked obesity" in terms of a morbid body composition may occur in cases of a high body fat percentage [2,14] and a high level of visceral adipose tissue despite normal BMI [2]. For these reasons, physical fitness is understudied and poorly addressed in the treatment of BN and BED. As a consequence, many treatment guidelines related to physical health are somewhat skewed towards the management and treatment of severe anorexia nervosa [12].

Cognitive-behavioral therapy (CBT) is recognized as a gold standard treatment for eating disorders due to its capacity to reduce concern for body weight and shape, to improve self-esteem, self-efficacy, and self-compassion, and to affect regulation [15,16]. Such cognitive-affective changes lead to behavioral changes like reduced bingeing and increased health-related physical activity [17,18]. However, in a previous clinical study on eating disorders, we showed that a CBT-based treatment approach, in fact, did not produce changes in physical fitness and body composition [19]. A possible explanation of such findings is that CBT for eating disorders lacks a specific focus on weight loss and physical fitness and how to improve it [20]. On the other hand, several studies as well as a systematic review have reported that including physical activity in treatment may reduce BN and BED symptoms [21–28]. However, these studies have not reported data on changes in physical fitness, body composition, and other variables related to NCDs. In sum then, with a lack of focus on addressing physical fitness in the CBT manuals, one may hypothesize that a CBT treatment for BN and BED may not lower the risk of NCDs. Consequently, it is reasonable to hypothesize that a treatment of BN and BED that has an explicit focus on physical activity and that has been found to reduce compulsive exercise [27] and to match CBT in overall treatment efficiency [28] may be more effective than a CBT treatment in terms of lowering the risk of NCDs.

In addition to investigating the effect of a new treatment program for BN and BED on ED-symptoms, i.e., bingeing/purging, and an overvaluation on the need to control food intake, body weight and shape (previously reported) [27,28], we also wanted to investigate the acute and long-term effects of physical exercise and dietary therapy (PED-t) or CBT on physical fitness, body composition (BC), and risk of NCDs. We hypothesized that PED-t improves physical fitness and BC more than CBT, hence resulting in a more favorable risk profile for NCDs.

2. Materials and Methods

2.1. Subjects

We recruited females with BN or a BED to a 16-week outpatient group treatment, arranged at the Norwegian School of Sport Sciences (NSSS) during 2014–2016 [28]. The recruitment was directed through general practitioners, national and regional media, and social media.

All interested were interviewed by telephone using the Eating Disorder Examination questionnaire (EDE-q) [29] and the mini international neuropsychiatric interview (MINI) [30]. To optimize group heterogeneity, only women aged 18–40 years with BN or a BED were eligible. Participation in the study was restricted to women who were not currently pregnant and who had a BMI to 17.5–35 in order to reduce the risk of injuries and other complications if being randomized to the PED-t, as women who do not meet these criteria may not be able to follow a standardized exercise and dietary treatment protocol or to follow group exercise with minor room for individual adjustments. The study also excluded competitive athletes, those with comorbid mental disorders in need of other treatments, or those living distances to the study site that prevented regular attendance.

As previously reported [31], power analysis indicted a need for a minimum of 144 (72 per group) participants. We randomized 164 of those 419 who initially responded to recruitment to either PED-t (n = 76) or CBT (n = 73) (Figure 1). A randomization list with block size of eight was produced by www.randomizer.org by a statistician not connected to the study, and a fellow worker with no involvement in the trial randomized participants to either CBT or PED-t. All participants were informed about the outcome of the randomization after they had completed all baseline measures.

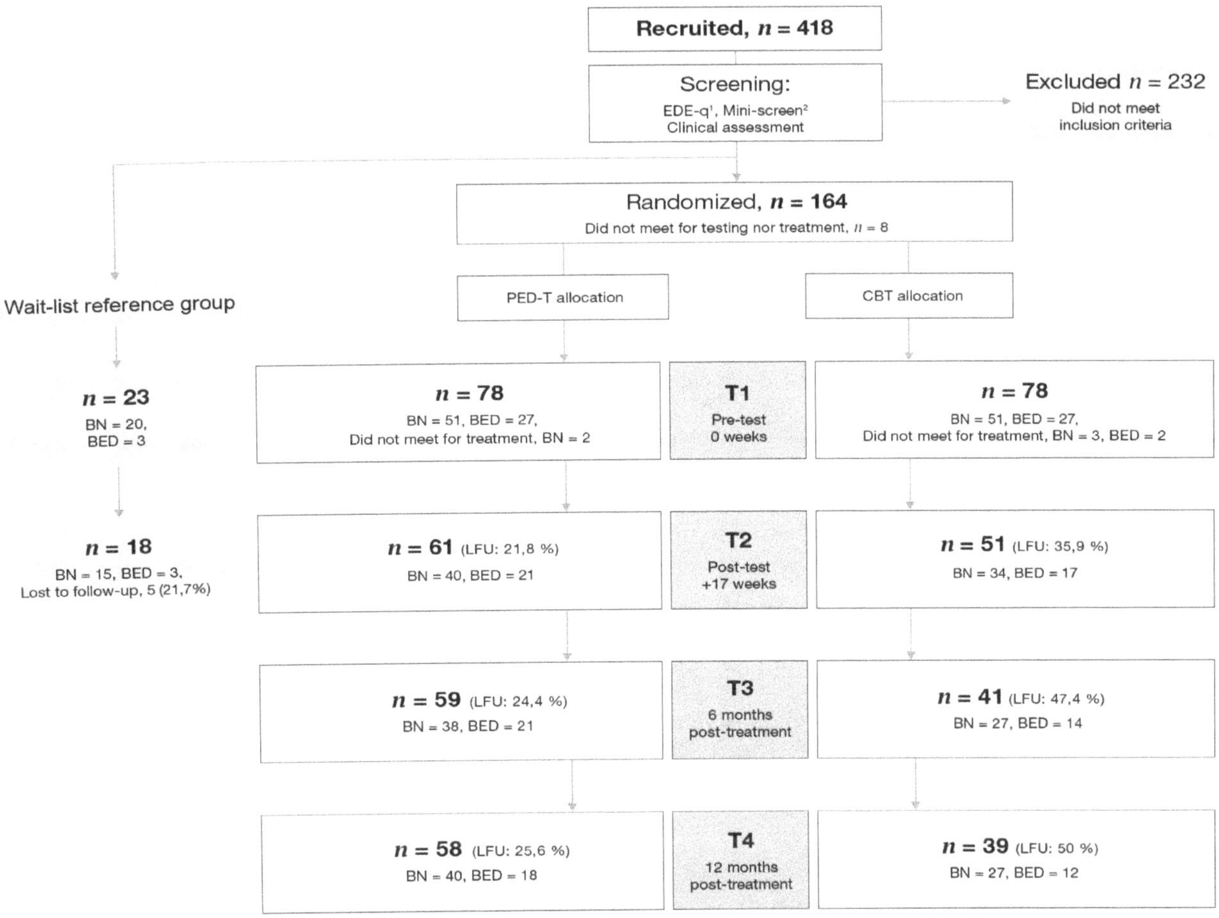

Figure 1. Recruitment, retention, and attrition during test periods. Overview of recruitment, screening, randomization, and attendance to the baseline (T1), post-treatment (T2), and follow-up measures (T3–T4). PED-t: physical exercise and dietary therapy; CBT: cognitive behavior therapy; BN: bulimia nervosa; BED: binge-eating disorder; EDE-q: eating disorder examination questionnaire; LFU: lost to follow up; [1] Fairburn and Beglin, 2008 [29]; [2] Sheehan, Lecrubier, Sheehan, et al., 1998 [30].

2.2. *Treatments*

The 16-week CBT and PED-t group-based therapies consisted of 20 sessions, each of 90 min duration, with five to eight participants in each group. A detailed account of the therapies and design are described elsewhere [31].

The manual-based CBT rests on a transdiagnostic model positing generic characteristics across ED-diagnoses [32]. Psychologists certified in CBT, with at least 10 years of experience, were conducting this therapy. The therapists were supervised by one senior therapist (PhD, psychologist and scientist) with more than 20 years of experience in CBT.

The PED-t consisted of a combination of dietary therapy and progressive resistance training (RET) and high intensity interval running (HIIT) [31]. The dietary manual focused on education on nutrition, group discussions, and practical skills in overcoming challenges in establishing regular daily eating patterns. We designed the whole-body, progressive resistance exercise program with two sessions per week arranged in three modules across the 16 weeks following basic principles for increases in maximal muscle strength (Table 1) [33]. The HIIT was designed with session intensity according to a pyramid structure, with progressive exercise load throughout the 16 weeks, following general recommendation for cardio respiratory fitness (CRF) improvement [34].

Table 1. Overview of the exercise module of the PED-t treatment. Resistance load is given as number of repetition maximum (RM).

		Supervised Exercise	Unsupervised Exercise	
Week	**Micro Cycle**	**Resistance Exercise**	**Interval Running**	**Resistance Exercise**
1–3	1	10RM	Pyramid interval (1–3 min intervals)	10RM
4–7	2	8RM	Pyramid interval (1–3 min intervals)	10RM
8–11	3	6RM	Pyramid interval (1–3 min intervals)	10RM
12–14	4	4RM	Pyramid interval (1–4 min intervals)	10RM
15–16	5	2RM	Pyramid interval (1–4 min intervals)	10RM

Specialists in physical exercise and in dietetics (MSc), all of whom were instructed by one experienced therapist (dietitian and exercise physiologist), were responsible for this therapy.

Participants were requested to complete training diaries throughout the treatment period in order to analyze adherence rate to training intervention.

2.3. Outcomes and Procedures

We measured body composition, physical activity, cardiorespiratory fitness (CRF), and maximal muscle strength during baseline and all follow-up test periods. Before all measure points, participants had to fast and to use passive transportation to the laboratories at the NSSS from 7:30 to 10:00 AM.

2.3.1. Body Composition

Participants were weighed in their underwear, and their height was measured with a fixed stadiometer (Seca scale, Mod: 8777021094, S/N: 5877248124885, Seca Deutschland, Hamburg, Germany). A dual-energy X-ray absorptiometry (Lunar iDXA, enCORE Software, version 14.10.022; GE Healthcare, Madison, WI, USA) performing a three-site scan was used to measure body composition (fat mass, percent body fat (%BF), lean body mass, visceral adipose tissue (VAT), android-to-gynoid fat mass ratio (AG ratio), and bone mineral density (lumbar area (L2–L4); femoral neck, trochanter, and shaft (proximal femur); whole body). All data were analyzed according to previously established guidelines [35].

We evaluated visceral adipose tissue (VAT) according to a cut-off for healthy VAT level of $\leq$300 g, based on previous findings of increased risk for high levels of triglycerides and fasting insulin levels with VAT above this threshold [36]. An optimal level of body fat percentage was defined as <33% [2,37], and masked obesity was defined as having a normal body weight according to the BMI scale (i.e., <25) but with high levels of body fat percentage (i.e., $\geq$33%) [2].

2.3.2. Cardio Respiratory Fitness (CRF)

After a breakfast meal, CRF was measured by performing a cardiopulmonary exercise test on a treadmill (ELG 90/200 Sports; Woodway, Weil am Rhein, Germany) with an incremental modified Balke protocol until exhaustion [38]. Gas exchange was measured using a breath-by-breath gas analysis system (OxyconPro analyzer; Jaeger, Würtzburg, Germany) with a Hans Rudolph two-way breathing mask (2700 series; Hans Rudolph, Kansas City, KS, USA). Measures of respiratory exchange ratio (RER) $\geq$ 1.10, and lactate concentration $\geq$ 7.0 mmol/L measured 1 min after test termination and analyzed immediately in a 1500-Sport-lactate analyzer (YSI, Yellow Springs Instruments, Yellow Springs, OH), were required to ensure a valid measure of peak oxygen uptake (VO_2 peak) [39]. A Borg scale rating $\geq$17 was additionally required to approve the test result [40,41].

We evaluated CRF as low according to the suggestion from a previous publication that found an increased risk of having a cluster of risk factors for cardiovascular diseases if VO2peak $\leq$ 35.1 mL$\times$kg BW$\times$min [42].

2.3.3. Maximal Muscle Strength

Maximal strength tests (one repetition maximum, 1RM) followed the cardiopulmonary exercise test in the following order: squats in Smith machine, bench press, and seated cable row. These three tests were performed according to predefined performance criteria and initiated with standardized warm-up sets of 10, 8, 6, and 4 repetitions.

2.3.4. NCD Risk Profile

We categorized participants into high-risk groups for NCD if they matched at least two out of three categories for high-risk evaluation: (1) having (either/or) high BMI, high body fat percentage, or masked obesity; (2) having high VAT levels; and/or (3) having low VO2peak.

2.4. Ethics

Active informed consent was required, and participants needed a conformation from their general practitioner that entering the study was medically safe. The study was approved by the Norwegian Regional Committee for Medical and Health Research Ethics (ID: 2013/1871) and registered in Clinical Trials (ID: NCT02079935).

2.5. Statistics

All analyses were conducted in SPSS version 24 (IBM, Armonk, NY, USA). Linear mixed regression models were built to estimate the between-group differences (PED-t vs. CBT) and the within-group changes (baseline vs. any of the three post-test measures). This analysis yields relatively unbiased estimates despite drop out (i.e., in the event that data are missing completely at random or missing at random). Moreover, it can be safely used without conducting multiple imputations beforehand [43]. Standard errors were estimated with the restricted maximum likelihood function, and type III *F*-tests were preferred. Dependency in the repeated outcome measures was accounted for by including a random intercept factor. The fixed factors were: *Group* (0-PED-t, 1-CBT), representing the overall treatment difference; *Time* (repeated measures), representing change across measurements; and the *Group*$\times$*Time* interaction, which was used in order to detect treatment differences at certain time points only. The between-group analyses used the baseline values as a covariate to increase the statistical power [44]. Differences between the treatment arms were examined with planned comparisons at each time point (least square difference tests). The within-group analyses included all four measurements in the *Time* factor. Due to the number of tests, differences with p-values < 0.01 were considered to be significant. A comparable statistical approach was used for the dichotomous outcome variables, replacing the analysis with a generalized linear model using a binominal distribution and logit link function (reference coded 0). Degrees of freedom were computed using Satterthwaite approximation. The outcome data are presented as estimated means including 99% confidence intervals.

Standardized Hedge's g effect sizes for continuous data were calculated as a ratio of the estimated means (extracted from the mixed model) to the observed pooled standard deviations (SDs). Values around 0.2, 0.5, and 0.8 were interpreted as weak, medium, and strong effect sizes, respectively [45].

Attrition rates were analyzed separately for each time (T2–T4) with independent t-test or chi-square analyses, as appropriate. A significance level of $p < 0.05$ were used for all t-tests or Mann-Whitney tests.

3. Results

3.1. Attrition Analysis

Drop-outs were less physically active (lower number of counts per minute in moderate-to-vigorous intensity of physical activity, MVPA, ($p = 0.02$)) and significantly more drop-outs had low femur bone mineral density (BMD) values ($p = 0.02$). Significantly more CBT-participants were lost to follow-up both at T3 (PED-t = 19 (24.4%), CBT = 37 (47.4%), $p = 0.005$) and T4 (PED-t = 20 (25.6%), CBT = 39 (50.0%), $p = 0.006$).

3.2. Demographics

Demographic information is presented in Table 2. The two treatment groups did not differ in any of the demographic variables. The mean (SD) attendance rate to therapist-lead PED-t sessions was 80.6% (11.4) and 82.1% (45.7) ($p = 0.79$) in CBT. In PED-t, the adherence rate to exercise sessions (supervised in therapy + unsupervised used for homework) was 69.8% for resistance exercise and 56.7% for HIIT.

Table 2. Demographic description of participants in therapy groups. Results are mean (SD).

	PED-t	CBT
Age, years	28.3 (6.2)	27.8 (5.3)
BMI, kg × height^{-1}	25.3 (5.1)	25.4 (4.6)
EDE-q, total score	3.7 (0.9)	3.7 (1.0)
Duration of illness, years	12.9 (7.5)	11.9 (6.7)
Bulimia nervosa, *n* (%)	51 (65.4)	50 (66.7)
Binge eating disorder, *n* (%)	27 (34.6)	25 (33.3)

Note: PED-t: Physical Exercise and Dietary therapy; CBT: Cognitive Behavior Therapy; BMI: Body Mass Index; EDE-q: Eating Disorder Examination questionnaire.

3.3. Body Composition

Changes in body composition are presented in Figures 2 and 3.

Mean BMI (99% CI) in PED-t increased to 25.64 (24.1, 27.1) at T2, 26.0 (24.5, 27.5) at T3, and 26.0 (24.5, 27.6) at T4. Only T3 ($g = -0.39$, $p = 0.001$) and T4 ($g = -0.4$, $p = 0.002$) were statistical different from baseline. There were corresponding findings in CBT, with levels of 25.2 (23.7, 26.8), 25.8 (24.3, 27.4), and 26.2 (24.6, 27.8), respectively, with only T4 different from baseline ($g = -0.36$, $p = 0.004$).

The within-group change in total body fat was significant at T3 ($g = -0.38$, $p = 0.003$) and T4 ($g = -0.31$, $p = 0.003$) in PED-t, and in CBT ($g = -0.34$, $p = 0.006$, and $g = -0.36$, $p = 0.002$, respectively). The numbers with masked obesity were 6.5% (99% CI: 2.0, 1.9) in PED-t and 5.3% (99% CI: 1.4, 1.8) in CBT, with no change by time in either group.

The within-group change in lean body mass (LBM) was significant at T2 ($g = -0.98$, $p < 0.001$) and T4 ($g = -0.47$, $p = 0.01$) in PED-t, while no change was found in CBT.

The within-group change in total VAT was significant at T4 in PED-t ($g = -0.29$, $p = 0.004$), with no significant change in CBT at any time. The numbers with VAT above recommended levels at T1 were 35.1% (99% CI: 22.4, 50.3) in PED-t and 36.0% (99% CI: 23.0, 51.5) in CBT, with no change by time in either group.

There were no between-group differences at any time in soft tissue body composition.

PED-t improved mean spine BMD at T3 ($g = -0.45$, $p = 0.004$) and T4 ($g = -0.31$, $p = 0.01$), and mean proximal femur BMD at T4 ($g = -0.37$, $p = 0.01$) (Figure 3). There were no changes in mean spine or proximal femur BMD after CBT. The occurrence of low proximal femur BMD at baseline was 1.3% (99% CI: 0.0, 55.7) in PED-t and 1.3% (99% CI: 0.2, 9.0) in CBT, with no change by time (T2–T4) in either group. There were corresponding findings for low spine BMD, with 5.2% (99% CI: 1.5, 16.8) in PED-t and 6.7% (99% CI: 2.2, 18.8) in CBT at T1, respectively.

No differences between groups were found at any time, other than a better score in proximal femur BMD ($g = 0.19$, $p = 0.01$) and proximal femur BMD Z-score ($g = 0.19$, $p = 0.007$) in PED-t compared to CBT at T4.

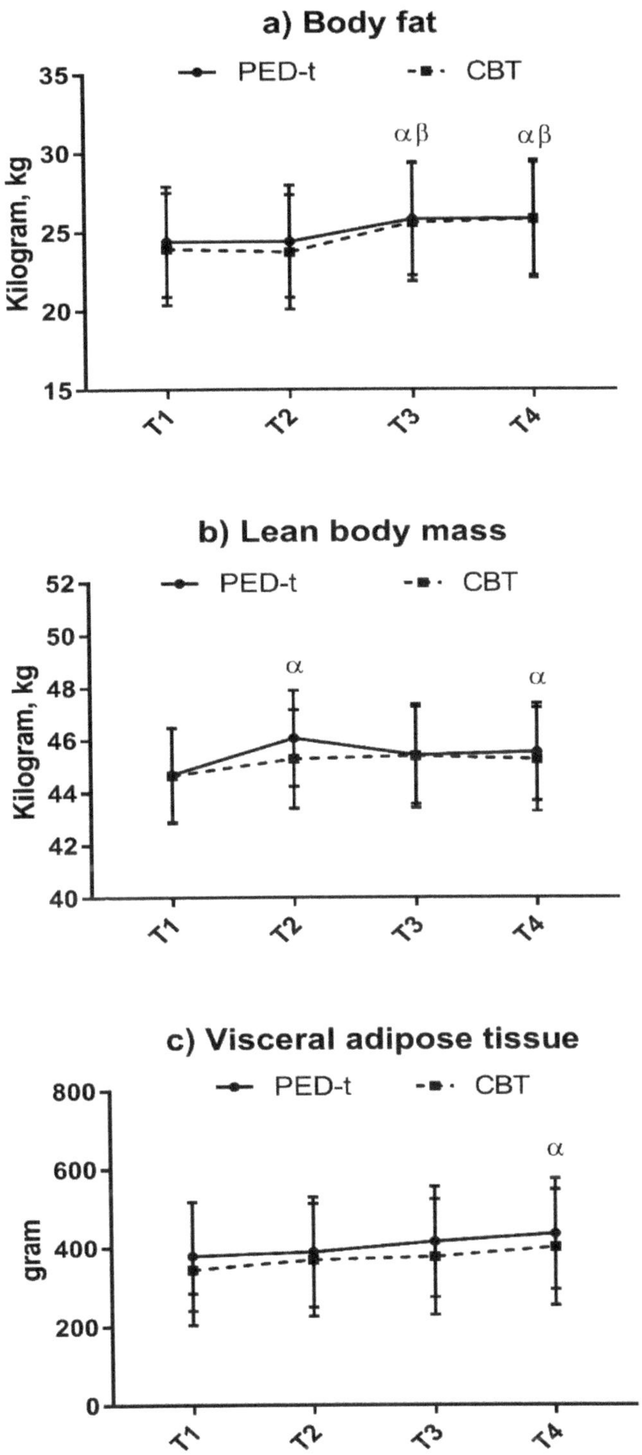

Figure 2. Changes in soft tissue body composition after PED-t or CBT. Results are estimated means (99% CI). (**a**) Changes in total body fat (kg); (**b**) changes in lean body mass (kg); (**c**) changes in visceral adipose tissue (gram). PED-t: Physical Exercise and Dietary therapy; CBT: Cognitive Behavior Therapy; 99% CI: 99% confidence interval; T1: baseline; T2: post-treatment; T3: 6 months post-treatment; T4: 12 months post-treatment; α: significant within-group change from T1 in PED-t ($p < 0.01$); β: significant within-group change from T1 in CBT ($p < 0.01$).

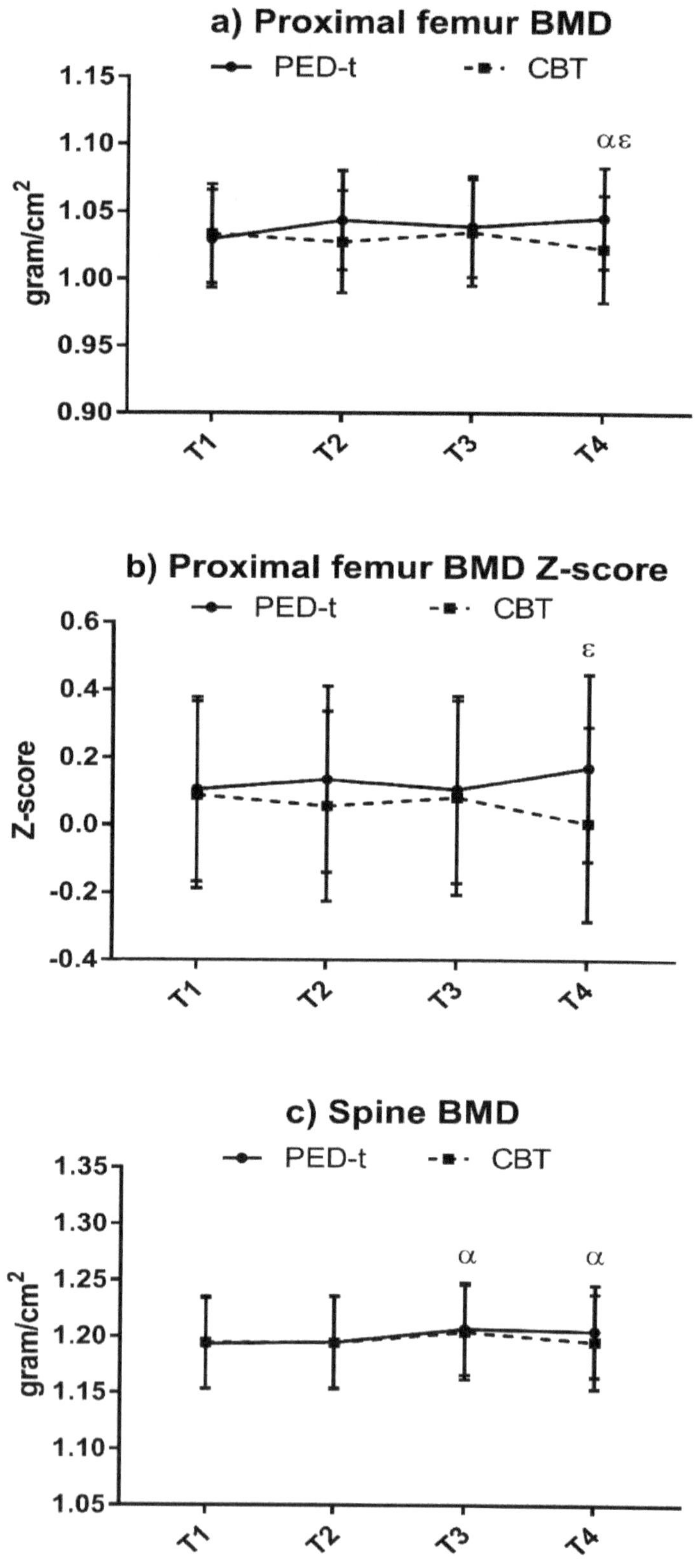

Figure 3. Changes in proximal femur bone mineral density (BMD), proximal femur BMD Z-score, and spine BMD after PED-t or CBT. Results are estimated means (99% CI). (**a**) Changes in proximal femur BMD (gram/cm^2); (**b**) changes in proximal femur BMD Z-score; (**c**) changes in spine BMD (gram/cm^2). PED-t: Physical Exercise and Dietary therapy; CBT: Cognitive Behavior Therapy; 99% CI: 99% confidence interval; BMD: bone mineral density; T1: baseline; T2: post-treatment; T3: 6 months post-treatment; T4: 12 months post-treatment; α: significant within-group change from T1 in PED-t ($p < 0.01$); ε: significant between-group difference ($p < 0.01$).

3.4. *Physical Fitness*

Effects from the two therapies on physical fitness are presented in Table 3.

3.4.1. 1RM

PED-t improved 1RM in squat, bench press, and seated row at all time points, with medium-to-large effect sizes. CBT improved in 1RM squat at all time points with small effect sizes, but resulted in no other observed 1RM improvements.

There were small-to-medium between-group differences for all strength tests at all time points, except no difference for 1RM squat at T3.

3.4.2. CRF

There was a small but significant within-group increase in CRF (in absolute terms; L × min)) after PED-t, but with no further effect from the PED-t during follow-up (T3–T4) (Table 3). No change in CRF after CBT occurred, and there were no between-group differences at any time.

Table 3. VO_2peak absolute, VO_2peak relative to BW, and maximal strength (1RM) in squats, bench press, and seated row at T1–T4. Results are estimated means (99% CI), and significant within-group changes are marked with asterisks.

					Between Effects, *p*-Value, Effect Size (g)		
	T1	T2	T3	T4	T2	T3	T4
$VO_2peak_{absolute}$ ($L \times min^{-1}$)							
PED-t	2.67 (2.53, 2.81)	2.78 * (2.63, 2.93) $g = 0.22$	2.72 (2.57, 2.87)	2.77 (2.61, 2.92)			
CBT	2.73 (2.59, 2.88)	2.77 (2.61, 2.93)	2.78 (2.59, 2.96)	2.80 (2.62, 2.98)	*n.s.*	*n.s.*	*n.s.*
$VO_2peak_{relative}$ ($mL \times kg^{-1} \times min^{-1}$)							
PED-t	38.25 (35.87, 40.63)	39.47 (36.92, 42.02)	38.35 (35.70, 41.00)	39.01 (36.30, 41.72)			
CBT	39.01 (36.49, 41.54)	40.35 (37.63, 43.08)	39.13 (35.95, 42.32)	39.24 (36.14, 42.33)	*n.s.*	*n.s.*	*n.s.*
Squat, 1RM (kg)							
PED-t	63.95 (58.33, 69.56)	78.60 * (72.81, 84.39) $g = -0.83$	73.89 * (67.94, 79.85) $g = -0.56$	74.98 * (68.96, 81.00) $g = -0.71$			
CBT	64.21 (58.37, 70.06)	67.15 * (61.06, 73.24) $g = -0.15$	70.07 ** (63.41, 76.72) $g = -0.30$	69.31 * (62.65, 75.97) $g = -0.26$	11.78 (7.42, 16.12) $g = 0.65$ $p < 0.001$	*n.s.*	6.10 (0.84, 11.36) $g = 0.31$ $p = 0.003$
Bench press, 1RM (kg)							
PED-t	37.02 (34.07, 39.97)	45.22 * (42.18, 48.26) $g = -0.86$	42.68 * (39.56, 45.79) $g = -0.62$	43.77 * (40.62, 46.93) $g = -0.74$			
CBT	38.32 (35.28, 41.37)	38.99 (35.80, 42.18)	39.81 (36.37, 43.26)	39.35 (35.90, 42.79)	7.28 (4.92, 9.63) $g = 0.63$ $p < 0.001$	4.12 (1.41, 6.84) $g = 0.30$ $p < 0.001$	5.60 (2.85, 8.35) $g = 0.43$ $p < 0.001$

Table 3. *Cont.*

					Between Effects, p-Value, Effect Size (g)		
Seated row, 1RM (kg)							
PED-t	34.38 (32.41, 36.34)	38.41 * (36.36, 40.46) $g = -0.65$	37.50 * (35.36, 39.64) $g = -0.52$	37.22 * (35.05, 39.40) $g = -0.46$			
CBT	34.56 (32.54, 36.58)	35.20 (33.06, 37.34)	35.03 (32.66, 37.41)	34.73 (32.31, 37.14)	3.39 (1.45, 5.34) $g = 0.52$ $p < 0.001$	2.58 (0.35, 4.81) $g = 0.41$ $p = 0.003$	2.74 (0.45, 5.02) $g = 0.40$ $p = 0.002$

PED-t: Physical Exercise and Dietary therapy; CBT: Cognitive Behavior Therapy; BW: Body Weight; 1RM: one repetition maximum; VO_2peak: peak maximal oxygen uptake; 99% CI: 99% confidence interval; g: Hedges g (effect size); T1: baseline; T2: post-treatment; T3: 6 months post-treatment; T4: 12 months post-treatment; n.s., non-significant; * $p < 0.001$; ** $p = 0.01$.

3.5. Risk of NCDs

In the evaluation of NCD risk, two participants impaired their risk profile during the treatment period in PED-t, while five participants improved. In total, 33 participants in PED-t remained without any high-risk NCD profile during treatment, while 19 participants remained in the high-risk group. The corresponding findings in CBT were one impairment, three improvements, 28 without any risk profile during treatment, and 17 remaining in the high-risk group.

4. Discussion

The aim of this study was to examine the immediate and long-term effects of CBT versus a physical exercise and dietary therapy (PED-t) on physical fitness, body composition, and the risk of NCDs. We found improvements in BMD, long-term increased maximal muscle strength, and short-term increased peak oxygen uptake after a treatment period with PED-t, while CBT did not result in comparable results. The overall study findings could not support the hypothesis that the PED-t provided sufficient improvements in physical fitness that actually lowered the risk of NCDs.

No improvement after CBT was expected. Here, healthy living was addressed, but the treatment did not consist of practical elements to help participants to improve nutrition and establish or maintain physical activity. It was unexpected, however, to observe no changes in soft BC and risk of NCDs after the PED-t; these results require some further considerations. First, it needs to be emphasized that the main aim of the PED-t was not to lower the risk of NCD, but to reduce eating disorder symptoms like irregular eating patterns and concerns about body and weight. Thus, learning how to achieve healthy living (i.e., adequate physical activity and a healthy diet composition) may be considered as positive side effects. To some extent, such side effects have been achieved through a shift of focus from overvaluation of the need to control body figure and weight towards attaining health and fitness [28]. In retrospect, however, given the low baseline values on parameters indicating an elevated risk of NCDs, it may have been overly optimistic to expect a change in physical activity and nutrition that really would lower this risk. Hence, findings that the PED-t may bring about a relaxation of dietary restrictions and compulsive physical exercise [27,28] may have counteracted any potential effect from PED-t on weight reduction and risk of NCDs. Secondly, the negative findings may, to some extent, also be explained by suboptimal treatment compliance. Thus, the participants in the PED-t, following an exercise program designed to affect BC (resistance exercise), as well as CRF and VAT (HIIT), reported unsatisfactory compliance to the program (i.e., ~70% of the RET and ~57% of the HIIT).

The deterioration of soft tissue BC, with increases in VAT, body fat, and BMI above recommendations [2,36,46] at the follow-ups, raises concern for the health of females under and after any kind of treatment for BN and BED, and the PED-t approach included herein. Such a concern highlights that the need to improve physical fitness and BC should be focused upon in the treatment of BN and BED. In a previous PED-t publication we showed that such a focus does not initiate or maintain excessive and obsessive physical exercise frequently observed in BN and BED [27]. Hence, there is empirical evidence refuting a main clinical reluctance to incorporate guided physical activity in the treatment of eating disorders.

An important limitation to our findings and conclusions is the skewed and high attrition rate during follow-up, with more participants being lost to follow-up in CBT compared to PED-t. The strengths of the study are the randomized design, the follow-up period, and the inclusion of participants from a real-life setting. As our findings show, maintaining lifestyle changes necessary for improvement of health is difficult in such real-life settings for persons suffering from BN or BED.

An important implication from the present study is that implementing guided physical exercise and dietary therapy is not sufficient to improve physical health in these patient groups. A recent systematic review of population-based studies on overweight has reported small but significant effects of combining CBT with a motivating interview (MI) [47]. Within the theoretical realm of self-determination theory, MI serves the purpose of internalizing treatment goals, while CBT may be effective in combating dysfunctional cognitions [48]. Such cognitions may comprise beliefs about not being able to reach treatment goals (i.e., low self-efficacy) as well as undue concerns about body, weight, and shape and the need to control eating as well as ambivalence towards change. The behavioral components of CBT serve the overall purpose of promoting self-regulation, a purpose that has been reported as being useful in the treatment of obesity [49]. However, future studies should examine if a combination of cognitive and behavioral approaches to lifestyle change improves long-term adherence to health-related exercise and eating behavior, and thus reduces risk of NCDs in persons with BN or BED to a greater extent than single-component interventions. A task for future randomized controlled studies may then be to explore the efficacy of various combinations of MI, CBT, and PED-t in the treatment of eating disorders as well as other disorders where poor physical fitness and a risk of NCDs is an issue of concern.

Author Contributions: Conceptualization, J.S.B., J.H.R., T.F.M. and S.B.S.; Methodology, J.S.B., J.H.R., T.F.M. and S.B.S.; Formal Analysis, T.F.M.; Investigation, T.F.M. and J.S.B.; Resources, T.F.M.; Writing-Original Draft Preparation, T.F.M. and S.B.S.; Writing-Review & Editing, J.S.B., J.H.R., T.F.M. and S.B.S.; Visualization, T.F.M.; Supervision, J.S.B. and J.H.R.; Project Administration, T.F.M.; Funding Acquisition, J.S.B., J.H.R., T.F.M. and S.B.S.

Acknowledgments: We would like to thank our master students in exercise is medicine for lab, exercise, and test services. We further would like to thank the head of the Sport Medicine department, Solveig Sunde, for taking care of concealed randomization.

References

1. Kaminsky, L.A.; Arena, R.; Myers, J. Reference Standards for Cardiorespiratory Fitness Measured with Cardiopulmonary Exercise Testing: Data From the Fitness Registry and the Importance of Exercise National Database. *Mayo. Clin. Proc.* **2015**, *90*, 1515–1523. [CrossRef] [PubMed]
2. Mathisen, T.F.; Rosenvinge, J.H.; Friborg, O.; Pettersen, G.; Stensrud, T.; Hansen, B.H.; Underhaug, K.E.; Teinung, E.; Vrabel, K.; Svendsen, M.; et al. Body composition and physical fitness in women with bulimia nervosa or binge-eating disorder. *Int. J. Eat. Disord.* **2018**, *51*, 331–342. [CrossRef] [PubMed]
3. Myers, J.; McAuley, P.; Lavie, C.J.; Despres, J.P.; Arena, R.; Kokkinos, P. Physical activity and cardiorespiratory fitness as major markers of cardiovascular risk: Their independent and interwoven importance to health status. *Prog. Cardiovasc. Dis.* **2015**, *57*, 306–314. [CrossRef] [PubMed]
4. Raevuori, A.; Suokas, J.; Haukka, J.; Gissler, M.; Linna, M.; Grainger, M.; Suvisaari, J. Highly increased risk of type 2 diabetes in patients with binge eating disorder and bulimia nervosa. *Int. J. Eat. Disord.* **2015**, *48*, 555–562. [CrossRef] [PubMed]
5. Hudson, J.I.; Lalonde, J.K.; Coit, C.E.; Tsuang, M.T.; McElroy, S.L.; Crow, S.J. Longitudinal study of the diagnosis of components of the metabolic syndrome in individuals with binge-eating disorder. *Am. J. Clin. Nutr.* **2010**, *91*, 1568–1573. [CrossRef] [PubMed]
6. Nieto-Martinez, R.; González-Rivas, J.P.; Medina-Inojosa, J.R.; Florez, H. Are Eating Disorders Risk Factors for Type 2 Diabetes? A Systematic Review and Meta-analysis. *Curr. Diab. Rep.* **2017**, *17*, 138. [CrossRef] [PubMed]
7. Villarejo, C.; Fernández-Aranda, F.; Jiménez-Murcia, S.; Peñas-Lledó, E.; Granero, R.; Penelo, E. Lifetime obesity in patients with eating disorders: Increasing prevalence, clinical and personality correlates. *Eur. Eat. Disord. Rev.* **2012**, *20*, 250–254. [CrossRef] [PubMed]
8. Nakai, Y.; Noma, S.I.; Fukusima, M.; Taniguchi, A.; Teramukai, S. Serum Lipid Levels in Patients with Eating Disorders. *Intern. Med.* **2016**, *55*, 1853–1857. [CrossRef]
9. Olguin, P.; Fuentes, M.; Gabler, G.; Guerdjikova, A.I.; Keck, P.E.; McElroy, S.L. Medical comorbidity of binge eating disorder. *Eat. Weight Disord. Stud. Anorex. Bulim. Obes.* **2017**, *22*, 13–26. [CrossRef]
10. Pedersen, B.K.; Saltin, B. Exercise as medicine—Evidence for prescribing exercise as therapy in 26 different chronic diseases. *Scand. J. Med. Sci. Sports* **2015**, *25*, 1–72. [CrossRef]

11. da Luz, F.Q.; Hay, P.; Touyz, S.; Sainsbury, A. Obesity with Comorbid Eating Disorders: Associated Health Risks and Treatment Approaches. *Nutrients* **2018**, *10*, 829. [CrossRef] [PubMed]
12. Hilbert, A.; Hoek, H.W.; Schmidt, R. Evidence-based clinical guidelines for eating disorders: International comparison. *Curr. Opin. Psychiatry* **2017**, *30*, 423–437. [CrossRef] [PubMed]
13. Norwegian Directorate of Health. *National Guidlines for Early Detection, Progress and Treatment of Eating Disorders*; Dahle, K.A., Ed.; Norwegian Directorate of Health: Oslo, Norway, 2016.
14. Davidson, L.E.; Hunt, S.C.; Adams, T.D. Fitness versus adiposity in cardiovascular disease risk. *Eur. J. Clin. Nutr.* 2018. [CrossRef]
15. Linardon, J.; Fairburn, C.G.; Fitzsimmons-Craft, E.E.; Wilfley, D.E.; Brennan, L. The empirical status of the third-wave behaviour therapies for the treatment of eating disorders: A systematic review. *Clin. Psychol. Rev.* **2017**, *58*, 125–140. [CrossRef] [PubMed]
16. de Jong, M.; Schoorl, M.; Hoek, H.W. Enhanced cognitive behavioural therapy for patients with eating disorders: A systematic review. *Curr. Opin. Psychiatry* **2018**, *31*, 436–444. [CrossRef] [PubMed]
17. Beck, A.T. Cognitive Therapy: Nature and Relation to Behavior Therapy—Republished Article. *Behav. Ther.* **2016**, *47*, 776–784. [CrossRef] [PubMed]
18. Denison, E.; Underland, V.; Mosdøl, A.; Vist, G.E. NIPH Systematic Reviews. In *Cognitive Therapies for Increasing Physical Activity*; The Norwegian Institute of Public Health (NIPH): Oslo, Norway, 2016.
19. Bratland-Sanda, S.; Martinsen, E.W.; Sundgot-Borgen, J. Changes in physical fitness, bone mineral density and body composition during inpatient treatment of underweight and normal weight females with longstanding eating disorders. *Int. J. Environ. Res. Public Health* **2012**, *9*, 315–330. [CrossRef]
20. Castelnuovo, G.; Pietrabissa, G.; Manzoni, G.M.; Cattivelli, R.; Rossi, A.; Novelli, M. Cognitive behavioral therapy to aid weight loss in obese patients: Current perspectives. *Psychol. Res. Behav. Manag.* **2017**, *10*, 165–173. [CrossRef] [PubMed]
21. Vancampfort, D.; Vanderlinden, J.; De Hert, M.; Adamkova, M.; Skjaerven, L.H.; Catalán-Matamoros, D. A systematic review on physical therapy interventions for patients with binge eating disorder. *Disabil. Rehabil.* **2013**, *35*, 2191–2196. [CrossRef] [PubMed]
22. Fossati, M.; Amati, F.; Painot, D.; Reiner, M.; Haenni, C.; Golay, A. Cognitive-behavioral therapy with simultaneous nutritional and physical activity education in obese patients with binge eating disorder. *Eat. Weight. Disord.* **2004**, *9*, 134–138. [CrossRef] [PubMed]
23. Levine, M.D.; Marcus, M.D.; Moulton, P. Exercise in the treatment of binge eating disorder. *Int. J. Eat. Disord.* **1996**, *19*, 171–177. [CrossRef]
24. Vancampfort, D.; Vanderlinden, J.; De Hert, M.; Soundy, A.; Adámkova, M.; Skjaerven, L.H. A systematic review of physical therapy interventions for patients with anorexia and bulemia nervosa. *Disabil. Rehabil.* **2014**, *36*, 628–634. [CrossRef] [PubMed]
25. Sundgot-Borgen, J.; Rosenvinge, J.H.; Bahr, R.; Schneider, L.S. The effect of exercise, cognitive therapy, and nutritional counseling in treating bulimia nervosa. *Med. Sci. Sports Exerc.* **2002**, *34*, 190–195. [CrossRef] [PubMed]
26. Hoie, L.H.; Myking, E.; Reine, E.C.; Bruusgaard, D. Diet and exercise in addition to psychotherapy, in the treatment of patients suffering from eating disorders with obesity. *Eat. Weight Disord.* **1997**, *2*, 207–210. [CrossRef] [PubMed]
27. Mathisen, T.F.; Bratland-Sanda, S.; Rosenvinge, J.H.; Friborg, O.; Pettersen, G.; Vrabel, K.A.; Sundgot-Borgen, J. Treatment effects on compulsive exercise and physical activity in eating disorders. *J. Eat. Disord.* **2018**, in press.
28. Mathisen, T.F. A randomized controlled trial of physical exercise- and dietary therapy versus cognitive behavior therapy: Treatment effects for women with bulimia nervosa or binge eating disorder. Ph.D. Thesis, Norwegian School of Sport Science, Oslo, Norway, September 2018. Available online: https://brage.bibsys.no/xmlui/handle/11250/2562679 (accessed on 28 November 2018).
29. Fairburn, C.; Beglin, S. Eating Disorder Examination Questionnaire (EDE-Q 6.0). In *Cognitive Behavior Therapy and Eating Disorders*; Fairburn, C., Ed.; Guilford Press: New York, NY, USA, 2008.
30. Sheehan, D.V.; Baker, R.; Dunbar, G.C. The Mini-International Neuropsychiatric Interview (M.I.N.I.): The development and validation of a structured diagnostic psychiatric interview for DSM-IV and ICD-10. *J. Clin. Psychiatry* **1998** *59*, 34–57.

31. Mathisen, T.F.; Rosenvinge, J.H.; Pettersen, G.; Friborg, O.; Vrabel, K.; Bratland-Sanda, S. The PED-t trial protocol: The effect of physical exercise –and dietary therapy compared with cognitive behavior therapy in treatment of bulimia nervosa and binge eating disorder. *BMC Psychiatry* **2017**, *17*, 180. [CrossRef]
32. Fairburn, C.G.; Cooper, Z.; Doll, H.A.; O'connor, M.E.; Bohn, K.; Hawker, D.M. Transdiagnostic Cognitive-Behavioral Therapy for Patients with Eating Disorders: A Two-Site Trial with 60-Week Follow-Up. *Am. J. Psychiatry* **2009**, *166*, 311–319. [CrossRef]
33. Ratamess, N.; Alvar, B.; Evetoch, T.; Housh, T.; Kibler, W.; Kraemer, W. Progression Models in Resistance Training for Healthy Adults. *Med. Sci. Sports Exerc.* **2009**, *41*, 687–708.
34. Garber, C.E.; Blissmer, B.; Deschenes, M.R.; Franklin, B.A.; Lamonte, M.J.; Lee, I.M. Quantity and Quality of Exercise for Developing and Maintaining Cardiorespiratory, Musculoskeletal, and Neuromotor Fitness in Apparently Healthy Adults: Guidance for Prescribing Exercise. *Med. Sci. Sports Exerc.* **2011**, *43*, 1334–1359.
35. Nana, A.; Slater, G.J.; Stewart, A.D.; Burke, L.M. Methodology Review: Using Dual-Energy X-Ray Absorptiometry (DXA) for the Assessment of Body Composition in Athletes and Active People. *Int. J. Sport Nutr. Exerc. Metab.* **2015**, *25*, 198–215. [CrossRef] [PubMed]
36. Bosch, T.A.; Steinberger, J.; Sinaiko, A.R.; Moran, A.; Jacobs Jr, D.R.; Kelly, A.S.; Dengel, D.R. Identification of sex-specific thresholds for accumulation of visceral adipose tissue in adults. *Obesity* **2015**, *23*, 375–382. [CrossRef] [PubMed]
37. Imboden, M.T.; Welch, W.A.; Swartz, A.M.; Montoye, A.H.; Finch, H.W.; Harber, M.P.; Kaminsky, L.A. Reference standards for body fat measures using GE dual energy x-ray absorptiometry in Caucasian adults. *PLoS ONE* **2017**, *12*, e0175110. [CrossRef]
38. Edvardsen, E.; Hansen, B.H.; Holme, I.M.; Dyrstad, S.M.; Anderssen, S.A. Reference Values for Cardiorespiratory Response and Fitness on the Treadmill in a 20- to 85-Year-Old Population. *Chest* **2013**, *144*, 241–248. [CrossRef] [PubMed]
39. Edvardsen, E.; Hem, E.; Anderssen, S.A. End Criteria for Reaching Maximal Oxygen Uptake Must Be Strict and Adjusted to Sex and Age: A Cross-Sectional Study. *PLoS ONE* **2014**, *9*, e85276. [CrossRef]
40. Borg, G. Psychophysical bases of perceived exertion. *Med. Sci. Sports Exerc.* **1982**, *14*, 377–381.
41. Haff, G.; Dumke, C. *Laboratory Manual for Exercise Physiology*, 2nd ed.; Human Kinetics: Champaign, IL, USA, 2012.
42. Aspenes, S.T.; Nilsen, T.I.; Skaug, E.A.; Bertheussen, G.F.; Ellingsen, Ø.; Vatten, L.; Wisløff, U. Peak Oxygen Uptake and Cardiovascular Risk Factors in 4631 Healthy Women and Men. *Med. Sci. Sports Exerc.* **2011**, *43*, 1465–1473.
43. Twisk, J.; de Boer, M.; de Vente, W.; Heymans, M. Multiple imputation of missing values was not necessary before performing a longitudinal mixed-model analysis. *J. Clin. Epidemiol.* **2013**, *66*, 1022–1028. [CrossRef]
44. Egbewale, B.E.; Lewis, M.; Sim, J. Bias, precision and statistical power of analysis of covariance in the analysis of randomized trials with baseline imbalance: A simulation study. *BMC Med. Res. Methodol.* **2014**, *14*, 49. [CrossRef]
45. Hedges, G.; Olkin, I. *Statistical Methods in Meta-Analysis*; Academic Press: Cambridge, MA, USA, 1985.
46. World Health Organization. Physical status: Theuse and interpretation of anthropometry. In *Technical Report Series*; World Health Organization: Geneva, Switherland, 1995; pp. 427–438.
47. Barrett, S.; Begg, S.; O'Halloran, P.; Kingsley, M. Integrated motivational interviewing and cognitive behaviour therapy for lifestyle mediators of overweight and obesity in community-dwelling adults: A systematic review and meta-analyses. *BMC Public Health* **2018**, *18*, 1160. [CrossRef]
48. Ryan, R.M.; Deci, E.L. Self-determination theory and the facilitation of intrinsic motivation, social development, and well-being. *Am. Psychol.* **2000**, *55*, 68. [CrossRef] [PubMed]
49. Samdal, G.B.; Eide, G.E.; Barth, T.; Williams, G.; Meland, E. Effective behaviour change techniques for physical activity and healthy eating in overweight and obese adults; systematic review and meta-regression analyses. *Int. J. Behav. Nutr. Phys. Act.* **2017**, *14*, 42. [CrossRef] [PubMed]

8

Efficacy of Web-Based Weight Loss Maintenance Programs: A Randomized Controlled Trial Comparing Standard Features Versus the Addition of Enhanced Personalized Feedback over 12 Months

Clare E. Collins [1,2,*], Philip J. Morgan [2,3], Melinda J. Hutchesson [1,2], Christopher Oldmeadow [4,5], Daniel Barker [4,5] and Robin Callister [2,6]

1 Nutrition and Dietetics, School of Health Sciences, Faculty of Health and Medicine, The University of Newcastle, Callaghan, NSW 2308, Australia; Melinda.Hutchesson@newcastle.edu.au
2 Priority Research Centre in Physical Activity and Nutrition, The University of Newcastle, Callaghan, NSW 2308, Australia; Philip.Morgan@newcastle.edu.au (P.J.M.); Robin.Callister@newcastle.edu.au (R.C.)
3 School of Education, Faculty of Education and Arts, The University of Newcastle, Callaghan, NSW 2308, Australia
4 Clinical Research Design, IT and Statistical Support Unit, Hunter Medical Research Institute, Level 3 Pod, HMRI building Lot 1, Kookaburra Circuit, New Lambton Heights, NSW 2305, Australia; Christopher.Oldmeadow@hmri.org.au (C.O.); Daniel.Barker@newcastle.edu.au (D.B.)
5 School of Medicine and Public Health, Faculty of Health and Medicine, The University of Newcastle, Callaghan, NSW 2308, Australia
6 School of Biomedical Sciences and Pharmacy, Faculty of Health and Medicine, The University of Newcastle, Callaghan, NSW 2308, Australia
* Correspondence: Clare.Collins@newcastle.edu.au

Abstract: Few randomized controlled trials (RCT) have evaluated the efficacy of web-based programs targeting maintenance of lost weight. The aims of this study were to evaluate two versions of a commercially available web-based weight loss maintenance (WLM) program and examine whether the provision of enhanced feedback was associated with better WLM. The study was an assessor-blinded RCT of change in body mass index (BMI) over 12 months WLM. Participants were 227 adults (44% male, 42.3 ± 10.1 years, BMI 30.4 ± 4.1 kg/m^2) randomized to either a basic (Basic WLM) or enhanced program with additional support (Enhanced WLM). Analysis was intention-to-treat with imputation using last observation carried forward. There was no significant weight rebound from the start of weight loss maintenance to 12 months for either group (mean: basic 1.3%, enhanced 1.5%) and limited change in secondary outcomes for either program. There were no significant between-group differences in the primary outcome of change in BMI (basic −0.5 (1.9) kg/m^2, enhanced −0.5 (1.6) kg/m^2, $p = 0.93$). In conclusion, a web-based WLM program was effective in preventing weight regain over one year following weight loss. However, the addition of personalized e-feedback provided limited additional benefits compared to a standard program. Given the potential reach of web-based approaches, further research examining which web-based program components optimize weight outcomes long-term is required.

Keywords: intervention; weight loss; web-based; randomized controlled trial; calorie restriction; eHealth

---

1. Introduction

Obesity rates are continuing to rise globally [1] in contrast to the limited access to treatment programs. While web-based approaches to treatment could potentially have broad reach, especially as households gain access to broadband internet, their evaluation in the context of longer-term follow-up has been limited.

Studies have shown that passive follow-up with no active intervention after weight loss is associated with weight gain [2], with 50–80% of participants gradually regaining weight lost following treatment, with most regain occurring in the first year [3–6]. A systematic review of weight loss maintenance (WLM) trials found that active WLM interventions facilitated a 1.56 kg (95% CI −2.27 to −0.86 kg) lower weight regain compared with passive follow-up after 12 months. Most WLM studies have required attendance at group sessions and have been hampered by methodological issues, such as mainly recruiting females or mid-aged adults and including only those with a good response to an initial weight loss phase, while excluding those with low adherence. [7]. Few studies have evaluated the use of eHealth technologies (e.g., websites, smartphone applications, text messages) to deliver WLM interventions. Furthermore, most research in this area has looked at short-term interventions (<6 months) without longer-term follow-up [8,9]. The small number of longer-term studies have reported a gradual regain of weight lost following treatment, with regain occurring after the first six months [10,11]. A recent randomized controlled trial examined the effectiveness of a 12-week short message service (SMS) based WLM program following an initial 12-week commercial weight loss program. At three and nine months follow-up, there was no significant difference in weight maintenance between the usual care control group who received a brief telephone call providing lifestyle information and a mailed leaflet with advice on weight loss maintenance and the intervention group who received a weekly SMS to remind them to self-weigh in addition to the call [12].

A systematic review published in 2017, evaluated the efficacy of web-based interventions on weight loss or WLM in adults with overweight or obesity and found web-based interventions were more effective than minimal treatments but less effective than face-to-face interventions [13]. Furthermore, a recent systematic review concluded that there was insufficient evidence to recommend the use of eHealth interventions for WLM [14]. There were however promising results from the eHealth weight loss trials with the addition of newer technologies including text messages, self-monitoring devices, and mobile applications, with meta-analysis demonstrating significantly greater weight loss (1.46 kg [0.80, 2.13], $p < 0.001$) in interventions with enhanced behavioral features (e.g., individualized counselling, feedback on dietary intake or weight change) or technologies (e.g., addition of text messaging) than standard eHealth interventions.

There is some evidence to suggest that these 'enhanced' interventions positively impact participant engagement, retention, and behavior change. We have previously published results of an online commercially available weight loss maintenance (WLM) program which demonstrated limited between-group differences for the basic and enhanced versions of the program after six months [15].

While the enhanced version resulted in greater retention (81.0% vs. 68.5%) and usage of the web-program, it did not result in a difference in weight loss [15].

A study using a 12-month intervention program (6-month weight loss plus a 6-month WLM) compared a self-directed web-based commercial program to a therapist-led behavioral web-based program and found greater weight loss in the behavioral web-based program than the therapist-led program at 12 months [16]. We have previously reported that adults randomized to this therapist-led web-based weight loss program initially lost more weight compared to wait list controls [17], and that there was no difference in weight loss between basic or enhanced versions of the weight loss program after either 12 weeks [17] or after 24 weeks [15] of participation.

To date, no WLM trials have specifically evaluated the inclusion of enhanced behavioral features in an eHealth WLM program, including those outlined in Table S1, such as automatically-generated personalized reports; personalized feedback on diet, physical activity, and weight loss, as well as reminders to use the online diary, visit the website, and weigh-in.

Therefore, the aim of the current study was to evaluate the impact of two versions of a WLM program on BMI in adults with overweight or obesity who had previously completed a weight loss program. The secondary aim was to compare differences in waist circumference and clinical measures including cholesterol, triglycerides, glucose and insulin between a standard version of a web-based WLM program (basic) and an enhanced version that provided additional personalized e-support.

2. Materials and Methods

2.1. Participants

Adults (BMI 25–40 kg/m^2), aged 18–60 years were initially recruited into a weight loss trial in 2009 from the Hunter community in NSW, Australia [18]. Written informed consent was obtained from all participants for the weight loss maintenance trial. The study was approved by the University of Newcastle Human Ethics Research Committee (H-2009-0245) on 10 September 2009. The trial was registered with the Australian New Zealand Clinical Trials Registry, anzctr.org.au ACTRN12610000197033.

2.2. Study Design

Participants who completed an initial 24-week web-based weight loss intervention (The Biggest Loser Club, SP Health Co Pty Ltd., North Sydney, Australia) were randomly assigned into one of two weight loss maintenance groups for 12 months using a stratified randomized block design. Participants were allocated to either a basic weight loss maintenance program (Basic WLM) or an enhanced version of the weight loss maintenance program (Enhanced WLM) (see Figure 1). Both participants and the outcome assessors were blinded to group allocation. Detailed methods of the RCT have been published elsewhere [18]. The WLM programs were developed to follow on directly after completion of 24 weeks of a web-based weight loss program [15]. Program features and differences between groups are summarized in Table S1 and also described in detail elsewhere [18]. The Basic WLM group received free access to the weight loss program, but the weekly meal plans were based on an energy intake target equivalent to weight maintenance. The Enhanced WLM group received access to these same meal plans and dietary information, but they also received personalized system-generated feedback on their progress. The feedback on progress was provided using system-generated personalized reports that were populated with the data entered into the platform by the participant. Feedback included progress in relation to weight maintenance goals; usage of the online diet and physical activity diary (which was recommended but not mandated); usage patterns for website features; and level of success with weight loss. Those allocated to the enhanced group also received an escalating scale of email reminders followed by SMS text message reminders (if no response) to use the diary, visit the website, to 'weigh-in' by recording their weekly weight in the online program, and a relapse phone call if their recorded weight rebounded by $\geq$3% to remind them to return to weight loss mode (Table S1).

2.3. Measures

Participants were assessed at baseline and 12 months [18] by blinded research assistants. Height, weight, waist circumference, and blood pressure were measured using standardized procedures [18] and BMI calculated. Following an overnight fast, blood samples were collected and analyzed for total cholesterol, low density lipoprotein (LDL), high density lipoprotein (HDL) cholesterol, triglycerides, glucose, and insulin by a single National Association of Testing Authorities accredited pathology service using standard automated techniques.

2.4. Data Analysis

Baseline variables were compared between treatment groups using analysis of variance (ANOVA) for continuous variables and chi-square tests for categorical variables. Analysis of covariance (ANCOVA) was used to test for group differences in outcomes at 12 months after adjusting for the baseline values of the outcome and sex. Analyses were performed in Stata v11 or SAS v9.2 (StataCorp, College Station, TX, USA). Intention-to-treat (ITT) analyses included all participants randomized at the weight loss management phase baseline, with missing follow-up data imputed using the last observation carried forward (LOCF).

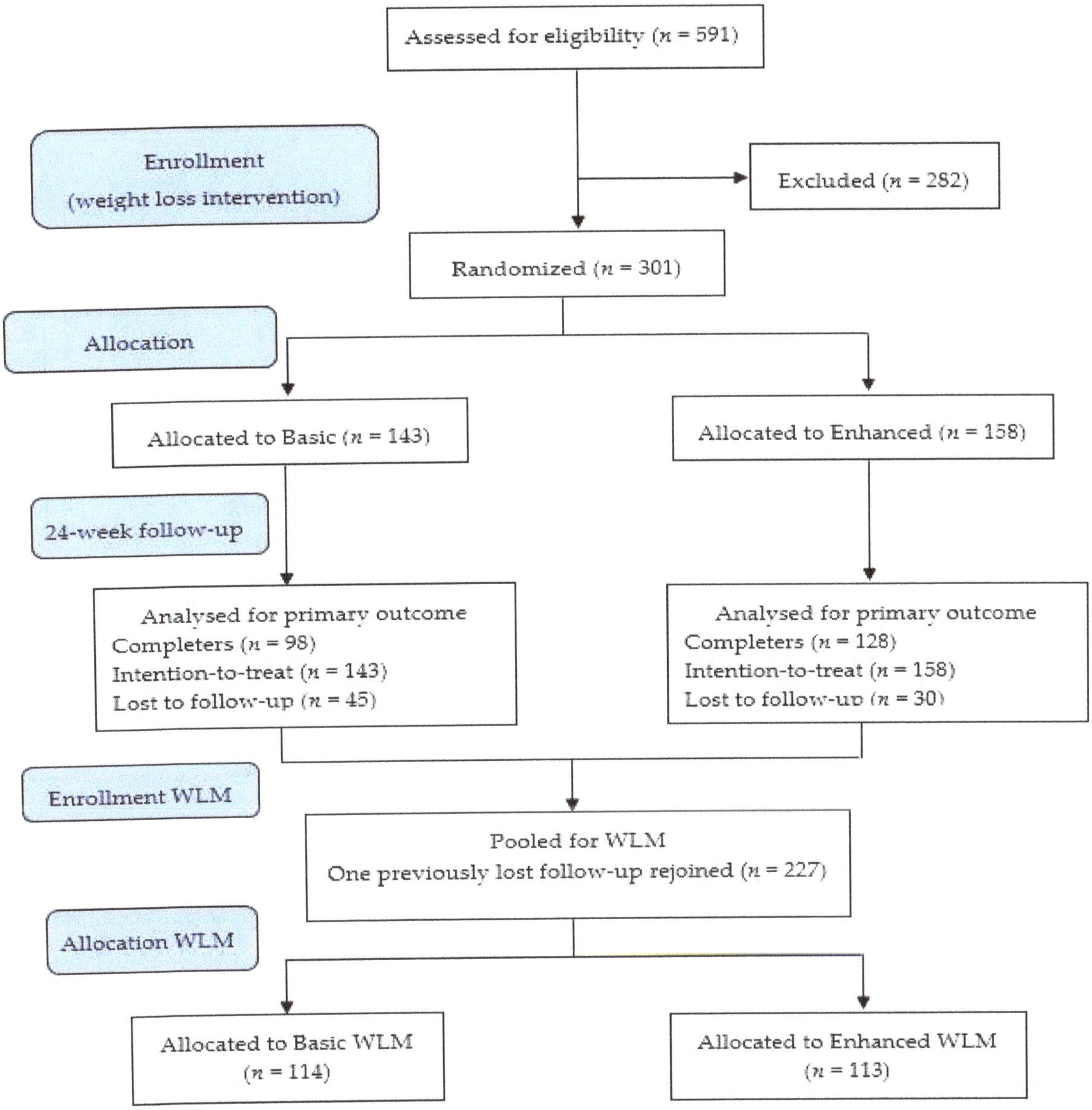

Figure 1. Participant flow from baseline of initial 24-week web-based weight loss intervention to group allocation in the WLM program. Further detail regarding participant flow has been published [15].

3. Results

At entry into WLM 227 participants were randomized to Basic WLM (n = 114) or Enhanced WLM (n = 113) program versions, with demographic data summarized in Table 1. Mean age was 43.3 (±9.7) years, with a mean BMI of 30.6 (±4.1) kg/m^2, 42% were male and 95% were Australian-born (Table 1). There was no significant between-group difference in attrition after 12 months, basic 18.4% and enhanced 23.9%, $p = 0.31$.

Both the Basic and Enhanced WLM groups successfully achieved WLM after 12 months with no significant rebound in weight. There were no significant between-group differences ($p > 0.05$) for the primary outcome of BMI with mean weight change (12 months—baseline) similar between the basic (−0.5 (1.9) kg/m^2) and enhanced groups (−0.5 (1.6) kg/m^2), $p > 0.05$ (Table 2). Table 2 shows that there were no significant differences in secondary outcomes between groups up to 12 months ($p > 0.05$).

Table 1. Demographic and other baseline characteristics of those randomized to 12 months of either a basic or enhanced features weight loss maintenance (WLM) web-based program.

Characteristic	Subgroup or Mean (SD)	Treatment Group			*p*-Value
		Basic WLM (n = 114)	Enhanced WLM (n = 113)	All (n = 227)	
Sex	Men	48 (42%)	52 (46%)	100 (44%)	0.55
Country of birth	Australia	108 (95%)	100 (88%)	208 (92%)	0.23
Highest level of education	School	37 (32%)	28 (25%)	65 (29%)	0.49
	Trade/Diploma	41 (36%)	40 (35%)	81 (35%)	
	University Degree	24 (21%)	28 (25%)	52 (23%)	
	Higher University Degree	12 (11%)	17 (15%)	29 (13%)	
Weekly household income (AUS$)	<$700	12 (11%)	7 (6.4%)	19 (8.8%)	0.60
	$700 to <$1000	6 (5.7%)	5 (4.5%)	11 (5.1%)	
	$1000 to <$1400	13 (12%)	11 (10%)	24 (11%)	
	$1500 or more	71 (67%)	84 (76%)	155 (72%)	
Age (years)	mean (SD)	43.3 (9.7)	41.3 (10.3)	42.3 (10.1)	0.14
Height (m)	mean (SD)	1.70 (0.09)	1.72 (0.09)	1.71 (0.09)	0.17
Weight (kg)	mean (SD)	88.5 (14.5)	89.3 (15.6)	88.9 (15.1)	0.70
Body mass index (kg/m^2)	mean (SD)	30.6 (4.1)	30.1 (4.1)	30.4 (4.1)	0.45
Waist circumference at umbilicus (cm)	mean (SD)	100.6 (11.1)	98.5 (11.7)	99.6 (11.4)	0.18
Waist circumference at narrowest point (cm)	mean (SD)	93.2 (11.5)	92.2 (11.9)	92.7 (11.7)	0.52
Waist to height ratio at umbilicus	mean (SD)	0.59 (0.07)	0.57 (0.07)	0.58 (0.07)	0.04
Waist to height ratio at narrowest point	mean (SD)	0.55 (0.07)	0.54 (0.06)	0.54 (0.06)	0.15
Weight loss at baseline entry to study (24 weeks)	mean (SD)	−4.38 (5.30)	−4.47 (6.37)	−4.42 (5.84)	0.91
Systolic blood pressure (mmHg)	mean (SD)	117.5 (13)	117.7 (12)	117.6 (12.5)	0.92
Diastolic blood pressure (mmHg)	mean (SD)	77.6 (10.6)	77.2 (9.2)	77.4 (9)	0.76
Resting heart rate (bpm)	mean (SD)	64.6 (9.5)	64.7 (10.2)	64.6 (9.8)	0.94
Total serum cholesterol (mmol/L)	mean (SD)	5.2 (1.1)	4.8(1.0)	5.0 (1.1)	0.03
LDL cholesterol (mmol/L)	mean (SD)	3.1 (1.0)	2.9 (0.8)	3.0 (0.9)	0.08
HDL cholesterol (mmol/L)	mean (SD)	1.3 (0.3)	1.3 (0.3)	1.3 (0.3)	0.41
Triglycerides (mmol/L)	mean (SD)	1.5 (1.0)	1.3 (0.7)	1.4 (0.9)	0.16
Glucose (mmol/L)	mean (SD)	4.6 (0.6)	4.5 (0.7)	4.6 (0.7)	0.08
Insulin (mIU/L)	mean (SD)	6.6 (5.5)	6.9 (6.2)	6.7 (5.9)	0.73

Table 2. Mean (SD) change in a anthropometric and clinical variables from WLM baseline to 12-month follow-up within each treatment group and least square mean (LSM) difference (95% CI) in change between treatments groups (Completed the six month Baseline, ITT/LOCF approach).

Characteristic	Treatment Group Mean Change (SD)		Absolute Difference between Groups LSM (95% CI)	p Values for Group Effect
	Basic	Enhanced	Enhanced vs. Basic	Difference at Specified Time
Weight (kg)	1.3 (5.1)	1.5 (4.4)	0.15 (−1.09, 1.39)	0.81
Systolic blood pressure (mmHg)	1.1 (12.1)	1.1 (10.2)	0.24 (−2.59, 3.08)	0.87
Diastolic blood pressure (mmHg)	−1.5 (8.1)	−0.1 (6.5)	1.15 (−0.76, 3.06)	0.24
Body mass index (kg/m^2)	0.5 (1.9)	0.5 (1.6)	0.02 (−0.46, 0.50)	0.93
Pulse rate (bpm)	−0.3 (6.7)	0.5 (5.8)	0.74 (−0.88, 2.35)	0.37
Waist circumference at umbilicus (cm)	3.8 (5.4)	3.3 (4.9)	0.76 (−0.63, 2.16)	0.28
Waist circumference at narrowest point (cm)	2.6 (4.6)	2.6 (4.6)	0.11 (−1.12, 1.35)	0.86
Waist to height ratio at umbilicus	0.0 (0.0)	0.0 (0.0)	0.01 (−0.00, 0.01)	0.21
Waist to height ratio at narrowest point	0.0 (0.0)	0.0 (0.0)	0.00 (−0.01, 0.01)	0.80
Total serum cholesterol (mmol/L)	0.1 (0.8)	0.2 (0.7)	0.07 (−0.12, 0.26)	0.50
LDL cholesterol (mmol/L)	0.0 (0.6)	0.1 (0.5)	0.01 (−0.15, 0.16)	0.94
HDL cholesterol (mmol/L)	0.0 (0.2)	0.0 (0.2)	0.00 (−0.06, 0.06)	0.88
Triglycerides (mmol/L)	0.0 (0.5)	0.2 (0.5)	0.13 (−0.02, 0.27)	0.10
Glucose (mmol/L)	0.1 (0.5)	0.2 (0.5)	0.08 (−0.05, 0.22)	0.20
Insulin (mIU/L)	1.6 (4.2)	0.89 (6.5)	0.61 (−0.719, 2.01)	0.39

4. Discussion

Whilst participants in both intervention arms of the current trial successfully maintained weight over one year of participating in a web-based program design to support maintenance of lost weight, those with access to the additional features designed to provide support and personalized feedback on diet, physical activity, and weight loss did not achieve better outcomes compared to those receiving access to the online program with minimal support. Both groups regained approximately one-and-a-half kilograms over the 12-month maintenance period, which was not significantly different between groups. This is comparable to results of the active intervention arms from a recent systematic review of all WLM intervention modes that included both food intake and physical activity advice, including group programs, face-to-face, and internet interventions [7]. The review included almost 3000 participants across 25 comparisons and found that the active intervention arms were associated with less weight regain of approximately 1.56 kg, up to 12 months [7]. This suggests that both active intervention arms in the current study were successful in achieving WLM. In our study, it appears that doing 'anything' was enough to support WLM, compared to the no-intervention arms in the systematic review, which also found no evidence that specific modes of intervention delivery were more effective than others. This suggests that having access to the level support provided in both the basic and enhanced versions of the current web-based WLM intervention, following a weight loss intervention did facilitate maintenance of lost weight. Given that it is well established that weight regain is common following initial weight loss [19], the results of the current study are important.

Our systematic review evaluating effectiveness of 56 interventions that included a specific dietary component within the WLM intervention found that 14 achieved significant between-group differences at follow-up [2]. Furthermore, our recent systematic review and meta-analysis which evaluated the effectiveness of 84 e-Health interventions, found that e-Health weight loss interventions that include extra support strategies including counselling, personalized feedback, motivational interviewing and/or personal contact, appear to achieve significantly greater weight loss compared with standard eHealth interventions [13]. However, five studies which focused specifically on WLM interventions found no significant difference in weight change between eHealth WLM programs vs. control [14]. The authors concluded that there is currently insufficient evidence to recommended eHealth interventions for WLM and that further high-quality research is required to determine their effectiveness [14]. Although the included studies were heterogeneous the typical intervention characteristics were WLM interventions that lasted 39 weeks on average, had approximately 180 participants and attrition of 26% compared to the current WLM study which lasted 52 weeks had 227 participants and an attrition rate of 21%.

The current study is important because individual studies to date suggest that face-to-face contact involving either weekly or monthly individual or group counseling sessions are more likely to achieve WLM than internet support in studies lasting 18 to 30 months. Recent systematic reviews on WLM interventions [7,14] suggest that there is a need for extended support for weight management following participation in weight loss programs internationally, as in-person attendance is not likely to be viable long-term. Hence, prolonged WLM support using eHealth technologies need to be evaluated for both feasibility, engagement, and cost-effectiveness in the long-term.

Limitations include the lack of a wait list control group, which is similar to the majority of WLM maintenance studies to date [2]. Although the small sample size and attrition likely reduced the power to detect significant differences between groups for the secondary outcomes, it is similar to other WLM trials lasting 12 or more months which had an average drop-out of 20% [7]. Furthermore. results from the current study need to be interpreted with caution given the meta-analysis within the systematic review [14] indicates that there is no significant difference between the support methods during WLM. This is also supported by our review of web-based interventions which also reported no difference between these two methods of delivery [20]. Strengths include the RCT design, use of blinded assessors, and the comparison of two versions of the WLM program for 12 months, following an initial period of weight loss. Future studies should consider evaluating cost-effectiveness and efficacy in specific population groups for whom access services may be a challenge, based on a range of issues related to time, cost, convenience, rurality, health conditions, or other socio-economic factors.

In conclusion, a commercial web-based weight loss maintenance program, with a specific intervention component targeting maintenance of lost weight can be effective at preventing weight re-gain up to one year following 24 weeks of weight loss. While the addition of enhanced features that provide additional feedback and social support did not provide additional benefits during maintenance, health professionals should advise clients that a specific WLM strategy does facilitate WLM up to one year following weight loss. Further research addressing level of feedback and support required to optimize weight status long-term in an online environment is required.

Acknowledgments: This trial was funded by an Australian Research Council Linkage Project grant (2009–2012) (LP0990414, G0189752), with SP Health as the Industry Partner Organization (G0189753). Clare E. Collins is supported by an NHMRC Senior Research Fellowship and a University of Newcastle, Faculty of Health and Medicine Senior Brawn Fellowship. Melinda J. Hutchesson is a University of Newcastle, Faculty of Health and Medicine Gladys M Brawn Career Development Fellow. We would like to thank the study subjects for participating in the trial and the research assistants for helping with data collection and D. Coyle for assistance with formatting the manuscript.

Author Contributions: Clare E. Collins, Philip J. Morgan., and Robin Callister were responsible for the design of study. Christopher Oldmeadow and Daniel Barker conducted the statistical analysis. Clare E. Collins drafted the paper, Melinda J. Hutchesson was responsible for data collection and management and critically reviewing the manuscript and providing feedback on intellectual content. All authors were responsible for revising the manuscript and have approved the final version.

References

1. NCD Risk Factor Collaboration. Worldwide trends in body-mass index, underweight, overweight, and obesity from 1975 to 2016: A pooled analysis of 2416 population-based measurement studies in 128·9 million children, adolescents, and adults. *Lancet* **2017**. [CrossRef]
2. Collins, C.E.; Neve, M.J.; Williams, R.; Young, M.; Morgan, P.J.; Fletcher, K.R.C. Effectiveness of interventions with a dietary component on weight loss maintenance: A systematic review. *JBI Database Syst. Rev. Implement. Rep.* **2013**, *11*, 317–414. [CrossRef]
3. Bond, D.S.; Phelan, S.; Leahey, T.M.; Hill, J.O.; Wing, R.R. Weight-loss maintenance in successful weight losers: Surgical vs non-surgical methods. *Int. J. Obes.* **2009**, *33*, 173–180. [CrossRef] [PubMed]
4. Burke, L.E.; Steenkiste, A.; Music, E.; Styn, M.A. A descriptive study of past experiences with weight-loss treatment. *J. Am. Diet. Assoc.* **2008**, *108*, 640–647. [CrossRef] [PubMed]
5. Douketis, J.D.; Macie, C.; Thabane, L.; Williamson, D.F. Systematic review of long-term weight loss studies in obese adults: Clinical significance and applicability to clinical practice. *Int. J. Obes.* **2005**, *29*, 1153–1167. [CrossRef] [PubMed]
6. Wadden, T.A.; Crerand, C.E.; Brock, J. Behavioral treatment of obesity. *Psychiatr. Clin. N. Am.* **2005**, *28*, 151–170. [CrossRef] [PubMed]
7. Dombrowski, S.; Knittle, K.; Avenell, A.; Araujo-Soares, V.; Sniehotta, F. Long term maintenance of weight loss with non-surgical interventions in obese adults: Systematic review and meta-analyses of randomised controlled trials. *BMJ* **2014**, *348*. [CrossRef] [PubMed]
8. Painter, S.L.; Ahmed, R.; Hill, J.O.; Kushner, R.F.; Lindquist, R.; Brunning, S.A.M. What matters in weight loss? An in-depth analysis of self-monitoring. *J. Med. Internet Res.* **2017**, *19*, e160. [CrossRef] [PubMed]
9. Balk-Møller, N.C.; Poulsen, S.K.; Larsen, T.M. Effect of a nine-month web- and app-based workplace intervention to promote healthy lifestyle and weight loss for employees in the social welfare and health care sector: A randomized controlled trial. *J. Med. Internet Res.* **2017**, *19*, e108. [CrossRef] [PubMed]
10. Watson, S.; Woodside, J.V.; Ware, L.J.; Hunter, S.J.; McGrath, A.; Cardwell, C.R.; Appleton, K.M.; Young, I.S.; Mckinley, M.C. Effect of a web-based behavior change program on weight loss and cardiovascular risk factors in overweight and obese adults at high risk of developing cardiovascular disease: Randomized controlled trial. *J. Med. Internet Res.* **2015**, *17*, e177. [CrossRef] [PubMed]

11. Hageman, P.A.; Pullen, C.H.; Hertzog, M.; Pozehl, B.; Eisenhauer, C.; Boeckner, L.S. Web-based interventions alone or supplemented with peer-led support or professional email counseling for weight loss and weight maintenance in women from rural communities: Results of a clinical trial. *J. Obes.* **2017**, *2017*. [CrossRef] [PubMed]
12. Sidhu, M.S.; Daley, A.; Jolly, K. Evaluation of a text supported weight maintenance programme 'lighten up plus' following a weight reduction programme: Randomised controlled trial. *Int. J. Behav. Nutr. Phys. Act.* **2016**, *13*. [CrossRef] [PubMed]
13. Sorgente, A.; Pietrabissa, G.; Manzoni, G.M.; Re, F.; Simpson, S.; Perona, S.; Rossi, A.; Cattivelli, R.; Innamorati, M.; Jackson, J.B.; et al. Web-based interventions for weight loss or weight loss maintenance in overweight and obese people: A systematic review of systematic reviews. *J. Med. Internet Res.* **2017**, *19*, e229. [CrossRef] [PubMed]
14. Hutchesson, M.J.; Rollo, M.; Krukowski, R.; Ells, L.; Harvey, J.; Morgan, P.J.; Callister, R.; Plotnikoff, R.; Collins, C.E. Ehealth interventions for the prevention and treatment of overweight and obesity in adults: A systematic review with meta-analysis. *Obes. Rev.* **2015**, *16*, 376–392. [CrossRef] [PubMed]
15. Collins, C.E.; Morgan, P.J.; Neve, M.J.; Callister, R. Efficacy of standard versus enhanced features in a web-based commercial weight-loss program for obese adults, part 2: Randomized controlled trial. *J. Med. Internet Res.* **2013**, *15*, e140. [CrossRef] [PubMed]
16. Gold, B.; Burke, S.; Pintauro, S.; Buzzell, P.; Harvey-Berino, J. Weight loss on the web: A pilot study comparing a structured behavioral intervention to a commercial program. *Obesity* **2007**, *15*, 155–164. [CrossRef] [PubMed]
17. Collins, C.E.; Morgan, P.J.; Jones, P.; Fletcher, K.; Martin, J.; Aguiar, E.J.; Lucas, A.; Neve, M.J.; Callister, R. A 12-week commercial web-based weight-loss program for overweight and obese adults: Randomized controlled trial comparing basic versus enhanced features. *J. Med. Internet Res.* **2012**, *14*, e57. [CrossRef] [PubMed]
18. Collins, C.E.; Morgan, P.J.; Jones, P.; Fletcher, K.; Martin, J.; Aguiar, E.J.; Lucas, A.; Neve, M.; McElduff, P.; Callister, R. Evaluation of a commercial web-based weight loss and weight loss maintenance program in overweight and obese adults: A randomised controlled trial. *BMC Public Health* **2010**, *10*, 669. [CrossRef] [PubMed]
19. Bamia, C.; Orfanos, P.; Ferrari, P.; Overvad, K.; Hundborg, H.H.; Tjønneland, A.; Olsen, A.; Kesse, E.; Boutron-Ruault, M.; Clavel-Chapelon, F.; et al. Dietary patterns among older europeans: The epic-elderly study. *Br. J. Nutr.* **2005**, *94*, 100–113. [CrossRef] [PubMed]
20. Neve, M.; Morgan, P.J.; Jones, P.R.; Collins, C.E. Effectiveness of web-based interventions in achieving weight loss and weight loss maintenance in overweight and obese adults: A systematic review with meta-analysis. *Obes. Rev.* **2010**, *11*, 306–321. [CrossRef] [PubMed]

9

Neuropsychological and Neurophysiological Indicators of General and Food-Specific Impulsivity in Children with Overweight and Obesity

Ricarda Schmidt [1,*], Caroline Sebert [1], Christine Kösling [1], Martin Grunwald [2], Anja Hilbert [1], Claudia Hübner [1,†] and Lisa Schäfer [1,†]

1 Integrated Research and Treatment Center Adiposity Diseases, Department of Medical Psychology and Medical Sociology and Psychosomatic Medicine and Psychotherapy, Leipzig University Medical Center, 04103 Leipzig, Germany; Caroline.Sebert@medizin.uni-leipzig.de (C.S.); Christine.Koesling@medizin.uni-leipzig.de (C.K.); Anja.Hilbert@medizin.uni-leipzig.de (A.H.); Claudia.Huebner@medizin.uni-leipzig.de (C.H.); Lisa.Schaefer@medizin.uni-leipzig.de (L.S.)

2 Haptic-Research Laboratory, Paul-Flechsig-Institute for Brain Research, University of Leipzig, 04103 Leipzig, Germany; mgrun@medizin.uni-leipzig.de

* Correspondence: ricarda.schmidt@medizin.uni-leipzig.de

† These authors contributed equally to this work.

Abstract: Impulsivity, particularly towards food, is a potential risk factor for increased energy intake and the development and maintenance of obesity in children. However, neuropsychological and neurophysiological indicators of general and food-specific impulsivity and their association with children's weight status are poorly understood. This pilot study examined electroencephalography (EEG) frequency band profiles during eyes-closed and eyes-open resting state in $n = 12$ children with overweight or obesity versus $n = 22$ normal-weight controls and their link to child- and parent-reported and experimentally assessed impulsivity of children (e.g., risk-taking behavior, approach-avoidance behavior towards food). The main results indicated that children with overweight/obesity versus normal weight showed significantly increased delta and decreased alpha band activity during eyes-closed resting state. Across the total sample, EEG slow-wave band activity was particularly linked to self- and parent-reported impulsivity and greater risk-taking behavior, but not to approach behavior towards food, after controlling for children's age and weight status. The identification of specific EEG patterns in children with excess weight may provide a new basis for developing neurophysiological diagnostic and treatment approaches for childhood obesity. Future studies with larger samples and longitudinal designs are needed to replicate the present findings and test their stability over time.

Keywords: EEG; frequency bands; obesity; brain activity; impulsivity; children

---

1. Introduction

During the last decades, an increasing number of studies focused on the neuronal basis of obesity, mostly based on functional magnet resonance imaging or electroencephalography (EEG, for reviews see References [1–3]). Consistently, neuroimaging studies revealed altered neurophysiological processes in the orbitofrontal cortex [4–6], a region crucial for reward and reinforcement processes [7], and the dorsolateral prefrontal cortex, which is known to be involved in cognitive control [8–10], particularly in the processing of food cues [11]. Processes of both reward and cognitive control are major determinants of human approach and avoidance behaviors and can be termed as facets of impulsivity, defined as spontaneous, unplanned behavior with lack of regard or diminished sensitivity towards negative or long-term consequences [12]. In line with neuronal measures, neuropsychological measures of impulsivity indicated abnormalities in a number of facets of impulsivity in individuals with overweight and obesity across the age range compared to normal-weight controls [13].

In the general population, longitudinal studies indicated poor inhibitory control to predict higher body mass index (BMI, kg/m^2) in children [14,15]. Recent research suggested that the association between impulsivity and weight status is driven by increased food intake [16,17]. In fact, experimental evidence revealed that children and adults with overweight and obesity were characterized by food-specific inhibition and interference deficits compared to normal-weight controls as measured by food-specific neuropsychological tasks (e.g., References [18–22]). However, while most evidence on impulsivity in children with obesity focused on the facets of inhibition or delay of gratification, there is little evidence on other dimensions of impulsivity, particularly decision-making, including risk-taking behavior [23] and automatic approach-avoidance tendencies towards food stimuli. Based on the Iowa Gambling Task (IGT) [24], an ecologically valid measure of decision-making under uncertainty in a context of punishment and reward, there is inconclusive evidence whether children and adolescents with excess weight show a general preference for disadvantageous, risky decisions compared to normal-weight controls [25,26] or not [27–29]. Similarly, studies applying other tasks than the IGT provided inconsistent findings on deviant decision-making in children and adolescents with excess versus normal weight [30,31]. As only two previous studies [25,30] used child-adapted tasks to examine decision-making in children and adolescents with excess weight, it is not clear whether methodological aspects accounted for the heterogeneity of findings.

Apart from behavioral measures, EEG profiles provide a more objective evaluation of pathological impulsivity across the age range [32]. The brain's functional states as measured by resting-state EEG are relatively stable over time and may be used as an indicator of arousal, cognitive activation, and psychopathology [32,33]. Based on spectral power analysis, the EEG waveform can be classified within different bands spanning the frequency spectrum, ranging from slow-wave frequencies (delta, theta) to moderate (alpha) and high frequency activity (beta). A vast number of studies found increased slow-wave EEG activity to be associated with behavioral impulsivity, including reduced inhibition [34] and increased risk-taking behavior in adults with attention-deficit/hyperactivity disorder (ADHD) or healthy university students [35–37]. Clinically, children with spectral elevations of resting-state slow-wave frequencies, mainly theta, and/or reduced alpha and beta activity were likely to have a diagnosis of externalizing behavior, including ADHD or antisocial symptomatology [34,38,39], which are common comorbidities in childhood obesity [40]. In contrast, the preponderance of fast-wave activity during resting-state EEG was found to be related to slower reaction times during a neuropsychological task in adults with ADHD [41]. In a sample of adults with a gambling disorder, frontal and central alpha band activity during eyes-closed resting state was negatively associated with self-reported impulsivity [42]. Thus, conditions characterized by increased impulsivity were found to show an EEG profile with increased slow-wave and decreased fast-wave band activity, suggesting cortical hypoarousal or a maturational lag in these individuals, respectively.

Despite the evidence that resting-state EEG brain activity is a marker of behavioral impulsivity, EEG studies in children did not explicitly consider child weight status so far, leaving the question whether the neurophysiological profile in children with obesity is actually deviant. EEG studies focusing on early, event-related information processing in children and adolescents with overweight and obesity versus normal weight found general and food-specific reductions in inhibitory processing during task performance [43,44], but nothing is known about the continuous brain activity at rest. Following the assumption of a proposed neuronal overlap between childhood obesity and ADHD [45], the EEG profile of children with obesity should be expected to resemble that of children with ADHD, at least to a certain extent. The only two studies analyzing EEG spectral power in relation to child's weight status revealed increased frontal beta in adolescent girls with overweight or obesity during a working memory task [46] and increased functional connectivity in the delta and beta band at eyes-closed rest [47] compared to normal-weight peers, but nothing is known about EEG spectral power at resting-state activity. Simultaneously, there is very little evidence on the EEG power spectrum and its associations with impulsivity in adults with obesity available [3]. Based on evidence from only two studies on the sources of resting-state EEG, adults with overweight and obesity showed lower parieto-occipital alpha oscillations during eyes-closed resting-state EEG [48], as well as posterior alpha desynchronization during eyes-open resting state compared to normal-weight adults [49] reflecting abnormal arousal/vigilance processes in these individuals.

Thus, the present pilot study sought to examine neuropsychological and neurophysiological indicators of impulsivity and their relation in children with overweight and obesity versus normal-weight controls. Specifically, this study aimed at investigating associations between eyes-closed and eyes-open resting-state EEG indices and neuropsychological, as well as questionnaire-based measures of general and food-specific impulsivity in children aged 8 to 13 years for the first time. Given the exploratory design of this study and the few available findings on EEG resting state activity in individuals with overweight and obesity, especially in children, both eyes-closed and eyes-open resting state were examined. It was hypothesized that children with overweight or obesity will exhibit greater slow-wave EEG band activity and lower fast-wave band activity during resting state than children with normal weight. According to previous findings in adults with ADHD [41] and the hypoarousal model of ADHD [50], it was expected that group differences would be more pronounced during eyes-closed resting-state, assuming that children with overweight and obesity are cortically under-aroused during eyes-closed resting condition and seeking for external stimulation. In order to assess children's impulsivity as detailed as possible and to reduce age-related biases in the context of self-report questionnaires, parent-report measures were used as well. Since EEG frequency band activity was evidenced to be a general indicator of impulsivity both in clinical child and non-clinical adult samples [36,41], the study aimed to evaluate the association between EEG resting-state activity and multiple indicators of impulsivity in a non-clinical child sample using the total sample. Specifically, it was expected that EEG resting-state slow-wave band activity would be positively and fast-wave band activity would be negatively related to experimentally assessed decision-making and automatic approach-avoidance tendencies towards foods, as well as self- and parent-reported general and food-specific impulsivity, respectively.

2. Materials and Methods

2.1. Participants

Eligible participants were German-speaking children aged 8 to 13 years with overweight or obesity, and normal weight, respectively, who were recruited from the population (e.g., via advertisements on the Internet, supermarkets) and clinical institutions (e.g., University Medical Center, outpatient weight reduction programs). Inclusion in the experimental group (EG) required objectively measured overweight or obesity based on age- and sex-specific German reference data [51]. Overweight and obesity were defined via BMI-standard deviation scores (SDS) ≥ 1.28 and ≥ 1.88, respectively. Children were assigned to the control group (CG) if they had normal weight ($-1.28 \leq$ BMI-SDS < 1.28). Exclusion criteria for both groups included parent-reported left-handedness, mental, neurological, or serious physical disorders (e.g., ADHD), medication intake affecting executive functions or brain activity, or mental retardation of the child. The pilot study was approved by the local Ethics Committee of the University of Leipzig.

The EG was comprised of $n = 5$ children with overweight and $n = 7$ children with obesity. The CG consisted of $n = 22$ children with normal weight, stratified to the EG for age and sex. By design, the groups significantly differed in their weight status, with the EG having a higher BMI-SDS than the CG ($p < 0.001$), but also in their socioeconomic status [52], with children of the EG having a lower socioeconomic status ($p < 0.01$) than the CG (Table 1).

Table 1. Sociodemographic description of the experimental group (EG) and control group (CG).

	EG (n = 12)	CG (n = 22)			
	n (%)	n (%)	χ^2	*df*	*p*
Sociodemographics					
Sex (female)	8 (66.7)	10 (45.5)	1.40	1	0.236
	M (SD)	*M (SD)*	*t*	*df*	*p*
Age (years)	10.9 (1.9)	10.1 (1.6)	1.26	1, 32	0.217
BMI percentile (0–100)	96.5 (3.3)	54.8 (20.7)	9.25	1, 22.9	<0.001
BMI-SDS	2.09 (0.49)	0.14 (0.60)	9.60	1, 32	<0.001
SES Winkler index (0–21)	12.3 (3.8)	15.8 (3.2)	−2.82	1, 32	0.008
Intelligence					
Matrix reasoning (1–19)	11.2 (2.8)	12.6 (1.8)	−1.55	1, 16.1	0.141

Note: BMI body mass index; CG control group; EG experimental group; *M* mean; *SD* standard deviation; SDS standard deviation score; SES socioeconomic status.

2.2. Procedure

The standardized experimental sessions were conducted by two highly trained PhD and MD students. In the beginning, written informed consent and assent were obtained from the parent and child, respectively, followed by children's intelligence assessment. During the subsequent EEG preparation, children completed self-report questionnaires, while parents were asked to do so at home beforehand. After EEG recordings and a 5-min break, neuropsychological tests were conducted. Subsequently, children's eating disorder psychopathology and mental comorbidities were assessed via separate clinical interviews with the child and one parent, respectively (Eating Disorder Examination adapted for Children [53,54], K-DIPS [55]). The experimental session ended with the objective assessment of children's weight and height. Altogether, the experimental session took approximately 3 h. Children and their parents received a financial compensation of 15€ for participation.

2.3. EEG Recording and Analysis

EEG recordings took place in an acoustically and electromagnetically shielded cabin with video control and were conducted using a 32 channel QuickAmp amplifier and Brain Vision Analyzer 2.1 software (Brain Products, Gilching, Germany). For all recordings, participants were grounded peripherally following the standard 10–20 International system with linked ear referencing to obtain EEG activity from 19 scalp sites (Fp1, Fp2, F3, F4, F7, F8, Fz, C3, C4, Cz, T3, T4, T5, T6, P3, P4, Pz, O1, and O2) at a sampling rate of 250 Hz. Eye movements and blinks were measured with two bipolar EOG electrodes placed 1 cm beyond the outer edge of both eyes and 1 cm below and above the right eye. EEG resting state was recorded for 300 s with eyes-open (EO) while looking at a fixation cross on the display and for 300 s with eyes-closed (EC). The order of EEG resting state with EO and EC was randomized.

A band-pass filter of 0.53–70 Hz and a notch filter of 50 Hz were used to filter EEG data. The continuous EEG was segmented in 2-s intervals and ocular artifact correction was conducted in accordance with Gratton et al. [56]. Further, automatic artifact rejection was applied to segments with voltage steps greater than 50 µV/ms and amplitudes exceeding ±100 µV. Subsequent to these automated procedures, two extensively trained researchers visually scanned all data in order to identify and remove residual contaminants (e.g., artifacts, focal abnormalities, drowsiness). At least 30 artifact-free segments (not necessarily consecutive) of the filtered EEG data were required for EO and EC to be included in the analysis. As a consequence, n = 10 children of the EG (*Mean [M]* = 57.8 segments; *Standard Deviation [SD]* = 19.8; range 36–88) and n = 19 children of the CG (M = 78.32 segments; SD = 28.1; range 39–127) were included in further analyses in the EO condition. Regarding EC, n = 11 children of the EG (M = 108.3 segments; SD = 38.0; range 41–150) and n = 22 children of the CG (M = 89.4 segments; SD = 30.9; range 40–156) were included in the subsequent analyses.

The filtered EEG data were Fourier transformed with a Hanning window length of 20% extracting delta (δ, 1.0–3.5 Hz), theta (θ, 3.5–7.5 Hz), alpha (α, 7.5–12.5 Hz), and beta (β, 12.5–30 Hz) frequency bands. The extracted absolute power for each frequency band was grouped for frontal (Fp1, Fp2, F3, F4, F7, F8, Fz), central (C3, C4, Cz), temporal (T3, T4, T5, T6), parietal (P3, P4, Pz), and occipital (O1, O2) regions, converted to relative band power (%), and ln-transformed before statistical hypotheses testing to obtain normally distributed data.

2.4. *Neuropsychological Tasks*

Approach-Avoidance Task (AAT). The study-specific AAT was adapted from Wiers et al. [57] and is a computerized measure for assessing approach and avoidance tendencies towards food in children. Following the principle of the AAT, children had to move the computer mouse as quickly and as accurately as possible in dependence of the format of pictures presented on a computer screen (portrait or landscape): By pulling the computer mouse to the bottom of the computer screen, the picture grows bigger (approach), while by pushing the computer mouse to the top of the screen, the picture size decreases (avoidance). After successful completion of a test run, including 10 grey rectangles, 40 pictures were presented in both landscape and portrait format in a randomized order, summing up to 80 trials. Specifically, there are four picture categories with 10 pictures each presenting high-calorie foods (e.g., burger), low-calorie foods (e.g., banana), pleasant neutral stimuli (e.g., smartphone), as well as boring neutral stimuli (e.g., ladder) to evaluate automatic responses depending on stimulus content. Boring neutral pictures and food pictures were pre-selected from a large, validated picture data base [58] based on the highest ratings of perceptibility and high familiarity. Finally, food pictures and pleasant neutral pictures were selected based on the criteria of high liking and perceptibility derived from a previous independent rating of food and pleasant neutral pictures in 38 children of two elementary schools aged between 8 and 12 years. In accordance to Wiers et al. [57], one child with overweight and two children with normal weight had to be excluded based on error percentages greater than 25%. Per each picture category, difference scores were computed based on mean reaction times in ms for the onset of correct responses to approach and avoidance trials, for example, "high calorie food/push—high calorie food/pull." Positive scores indicate relatively faster reaction times for approach responses compared to avoidance, hence an approach behavior. In the present study, only approach-avoidance tendencies for low-calorie and high-calorie food pictures were analyzed.

Youth Version of the Balloon Analogue Risk Task (BART-Y). The BART-Y [59] is a computerized task for the assessment of risk-taking behavior through balancing reward versus loss of points. Children were instructed to pump up 30 computer-generated balloons by clicking a button. With each click, the balloon was inflated further, and points were added to a counter up to a certain threshold at which the balloon explodes. If the child decided to cash-out before the balloon explodes, the accumulated points for that trial were added to the counter. However, if the balloon exploded, the child lost the points earned so far for that trial. Children were not informed about the balloons' break point that varied across each of the 30 trials. Thus, each pump confers greater risk, but also greater potential reward. After balloon explosion or saving of points, a new balloon appeared. At the end of the task, collected points were exchanged to differently sized prizes (small, medium, large, and bonus toy). Risk-taking behavior was measured by the average number of pumps on balloons that did not explode, with higher scores indicating higher risk-taking behavior.

2.5. *Self-Report Questionnaires*

To assess children's eating behavior and food-specific approach-behaviors, the subscales 'enjoyment of food' (α = Cronbach's α in this study's sample = 0.81) and 'food responsiveness' (α = 0.91) of the Children's Eating Behavior Questionnaire (CEBQ) [60] were administrated to parents and mean scores were computed for each subscale. Sum scores of the subscale 'hyperactivity' from the parent version of the Strength and Difficulties Questionnaire (SDQ; α = 0.72, [61]) were used to determine children's general impulsivity. Additionally, children's self-reported general impulsivity was measured using the sum score of the subscale 'impulsivity' of the Inventory for the Assessment of Impulsivity, Venturesomeness and Empathy in 9–14 years old children (IVE, $\alpha = 0.62$, [62]) which is an adapted German version of the Impulsivity Questionnaire I6 by Eysenck and Eysenck [63].

2.6. Intelligence

Children's intelligence was estimated using the 'matrix reasoning subtest' of the Wechsler Intelligence Scale for Children—Fourth edition (WISC-IV; [64,65]) which nonverbally assesses abstract-logical reasoning. Subtest scores were converted into age-specific standard values ranging between 1 and 19, with higher scores indicating higher levels of intelligence.

2.7. Data Analytic Plan

Statistical analyses were performed using IBM SPSS Statistics version 23 (IBM Corp. Released 2015. IBM SPSS Statistics for Windows, Version 23.0. Armonk, NY: IBM Corp) and consisted of two steps. First, group differences between the EG and CG regarding impulsivity measures and resting-state EEG activity measured during EC and EO were examined using two-tailed independent sample t tests. In order to correct for possible inflations of the Type I error rate due to multiple testing, an adjusted significance level of $p < 0.05/20 = 0.0025$ was considered to indicate statistical significance. In terms of violation of normality and homogeneity of variances, non-parametric tests were used and reported if results differed from the parametric tests. Effect sizes of group differences were reported by Cohen's d, whereby values ≥ 0.20 refer to small, ≥ 0.50 to medium, and ≥ 0.80 to large effects [66].

Second, associations between children's EEG activity and various impulsivity indicators (AAT, BART-Y, CEBQ, SDQ, IVE) over and above group status (EG vs. CG) were examined via partial correlations (Pearson) with children's weight status (BMI-SDS) and age serving as control variables to exclude weight- and development-related effects on measured EEG activity [67]. Effect sizes of correlations were interpreted according to Cohen with values $r \geq 0.10$ referring to small, $r \geq 0.30$ to medium, and $r \geq 0.50$ to large effects [66]. Statistical significance for correlation analyses was set at $\alpha < 0.05$. Post-hoc power analyses revealed adequate power ($1 - \beta = 0.80$) for detecting large-sized group differences ($d > 1$) in EEG resting state and medium-to-large-sized effects ($r > 0.40$) in correlation analyses.

3. Results

3.1. Neuropsychological Tasks

While the EG showed an avoidance behavior and the CG an approach behavior of medium effect size regarding high-calorie foods, an approach behavior to low-calorie foods was found in both groups; however, biases were not significantly different from 0 ($p > 0.05$). The EG and CG did not significantly differ in approach or avoidance behaviors to high- or low-calorie foods in the AAT ($p > 0.05$, Table 2).

A non-significant ($p > 0.05$), but medium-sized group difference was found for the number of pumps in the BART-Y, with the EG presenting a lower average number of pumps than the CG, indicating lower risk-taking behavior.

3.2. Self-Report Questionnaires

Parents of children of the EG reported significantly higher levels of 'food responsiveness' ($p < 0.01$, large effect) and marginally significantly higher levels on the subscale 'enjoyment of food' ($p < 0.100$, medium effect) of the CEBQ compared to the CG.

For general self- and parent-reported impulsivity, small-to-medium-sized, but non-significant group differences were revealed ($p > 0.05$) indicating descriptively higher levels of impulsivity in the EG than the CG.

Table 2. Self-reported and neuropsychological measures of general and food-specific impulsivity as a function of weight status.

	EG	CG				
Neuropsychological Tasks	*M (SD)*	*M (SD)*	*t*	*df*	*p*	*d*
AAT (ms)						
High-calorie food	−12.2 (134.5)	70.6 (171.3)	−1.38	1, 29	0.177	−0.52
Low-calorie food	39.2 (272.1)	82.2 (230.6)	−0.46	1, 28	0.649	−0.18
BART-Y						
N pumps	17.9 (9.0)	24.0 (10.8)	−1.66	1, 31	0.108	−0.60
Self-report questionnaires	*M (SD)*	*M (SD)*	*t*	*df*	*p*	*d*
CEBQ						
Enjoyment of Food	3.2 (0.7)	2.9 (0.5)	1.79	1, 32	0.083	0.52
Food Responsiveness	2.2 (1.2)	0.9 (0.5)	3.54	1, 13.2	0.004	1.60
IVE						
Impulsivity	8.1 (3.2)	6.7 (2.8)	1.35	1, 32	0.188	0.48
SDQ						
Hyperactivity	3.3 (2.1)	2.6 (1.9)	0.94	1, 32	0.357	0.36

Note. AAT Approach Avoidance Task; BART-Y Youth Version of the Balloon Analogue Risk Task; CEBQ Children's Eating Behavior Questionnaire; CG control group; EG experimental group; IVE Inventory for the Assessment of Impulsivity, Venturesomeness and Empathy in 9–14 years old children; *M* mean; *SD* standard deviation; SDQ Strengths and Difficulties Questionnaire. Negative *d* values indicate that the EG scored lower in the respective measure than the CG.

3.3. Resting-State EEG Activity

As depicted in Table 3, the EG showed significantly higher delta band activity than the CG during EC resting state with large-sized effects for parietal and occipital regions ($p \leq 0.003$), while greater delta band activity in the EG versus CG did not reach significance for other regions ($0.022 \leq ps \leq 0.149$). Although non-significant, large-sized group effects were found for greater occipital theta band activity and lower alpha band activity in all brain regions in the EG versus CG ($0.007 \leq ps \leq 0.036$). Descriptively higher theta and beta band activity in the EG versus CG did not reach significance ($ps \geq 0.027$).

Table 3. Eyes-closed resting-state electroencephalography (EEG) activity as a function of weight status.

	EG	CG				
	M (SD)	*M (SD)*	*t*	*df*	*p*	*d*
Delta (μV^2)						
Frontal	−1.07 (0.18)	−1.18 (0.21)	1.48	1, 31	0.149	0.55
Central	−1.19 (0.15)	−1.34 (0.19)	2.41	1, 31	0.022	0.84
Parietal	−1.25 (0.19)	−1.51 (0.23)	3.26	1, 31	0.003	1.19
Temporal	−1.22 (0.17)	−1.35 (0.17)	2.13	1, 31	0.041	0.77
Occipital	−1.29 (0.23)	−1.71 (0.38)	3.31	1, 31	0.002	1.24
Theta (μV^2)						
Frontal	−1.27 (0.16)	−1.37 (0.26)	1.21	1, 31	0.235	0.43
Central	−1.16 (0.12)	−1.30 (0.25)	1.84	1, 31	0.975	0.65
Parietal	−1.31 (0.15)	−1.51 (0.32)	1.96	1, 31	0.059	0.72
Temporal	−1.23 (0.13)	−1.38 (0.24)	1.88	1, 31	0.069	0.71
Occipital	−1.48 (0.23)	−1.83 (0.46)	2.33	1, 31	0.027	0.87
Alpha (μV^2)						
Frontal	−1.54 (0.32)	−1.26 (0.34)	−2.29	1, 31	0.029	−0.84
Central	−1.41 (0.34)	−1.06 (0.36)	−2.73	1, 31	0.010	−0.99
Parietal	−1.26 (0.30)	−0.94 (0.30)	−2.88	1, 31	0.007	−1.07
Temporal	−1.33 (0.31)	−1.09 (0.30)	−2.19	1, 31	0.036	−0.79
Occipital	−1.00 (0.33)	−0.69 (0.36)	−2.36	1, 31	0.025	−0.88
Beta (μV^2)						
Frontal	−1.95 (0.22)	−2.11 (0.34)	1.41	1, 31	0.167	0.52
Central	−2.06 (0.12)	−2.19 (0.34)	1.27	1, 31	0.214	0.45
Parietal	−2.25 (0.26)	−2.36 (0.33)	0.93	1, 31	0.360	0.36
Temporal	−2.05 (0.19)	−2.12 (0.34)	0.62	1, 31	0.538	0.23
Occipital	−2.37 (0.37)	−2.43 (0.43)	0.39	1, 31	0.703	0.15

Note: Percentage EEG activity at a particular location increases as the mean of the ln-transformed data becomes less negative. Negative *d* values indicate that the EG scored lower in the respective measure than the CG. *M* mean; *SD* standard deviation.

For resting-state EEG activity measured during EO, no significant group differences were found for any frequency band and any brain region ($0.333 \leq ps \leq 0.998$).

3.4. *Associations between Resting-State EEG Activity and Impulsivity Measures*

Eyes-open. Results of the correlation analyses between frequency band activities measured during EO resting-state EEG and neuropsychological indices of impulsivity are presented in Figure 1. After controlling for children's age and weight status, increased slow-wave band activity (i.e., delta and theta) found in frontal, central, parietal, and temporal regions was significantly associated with higher scores in the CEBQ subscale 'enjoyment of food' with medium-to-large-sized effects ($0.002 \leq ps \leq 0.043$). Additionally, significant positive correlations of medium effect size were detected between frontal, central, and temporal theta band activity and average numbers of pumps in the BART-Y ($0.038 \leq ps \leq 0.046$).

Regarding fast-wave band activity (i.e., alpha and beta), increased frontal and central alpha band activity was significantly associated with lower scores in the CEBQ subscale 'enjoyment of food' with medium-to-large-sized effects ($0.004 \leq ps \leq 0.005$). Increased central and temporal beta band activity was significantly associated with approach behavior for low-calorie food in the AAT with medium-to-large-sized effects ($0.023 \leq ps \leq 0.024$). Medium-sized significant positive correlations were revealed between occipital beta band activity and the SDQ subscale 'hyperactivity' ($p = 0.044$). No other significant correlations were found during EO.

Eyes-closed. After controlling for children's age and weight status, occipital delta band activity and average numbers of pumps in the BART-Y were negatively correlated with medium-sized effects ($p = 0.028$).

Regarding fast-wave band activity, increased beta band activity in frontal regions was associated with lower scores on the IVE subscale 'impulsivity' ($p = 0.021$, medium-to-large-sized effect). Other correlations between EC resting-state EEG and impulsivity indices were not significant.

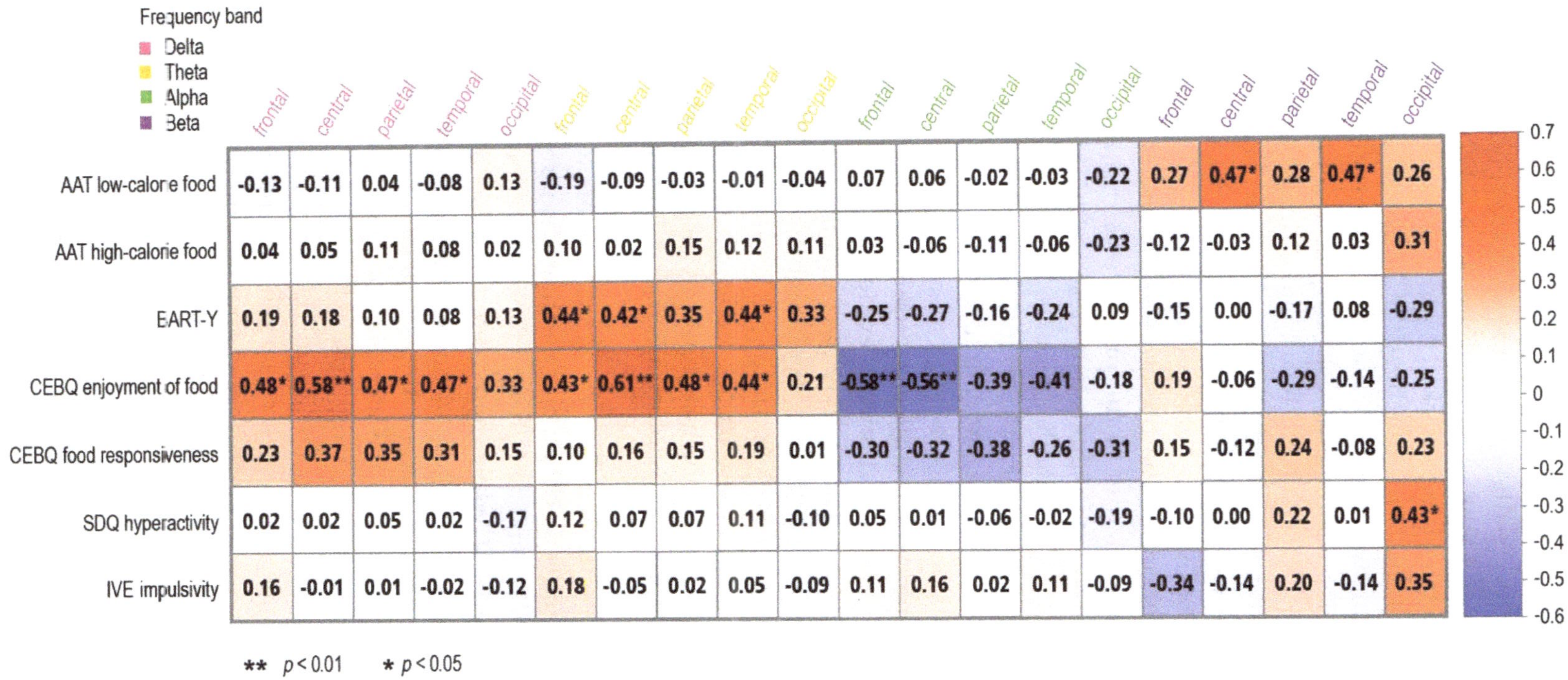

Figure 1. Matrix of correlations between eyes-open EEG resting-state activity, Approach-Avoidance-Task (AAT), the Youth Version of the Balloon Analogue Risk Task (BART-Y), parent-reported Child Eating Behavior Questionnaire (CEBQ), Strengths and Difficulties Questionnaire (SDQ), and child-reported Inventory of Venturesomeness and Empathy in 9–14 years old children (IVE) across the total sample with valid EEG data ($n = 29$), while controlling for child age and weight status.

4. Discussion

To our knowledge, this is the first study that investigated both eyes-closed (EC) and eyes-open (EO) resting-state EEG activity in 8-to-13-year-old children with overweight and obesity versus normal weight and its associations with general and food-specific impulsivity measured experimentally and via self- and parent-report. The results revealed an obesity-specific EEG profile characterized by greater slow-wave and decreased alpha band activity during EC resting-state EEG, congruent with EEG patterns found in other conditions marked by increased impulsivity, such as ADHD (e.g., References [68,69]). Independent of children's weight status, increased slow-wave and decreased alpha band activity during EO resting state were associated with higher impulsivity, characterized by greater risk-taking behavior during a neuropsychological task and parent-reported food-approach behaviors, mirroring findings in youth with ADHD [70] and healthy individuals [35,36].

The preponderance of slow-wave band activity and reductions of alpha band activity during EC resting state in children with overweight and obesity suggested neuronal similarities with ADHD, a highly comorbid disorder to obesity across the age range [40]. Because a concurrent diagnosis of ADHD was an exclusion criterion for the present sample, the results were not contaminated by underlying neuronal abnormalities due to the presence of this neurodevelopmental disorder. Notably, disorder-specific symptoms in individuals with deviant EEG patterns are considered to reflect compensatory mechanisms to counter-regulate the vigilance level, either via withdrawal and sensation avoidance (depression) or inattention, hyperactivity/impulsivity [71]. Thus, general deficiencies in self-control in children with obesity might be attributable to cortical hypoarousal, as in those with ADHD or other externalizing behavior [39]. Although there are no studies available addressing the particular aspect of the association between cortical arousal and self-regulation neither in adults nor in children with overweight and obesity, preliminary evidence in adults with obesity indicated that stimulant treatment, such as methylphenidate, may have an effect on the reduction of food intake, at least in some individuals [72] proposing that there might be an EEG phenotype of slow-wave preponderance in individuals with obesity. According to Knyazev (2012) [73], delta band activity represents the most basic evolutionary old oscillatory mode in animals and humans and is especially associated with motivational processes and biological rewards, including food, suggesting that children with overweight and obesity may be neurophysiologically characterized by persistent states of attention to motivationally rewarding stimuli.

Existing evidence on resting-state EEG activity in individuals with obesity was based on two studies in adults with obesity and comorbid binge-eating disorder (BED) [74,75]. Consistently, these studies revealed increased beta band activity and functional connectivity, respectively, in adults with obesity with versus without BED, while there were no group differences for other frequency bands [74,75]. However, the present study did not reveal significant differences in the beta band in either resting-state condition between children with overweight and obesity versus normal weight suggesting that increased beta band activity has a crucial role for individuals with obesity and high levels of food-specific impulsivity characterizing those with comorbid BED, but not children with obesity only. Notably, none of these previous studies on EEG resting-state activity included a control group of normal-weight individuals so far, making specific comparisons to these previous studies difficult [74,75]. It therefore remains to be further examined whether there are EEG subtypes in individuals with obesity and/or BED, possibly reflecting the heterogeneity in eating disorder and general psychopathology, including impulsivity in this population [76,77], in accordance with findings in ADHD research [78,79].

The fact that children with overweight and obesity versus those with normal weight did not show greater approach behavior towards high-calorie foods during the AAT is contrary to expectations, but fits into the inconsistent findings of previous studies in child and adult samples (e.g., References [80,81]). Within an intervention study in 276 8–16 years old youth, baseline AAT data already indicated avoidance tendencies for snack foods in children with obesity, much like in the present study; however, there were no data of a normal-weight control group available [82]. Similarly, the only study investigating adults with obesity did not find an approach bias towards high- or low-calorie foods [81], while university students with high levels of food cravings showed greater approach behavior towards food cues than adults with low levels of food craving [83]. The lack of effects may mirror conditioned responses towards high-calorie foods, the anticipation of punishment, or repeated reminders to avoid high-calorie foods, because children with obesity were mainly recruited via weight loss facilities. As the AAT is a reaction time task, socially desirable response behavior can be ruled out. In contrast, the BART-Y does not include any time component, but reflexive decision-making. The results of the BART-Y were unexpected as well, because children with overweight and obesity were not found to decide highly risky and did not strive for a large reward. Thus, the present results add to the inconsistent evidence on decision-making and risk-taking behavior in children with obesity (e.g., References [25,28]). Compared to the IGT or its age-adapted versions, such as the Hungry Donkey Task [25], the component of punishment in the BART-Y is more emotionally intensive as it is presented by an annoying tone when the balloon explodes. Thus, the results obtained from the BART-Y may rather mirror sensitivity to punishment or increased levels of anxiety (e.g., Reference [84]) than risk-taking behavior in children with obesity. Importantly, the questionnaire-based measures indicated higher levels of food-specific and general impulsivity in children with overweight and obesity versus normal-weight controls, consistent with recent findings [85].

Given that EEG resting-state frequency band activity serves as an electrophysiological signature for a range of impulsivity facets [32], correlational analyses between these measures were conducted across the total sample of children with normal weight, overweight, and obesity. In line with expectations and previous findings [34–37], delta and theta band activity during EO was positively related to parent-reported levels of enjoyment of food, describing strong approach behaviors towards foods. In contrast, but as expected [42], the direction of the association between alpha band activity and parent-reported food approach tendencies was the opposite (i.e., negative). After controlling for children's weight status and age, children's theta band activity and risk-taking behavior in the BART-Y were positively associated, as found in previous studies using the IGT in university student samples [35–37]. Notably, these associations were consistently found across many brain regions underlying the strength and connectivity of findings. For fast-wave band activity, positive relations between occipital beta band activity and children's level of hyperactivity were revealed, which goes in line with studies in adult and adolescent samples with obesity, although these findings were particularly relevant for frontal brain regions (for a review, see Reference [3]).

Compared to the associations found between EO resting-state frequency band activity and impulsivity measures the results on EC resting-state correlates were more selective regarding brain region and the direction of the association. For example, occipital delta band activity was negatively associated with risk-taking decisions during the BART-Y. These localized changes in the direction and topography of effects might be related to task-specific activation processes or the differential cortical processing of visual input, as EO and EC conditions generally produce differences in power and topography levels in children and adults [86,87].

A major strength of this pilot study is the standardized record of children's resting-state EEG activity in an acoustically and electromagnetically shielded cabin with video control. To increase the validity of the present results, EEG data were cleaned from artifacts by two independent experts. Furthermore, behavioral parameters of impulsivity were multimodally assessed via neuropsychological tasks with child-adapted food-specific and neutral stimuli and state-of-the-art questionnaires. For the first time, children's weight status was considered to describe specific EEG patterns in children with overweight and obesity under exclusion of ADHD and eating disorders.

However, some limitations must be considered when interpreting the results. Only large effects could be detected with sufficient power, due to the small sample size. For this reason, non-parametric tests were used where necessary and the corresponding effect sizes were reported. In addition to children with obesity, children with overweight were included in the EG, possibly attenuating between-group differences in EEG profiles related to obesity only. Due to the cross-sectional design, no conclusions can be drawn about the predictive value of EEG profiles on children's eating behavior and weight status.

Clinically, the identification of EEG profiles specific to childhood overweight and obesity may allow for taking a neurophysiological approach to target insufficient self-regulation in obesity, for example via EEG neurofeedback. Recent studies revealed promising effects of a specific EEG frequency band training for reducing the number of binge-eating episodes in women with obesity [88]. From a research point of view, this study implicates the need for further EEG studies in childhood obesity using larger sample sizes for detecting small-to-medium-sized group differences and longitudinal designs to evaluate the stability of EEG profiles over time. In this context, future studies should consider using alternative measures of impulsivity to cover its multifaceted nature, for example, via the stop signal task [89], a measure of response inhibition. Finally, research is warranted to determine the presence of EEG subtypes in children with obesity in order to account for the expected neurophysiological heterogeneity similar to that in ADHD (e.g., Reference [90]).

Author Contributions: Conceptualization, R.S. and C.H.; methodology, R.S., C.H., M.G., and L.S.; formal analysis, L.S. and C.H.; investigation, C.S., C.K., C.H.; resources, M.G. and A.H.; writing—original draft preparation, R.S., C.H. and L.S.; writing—review and editing, all authors; supervision, M.G.; funding acquisition, R.S. and A.H.

Acknowledgments: We are grateful to all children and their families for participating in the study and to Sabine Schäfer for her help in data visualization.

References

1. Carnell, S.; Gibson, C.; Benson, L.; Ochner, C.N.; Geliebter, A. Neuroimaging and obesity: Current knowledge and future directions. *Obes. Rev.* **2012**, *13*, 43–56. [CrossRef] [PubMed]
2. Makaronidis, J.M.; Batterham, R.L. Obesity, body weight regulation and the brain: Insights from fMRI. *Br. J. Radiol.* **2018**. [CrossRef] [PubMed]
3. Blume, M.; Schmidt, R.; Hilbert, A. Abnormalities in the EEG power spectrum in bulimia nervosa, binge-eating disorder, and obesity: A systematic review. *Eur. Eat. Disord. Rev.* **2018**. [CrossRef] [PubMed]
4. Tang, D.W.; Fellows, L.K.; Small, D.M.; Dagher, A. Food and drug cues activate similar brain regions: A meta-analysis of functional MRI studies. *Physiol. Behav.* **2012**, *106*, 317–324. [CrossRef] [PubMed]
5. Bruce, A.S.; Holsen, L.M.; Chambers, R.J.; Martin, L.E.; Brooks, W.M.; Zarcone, J.R.; Butler, M.G.; Savage, C.R. Obese children show hyperactivation to food pictures in brain networks linked to motivation, reward and cognitive control. *Int. J. Obes. (Lond.)* **2010**, *34*, 1494–1500. [CrossRef] [PubMed]
6. Pursey, K.M.; Stanwell, P.; Callister, R.J.; Brain, K.; Collins, C.E.; Burrows, T.L. Neuronal responses to visual food cues according to weight status: A systematic review of functional magnetic resonance imaging studies. *Front. Nutr.* **2014**, *1*, 7. [CrossRef] [PubMed]
7. Volkow, N.D.; Baler, R.D. Now vs. later brain circuits: Implications for obesity and addiction. *Trends Neurosci.* **2015**, *38*, 345–352. [CrossRef]
8. Aron, A.R.; Robbins, T.W.; Poldrack, R.A. Inhibition and the right inferior frontal cortex. *Trends Cogn. Sci.* **2004**, *8*, 170–177. [CrossRef]
9. Aron, A.R.; Robbins, T.W.; Poldrack, R.A. Inhibition and the right inferior frontal cortex: One decade on. *Trends Cogn. Sci.* **2014**, *18*, 177–185. [CrossRef]
10. Ridderinkhof, K.R.; van den Wildenberg, W.P.; Segalowitz, S.J.; Carter, C.S. Neurocognitive mechanisms of cognitive control: The role of prefrontal cortex on action selection, response inhibition, performance monitoring, and reward-based learning. *Brain Cogn.* **2004**, *56*, 129–140. [CrossRef]
11. Burger, K.S.; Berner, L.A. A functional neuroimaging review of obesity, appetitive hormones and ingestive behavior. *Physiol. Behav.* **2014**, *136*, 121–127. [CrossRef] [PubMed]
12. Moeller, F.G.; Barratt, E.S.; Dougherty, D.M.; Schmitz, J.M.; Swann, A.C. Psychiatric aspects of impulsivity. *Am. J. Psychiatry* **2001**, *158*, 1783–1793. [CrossRef] [PubMed]

13. Yang, Y.; Shields, G.S.; Guo, C.; Liu, Y. Executive function performance in obesity and overweight individuals: A meta-analysis and review. *Neurosci. Biobehav. Rev.* **2018**, *84*, 225–244. [CrossRef] [PubMed]
14. Graziano, P.A.; Kelleher, R.; Calkins, S.D.; Keane, S.P.; Brien, M.O. Predicting weight outcomes in preadolescence: The role of toddlers' self-regulation skills and the temperament dimension of pleasure. *Int. J. Obes.* **2013**, *37*, 937–942. [CrossRef] [PubMed]
15. Francis, L.A.; Susman, E.J. Self-regulation and rapid weight gain in children from age 3 to 12 years. *Arch. Pediatr. Adolesc. Med.* **2009**, *163*, 297–302. [CrossRef] [PubMed]
16. Nederkoorn, C.; Dassen, F.C.; Franken, L.; Resch, C.; Hauben, K. Impulsivity and overeating in children in the absence and presence of hunger. *Appetite* **2015**, *93*, 57–61. [CrossRef] [PubMed]
17. Van den Berg, L.; Pieterse, K.; Malik, J.A.; Luman, M.; Willems van Dijk, K.; Oosterlaan, J.; Delemarre-van de Waal, H.A. Association between impulsivity, reward responsiveness and body mass index in children. *Int. J. Obes.* **2011**, *35*, 1301–1307. [CrossRef]
18. Batterink, L.; Yokum, S.; Stice, E. Body mass correlates inversely with inhibitory control in response to food among adolescent girls: An fMRI study. *Neuroimage* **2010**, *52*, 1696–1703. [CrossRef]
19. Houben, K.; Nederkoorn, C.; Jansen, A. Eating on impulse: The relation between overweight and food-specific inhibitory control. *Obesity (Silver Spring)* **2014**, *22*, E6–E8. [CrossRef]
20. Nederkoorn, C.; Coelho, J.S.; Guerrieri, R.; Houben, K.; Jansen, A. Specificity of the failure to inhibit responses in overweight children. *Appetite* **2012**, *59*, 409–413. [CrossRef]
21. Braet, C.; Crombez, G. Cognitive interference due to food cues in childhood obesity. *J. Clin. Child Adolesc. Psychol.* **2003**, *32*, 32–39. [CrossRef] [PubMed]
22. Koch, A.; Matthias, E.; Pollatos, O. Increased attentional bias towards food pictures in overweight and obese children. *J. Child Adolesc. Behav.* **2014**, *2*, 130. [CrossRef]
23. Liang, J.; Matheson, B.E.; Kaye, W.H.; Boutelle, K.N. Neurocognitive correlates of obesity and obesity-related behaviors in children and adolescents. *Int. J. Obes. (Lond.)* **2014**, *38*, 494–506. [CrossRef] [PubMed]
24. Bechara, A.; Damasio, A.R.; Damasio, H.; Anderson, S.W. Insensitivity to future consequences following damage to human prefrontal cortex. *Cognition* **1994**, *50*, 7–15. [CrossRef]
25. Verbeken, S.; Braet, C.; Bosmans, G.; Goossens, L. Comparing decision making in average and overweight children and adolescents. *Int. J. Obes. (Lond.)* **2014**, *38*, 547–551. [CrossRef] [PubMed]
26. Verdejo-García, A.; Pérez-Expósito, M.; Schmidt-Río-Valle, J.; Fernández-Serrano, M.J.; Cruz, F.; Pérez-García, M.; López-Belmonte, G.; Martín-Matillas, M.; Martín-Lagos, J.A.; Marcos, A.; et al. Selective alterations within executive functions in adolescents with excess weight. *Obesity (Silver Spring)* **2010**, *18*, 1572–1578. [CrossRef] [PubMed]
27. Delgado-Rico, E.; Río-Valle, J.S.; González-Jiménez, E.; Campoy, C.; Verdejo-García, A. BMI predicts emotion-driven impulsivity and cognitive inflexibility in adolescents with excess weight. *Obesity* **2012**, *20*, 1604–1610. [CrossRef]
28. Goldschmidt, A.B.; O'Brien, S.; Lavender, J.M.; Pearson, C.M.; Le Grange, D.; Hunter, S.J. Executive functioning in a racially diverse sample of children who are overweight and at risk for eating disorders. *Appetite* **2018**, *124*, 43–49. [CrossRef]
29. Kittel, R.; Schmidt, R.; Hilbert, A. Executive functions in adolescents with binge-eating disorder and obesity. *Int. J. Eat. Disord.* **2017**, *50*, 933–941. [CrossRef]
30. Nederkoorn, C.; Braet, C.; Van Eijs, Y.; Tanghe, A.; Jansen, A. Why obese children cannot resist food: The role of impulsivity. *Eat. Behav.* **2006**, *7*, 315–322. [CrossRef]
31. Mata, F.; Verdejo-Roman, J.; Soriano-Mas, C.; Verdejo-Garcia, A. Insula tuning towards external eating versus interoceptive input in adolescents with overweight and obesity. *Appetite* **2015**, *93*, 24–30. [CrossRef] [PubMed]
32. Andreassi, J.L. *Psychophysiology: Human Behavior and Physiological Response*, 5th ed.; Taylor & Francis Inc.: New York, NY, USA, 2006.
33. Loo, S.K.; Lenartowicz, A.; Makeig, S. Use of EEG biomarkers in child psychiatry research: Current state and future directions. *J. Child Psychol. Psychiatry* **2016**, *57*, 4–17. [CrossRef] [PubMed]
34. Loo, S.K.; McGough, J.J.; McCracken, J.T.; Smalley, S.L. Parsing heterogeneity in attention-deficit hyperactivity disorder using EEG-based subgroups. *J. Child Psychol. Psychiatry* **2018**, *59*, 223–231. [CrossRef]

35. Massar, S.A.A.; Rossi, V.; Schutter, D.J.L.G.; Kenemans, J.L. Baseline EEG theta/beta ratio and punishment sensitivity as biomarkers for feedback-related negativity (FRN) and risk-taking. *Clin. Neurophysiol.* **2012**, *10*, 1958–1965. [CrossRef] [PubMed]
36. Massar, S.A.A.; Kenemans, J.L.; Schutter, D.J.L.G. Resting-state EEG theta activity and risk learning: Sensitivity to reward or punishment? *Int. J. Psychophysiol.* **2014**, *3*, 172–177. [CrossRef] [PubMed]
37. Schutter, D.J.L.G.; Van Honk, J. Electrophysiological ratio markers for the balance between reward and punishment. *Brain Res. Cogn. Brain Res.* **2005**, *24*, 685–690. [CrossRef] [PubMed]
38. Ogrim, G.; Kropotov, J.; Hestad, K. The quantitative EEG theta/beta ratio in attention deficit/hyperactivity disorder and normal controls: Sensitivity, specificity, and behavioral correlates. *Psychiatry Res.* **2012**, *198*, 482–488. [CrossRef]
39. Rudo-Hutt, A.S. Electroencephalography and externalizing behavior: A meta-analysis. *Biol. Psychol.* **2015**, *105*, 1–19. [CrossRef]
40. Cortese, S.; Moreira-Maia, C.R.; St Fleur, D.; Morcillo-Peñalver, C.; Rohde, L.A.; Faraone, S.V. Associations between ADHD and obesity: A systematic review and meta-analysis. *Am. J. Psychiatry* **2016**, *173*, 34–43. [CrossRef]
41. Van Dongen-Boomsma, M.; Lansbergen, M.M.; Bekker, E.M.; Kooij, J.J.; van der Molen, M.; Kenemans, J.L.; Buitelaar, J.K. Relation between resting EEG to cognitive performance and clinical symptoms in adults with attention-deficit/hyperactivity disorder. *Neurosci. Lett.* **2010**, *469*, 102–106. [CrossRef]
42. Lee, J.Y.; Park, S.M.; Kim, Y.J.; Kim, D.J.; Choi, S.W.; Kwon, J.S.; Choi, J.S. Resting-state EEG activity related to impulsivity in gambling disorder. *J. Behav. Addict.* **2017**, *6*, 387–395. [CrossRef] [PubMed]
43. Chen, S.; Jia, Y.; Woltering, S. Neural differences of inhibitory control between adolescents with obesity and their peers. *Int. J. Obes.* **2018**, *42*, 1753–1761. [CrossRef] [PubMed]
44. Hill, C.; Wu, J.; Crowley, M.J.; Fearon, P. Restrictive feeding practices and adiposity are differentially related to P3b cortical responses to food stimuli in children. *Appetite* **2013**, *63*, 7–17. [CrossRef] [PubMed]
45. Seymour, K.E.; Reinblatt, S.P.; Benson, L.; Carnell, S. Overlapping neurobehavioral circuits in ADHD, obesity, and binge eating: Evidence from neuroimaging research. *CNS Spectr.* **2015**, *20*, 401–411. [CrossRef] [PubMed]
46. Bauer, L.O.; Manning, K.J. Challenges in the detection of working memory and attention decrements among overweight adolescent girls. *Neuropsychobiology* **2016**, *73*, 43–51. [CrossRef] [PubMed]
47. Olde Dubbelink, K.T.E.; Felius, A.; Verbunt, J.P.A.; van Dijk, B.W.; Berendse, H.W.; Stam, C.J.; Delemarre-van de Waal, H. Increased resting-state functional connectivity in obese adolescents: A magnetoencephalographic pilot study. *PLoS ONE* **2008**, *3*, e2827. [CrossRef] [PubMed]
48. Babiloni, C.; Marzano, N.; Lizio, R.; Valenzano, A.; Triggiani, A.I.; Petito, A.; Bellomo, A.; Lecce, B.; Mundi, C.; Soricelli, A.; et al. Resting state cortical electroencephalographic rhythms in subjects with normal and abnormal body weight. *Neuroimage* **2011**, *58*, 698–707. [CrossRef] [PubMed]
49. Del Percio, C.; Triggiani, A.I.; Marzano, N.; Valenzano, A.; De Rosas, M.; Petito, A.; Bellomo, A.; Lecce, B.; Muni, C.; Infarinato, F.; et al. Poor desynchronisation of resting-state eyes-open cortical alpha rhythms in obese subjects without eating disorders. *Clin. Neurophysiol.* **2013**, *124*, 1095–1105. [CrossRef]
50. Satterfield, J.H.; Cantwell, D.P.; Satterfield, B.T. Pathophysiology of the hyperactive child syndrome. *Arch. Gen. Psychiatry* **1974**, *31*, 839–844. [CrossRef]
51. Kurth, B.M.; Schaffrath Rosario, A. Overweight and obesity in children and adolescents in Germany. *Bundesgesundheitsblatt Gesundheitsforschung Gesundheitsschutz* **2010**, *53*, 643–652. [CrossRef]
52. Lange, M.; Kamtsiuris, P.; Lange, C.; Schaffrath Rosario, A.; Stolzenberg, H.; Lampert, T. Sociodemographic characteristics in the German health interview and examination survey for children and adolescents (KiGGS)—Operationalization and public health significance, taking as an example the assessment of general state of health. *Bundesgesundheitsblatt Gesundheitsforschung Gesundheitsschutz* **2007**, *50*, 578–589. [CrossRef] [PubMed]
53. Bryant-Waugh, R.J.; Cooper, P.J.; Taylor, C.L.; Lask, B.D. The use of the eating disorder examination with children: A pilot study. *Int. J. Eat. Disord.* **1996**, *19*, 391–397. [CrossRef]
54. Hilbert, A. *Eating Disorder Examination für Kinder: Deutschsprachige Übersetzung [Eating Disorder Examination for Children: German translation]*; DGVT-Verlag: Tübingen, Germany, 2016; ISBN 978-3-87159-413-7.
55. Schneider, S.; Unnewehr, S.; Margraf, J. *Kinder-DIPS: Diagnostisches Interview bei Psychischen Störungen im Kindes- und Jugendalter [Diagnostic Interview for Mental Disorders in Childhood and Adolescence]*, 2nd ed.; Springer: Berlin, Germany, 2009; ISBN 978-3540782100.

56. Gratton, G.; Coles, M.G.; Donchin, E. A new method for off-line removal of ocular artifact. *Electroencephalogr. Clin. Neurophysiol.* **1983**, *55*, 468–484. [CrossRef]
57. Wiers, R.W.; Rinck, M.; Dictus, M.; van den Wildenberg, E. Relatively strong automatic appetitive action-tendencies in male carriers of the OPRM1 G-allele. *Genes Brain Behav.* **2009**, *8*, 101–106. [CrossRef] [PubMed]
58. Blechert, J.; Meule, A.; Busch, N.A.; Ohla, K. Food-pics: An image database for experimental research on eating and appetite. *Front. Psychol.* **2014**, *5*, 617. [CrossRef] [PubMed]
59. Lejuez, C.; Aklin, W.; Daughters, S.; Zvolensky, M.; Kahler, C.; Gwadz, M. Reliability and validity of the youth version of the Balloon Analogue Risk Task (BART-Y) in the assessment of risk-taking behavior among inner-city adolescents. *J. Clin. Child Adolesc. Psychol.* **2007**, *36*, 106–111. [CrossRef] [PubMed]
60. Wardle, J.; Guthrie, C.A.; Sanderson, S.; Rapoport, L. Development of the Children's Eating Behavior Questionnaire. *J. Child Psychol. Psychiatry* **2001**, *42*, 963–970. [CrossRef]
61. Klasen, H.; Woerner, W.; Rothenberger, A.; Goodman, R. The German version of the Strengths and Difficulties Questionnaire (SDQ-Deu)—Overview over first validation and normative studies. *Prax. Kinderpsychol. Kinderpsychiat.* **2003**, *52*, 491–502.
62. Stadler, C.; Janke, W.; Schmeck, K. *Inventar zur Erfassung von Impulsivität, Risikoverhalten und Empathie bei 9-bis 14-Jährigen Kindern [Inventory for Assessing Impulsivity, Risk Behavior, and Empathy]*; Hogrefe: Göttingen, Germany, 2004.
63. Eysenck, S.B.G.; Eysenck, H.J. Impulsiveness and venturesomeness in children. *Personal. Individ. Differ.* **1980**, *1*, 73–78. [CrossRef]
64. Wechsler, D. *The Wechsler Intelligence Scale for Children-Fourth Edition*; Pearson: London, UK, 2003.
65. Petermann, F.; Petermann, U. *Wechsler Intelligence Scale for Children—Fourth Edition (WISC-IV)*; Pearson: Frankfurt, Germany, 2011; ISBN 978-3-943274-00-4.
66. Cohen, J. *Statistical Power Analysis for the Behavioral Sciences*, 2nd ed.; Erlbaum: Hillsdale, NJ, USA, 1988; ISBN 9780805802832.
67. Clarke, A.R.; Barry, R.J.; McCarthy, R.; Selikowitz, M. Age and sex effects in the EEG: Development of the normal child. *Clin. Neurophysiol.* **2001**, *112*, 806–814. [CrossRef]
68. Clarke, A.R.; Barry, R.J.; McCarthy, R.; Selikowitz, M. EEG-defined subtypes of children with attention-deficit/hyperactivity disorder. *Clin. Neurophysiol.* **2001**, *112*, 2098–2105. [CrossRef]
69. Markovska-Simoska, S.; Pop-Jordanova, N. Quantitative EEG in children and adults with attention deficit hyperactivity disorder: Comparison of absolute and relative power spectra and theta/beta ratio. *Clin. EEG Neurosci.* **2017**, *48*, 20–32. [CrossRef] [PubMed]
70. Rommel, A.-S.; James, S. N.; McLoughlin, G.; Brandeis, D.; Banaschewski, T.; Asherson, P.; Kuntsi, J. Altered EEG spectral power during rest and cognitive performance: A comparison of preterm-born adolescents to adolescents with ADHD. *Eur. Child Adolesc. Psychiatry* **2017**, *26*, 1511–1522. [CrossRef]
71. Hegerl, U.; Hensch, T. The vigilance reduction model of affective disorders and ADHD. *Neurosci. Biobehav. Rev.* **2014**, *44*, 45–57. [CrossRef]
72. Leddy, J.J.; Epstein, L.H.; Jaroni, J.L.; Roemmich, J.N.; Paluch, R.A.; Goldfield, G.S.; Lerman, C. Influence of methylphenidate on eating in obese men. *Obes. Res.* **2004**, *12*, 224–232. [CrossRef] [PubMed]
73. Knyazev, G.G. EEG delta oscillations as a correlate of basic homeostatic and motivational processes. *Neurosci. Biobehav. Rev.* **2012**, *36*, 677–695. [CrossRef] [PubMed]
74. Imperatori, C.; Fabbricatore, M.; Farina, M.; Innamorati, M.; Quintiliani, M.I.; Lamis, D.A.; Contardi, A.; Della Marca, G.; Speranza, A.M. Alterations of EEG functional connectivity in resting state obese and overweight patients with binge eating disorder: A preliminary report. *Neurosci. Lett.* **2015**, *607*, 120–124. [CrossRef]
75. Tammela, L.I.; Pääkkönen, A.; Karhunen, L.J.; Karhu, J.; Uusitupa, I.J.; Kuikka, J.T. Brain electrical activity during food presentation in obese binge-eating women. *Clin. Physiol. Funct. Imaging* **2010**, *30*, 135–140. [CrossRef]
76. Braet, C.; Beyers, W.; Goossens, L.; Verbeken, S.; Moens, E. Subtyping children and adolescents who are overweight based on eating pathology and psychopathology. *Eur. Eat. Disord. Rev.* **2012**, *20*, 279–286. [CrossRef]

77. Sysko, R.; Blake Zakarin, E.B.; Devlin, M.J.; Bush, J.; Walsh, B.T. A latent class analysis of psychiatric symptoms among 125 adolescents in a bariatric surgery program. *Int. J. Pediatr. Obes.* **2011**, *6*, 289–297. [CrossRef]
78. Sander, C.; Arns, M.; Olbrich, S.; Hegerl, U. EEG-vigilance and response to stimulants in paediatric patients with attention deficit/hyperactivity disorder. *Clin. Neurophysiol.* **2010**, *121*, 1511–1518. [CrossRef] [PubMed]
79. Arns, M.; Gunkelman, J.; Breteler, M.; Spronk, D. EEG phenotypes predict treatment outcome to stimulants in children with ADHD. *J. Integr. Neurosci.* **2008**, *7*, 421–438. [CrossRef] [PubMed]
80. Becker, D.; Jostmann, N.B.; Wiers, R.W.; Holland, R.W. Approach avoidance training in the eating domain: Testing the effectiveness across three single session studies. *Appetite* **2015**, *85*, 58–65. [CrossRef] [PubMed]
81. Paslakis, G.; Kühn, S.; Grunert, S.; Erim, Y. Explicit and implicit approach vs. avoidance tendencies towards high vs. low calorie food cues in patients with obesity and active binge eating disorder. *Nutrients* **2017**, *9*, 1068. [CrossRef] [PubMed]
82. Warschburger, P.; Gmeiner, M.; Morawietz, M.; Rinck, M. Battle of plates: A pilot study of an approch-avoidance training for overweight children and adolescents. *Public Health Nutr.* **2018**, *21*, 426–434. [CrossRef] [PubMed]
83. Brockmeyer, T.; Hahn, C.; Reetz, C.; Schmidt, U.; Friederich, H.-C. Approach bias and cue reactivity towards food in people with high versus low levels of food craving. *Appetite* **2015**, *95*, 197–202. [CrossRef]
84. Esposito, M.; Gallai, B.; Roccella, M.; Marotta, R.; Lavano, F.; Lavano, S.M.; Mazzotta, G.; Bove, D.; Sorrentino, M.; Precenzano, F.; et al. Anxiety and depression levels in prepubertal obese children: A case-control study. *Neuropsychiatr. Dis. Treat.* **2014**, *10*, 1897–1902. [CrossRef]
85. Webber, L.; Hill, C.; Saxton, J.; Van Jaarsveld, C.H.; Wardle, J. Eating behaviour and weight in children. *Int. J. Obes. (Lond.)* **2009**, *33*, 21–28. [CrossRef]
86. Barry, R.J.; Clarke, A.R.; Johnstone, S.J.; Magee, C.A.; Rushby, J.A. EEG differences between eyes-closed and eyes-open resting conditions. *Clin. Neurophysiol.* **2007**, *118*, 2765–2773. [CrossRef]
87. Barry, R.J.; Clarke, A.R.; Johnstone, S.J.; Brown, C.R. EEG differences in children between eyes-closed and eyes-open resting conditions. *Clin. Neurophysiol.* **2009**, 1806–1811. [CrossRef]
88. Schmidt, J.; Martin, A. Neurofeedback against binge eating: A randomized controlled trial in a female subclinical threshold sample. *Eur. Eat. Disord. Rev.* **2016**, *24*, 406–416. [CrossRef] [PubMed]
89. Logan, G.D.; Dagenbach, D.; Carr, T.H. On the ability to inhibit thought and action. A users' guide to the stop signal paradigm. In *Inhibitory Processes in Attention, Memory and Language*, 1st ed.; Dagenbach, D., Carr, T.H., Eds.; Academic Press: San Diego, CA, USA, 1994; pp. 189–236, ISBN 9780122004100.
90. Barth, B.; Mayer-Carius, K.; Strehl, U.; Kelava, A.; Häußinger, F.B.; Fallgatter, A.J.; Ehlis, A.C. Identification of neurophysiological biotypes in attention deficit hyperactivity disorder. *Psychiatry Clin. Neurosci.* **2018**, *72*, 836–848. [CrossRef] [PubMed]

10

The Distribution of Obesity Phenotypes in HIV-Infected African Population

Kim Anh Nguyen [1,2], Nasheeta Peer [1,2], Anniza de Villiers [1], Barbara Mukasa [3], Tandi E. Matsha [4], Edward J. Mills [5] and Andre Pascal Kengne [1,2,*]

1 Non-Communicable Diseases Research Unit, South African Medical Research Council, Cape Town 7505, South Africa; Kim.Nguyen@mrc.ac.za (K.A.N.); nasheeta.peer@mrc.ac.za (N.P.); Anniza.DeVilliers@mrc.ac.za (A.d.V.)
2 Department of Medicine, University of Cape Town, Cape Town 7935, South Africa
3 United Nations Population Fund (UNFPA), Mildmay Uganda PO Box 24985, Lweza, Uganda; barbara.mukasa@mildmay.or.ug
4 Department of Biomedical Sciences, Faculty of Health and Wellness Science, Cape Peninsula University of Technology, Cape Town 7535, South Africa; matshat@cput.ac.za
5 Global Evaluation Science, Vancouver, BC V6H 3X4, Canada; emills@redwoodoutcomes.com
* Correspondence: andre.kengne@mrc.ac.za

Abstract: The distribution of body size phenotypes in people with human immunodeficiency virus (HIV) infection has yet to be characterized. We assessed the distribution of body size phenotypes overall, and according to antiretroviral therapy (ART), diagnosed duration of the infection and CD4 count in a sample of HIV infected people recruited across primary care facilities in the Western Cape Province, South Africa. Adults aged $\geqslant$ 18 years were consecutively recruited using random sampling procedures, and their cardio-metabolic profile were assessed during March 2014 and February 2015. They were classified across body mass index (BMI) categories as normal-weight (BMI < 25 kg/m^2), overweight (25 $\leqslant$ BMI < 30 kg/m^2), and obese (BMI $\geqslant$ 30 kg/m^2), and further classified according to their metabolic status as "metabolically healthy" *vs.* "metabolically abnormal" if they had less than two *vs.* two or more of the following abnormalities: high blood glucose, raised blood pressure, raised triglycerides, and low HDL-cholesterol. Their cross-classification gave the following six phenotypes: normal-weight metabolically healthy (NWMH), normal-weight metabolically abnormal (NWMA), overweight metabolically healthy (OvMH), overweight metabolically abnormal (OvMA), obese metabolically healthy (OMH), and obese metabolically abnormal (OMA). Among the 748 participants included (median age 38 years (25th–75th percentiles: 32–44)), 79% were women. The median diagnosed duration of HIV was five years; the median CD4 count was 392 cells/mm^3 and most participants were on ART. The overall distribution of body size phenotypes was the following: 31.7% (NWMH), 11.7% (NWMA), 13.4% (OvMH), 9.5% (OvMA), 18.6% (OMH), and 15.1% (OMA). The distribution of metabolic phenotypes across BMI levels did not differ significantly in men *vs.* women (p = 0.062), in participants below *vs.* those at or above median diagnosed duration of HIV infection (p = 0.897), in participants below *vs.* those at or above median CD4 count (p = 0.447), and by ART regimens (p = 0.205). In this relatively young sample of HIV-infected individuals, metabolically abnormal phenotypes are frequent across BMI categories. This highlights the importance of general measures targeting an overall improvement in cardiometabolic risk profile across the spectrum of BMI distribution in all adults with HIV.

Keywords: obesity phenotype; metabolic abnormalities; HIV infection

1. Introduction

People living with HIV infection constitute a sizable proportion of the world population and the number is increasing [1]. The advent and uptake of antiretroviral therapy (ART) has turned HIV infection from a highly fatal infectious disease into a chronic manageable condition [2]. Consequently, the lifespan of HIV infected patients receiving ART is now close to that of the general population [3]. This has led to a rise in chronic and age-related conditions such as cardio-metabolic disorders in HIV-infected people [4,5], that is contributing substantially to the overall morbidity and mortality in this population [6,7].

A major contributor to cardio-metabolic diseases is the global obesity epidemic with 52% (1.9 millions) of the worldwide adult population being either overweight or obese in 2014 [8]. Obesity contributes to cardio-metabolic abnormalities by impairing metabolic functions that promote dyslipidemia, insulin resistance, as well as chronic inflammation [9]. Consequently, concepts such as "metabolically healthy" and "metabolically abnormal" have been used to characterize individuals across the distribution of body mass index (BMI) as a function of the underlying burden of metabolic abnormalities [10].

The changes in body fat distribution associated with HIV infection are well-described [11]. The advanced stage of untreated HIV infection is associated with changes in body fat content and distribution, which are partially and perhaps non-optimally restored following treatment with ART [12]. ART extends the lifespan of HIV-infected people by reducing the viral load with a subsequent strengthening of the immune system; notably, it does not eliminate the HIV infection. Hence, chronic inflammation persists and there is incomplete restoration of the immune system [13]. Additionally, various metabolic abnormalities are associated with HIV infection and its related treatments [14,15]. These include dyslipidemia, insulin resistance, and abnormal blood pressure levels, [13], which contribute to cardiovascular diseases (CVDs) and type 2 diabetes mellitus (T2DM) [13,16].

While obesity and HIV infection have been extensively researched separately, there is a dearth of data on the distribution of obesity phenotypes in HIV-infected people [17]. Therefore, in the current study, we assessed the distribution of obesity phenotypes, and the effects if any, of ART and other major distinctive characteristics of HIV infection, in a representative sample of people with HIV recruited across primary healthcare facilities in the Western Cape Province, South Africa.

2. Materials and Methods

2.1. Study Design and Sampling Procedure

A cross-sectional survey was conducted from March 2014 to February 2015 in a random sample of HIV-infected adults aged 18 years and older being treated at public healthcare facilities across the Western Cape Province in South Africa. Permission to conduct the survey was obtained from Health Research Office of the Western Cape Department of Health, and the relevant healthcare facilities.

The healthcare facilities considered for this study needed to provide ART to at least 325 HIV-infected patients per month to ensure adequate recruitment within a reasonable period. Thus, the sample frame comprised a total of 62 healthcare facilities with 42 across Cape Town and 20 in the surrounding rural municipalities. Of these, 17 facilities, including four rural, were randomly selected for inclusion in this study. At each participating healthcare facility, 15–60 patients were randomly sampled.

The study was approved by the South African Medical Research Council Ethics Committee and conducted in accordance with the principles of the Declaration of Helsinki.

2.2. Data Collection

A team of trained clinicians, nurses, and field workers collected data by administering questionnaires, clinical measurements, and biochemical analyses. Data were captured on electronic case report forms, which were available on personal digital assistants (PDAs), with built-in checks for quality control. Data were encrypted at the point of collection and sent via mobile connection to a dedicated server, from which it was further checked, downloaded, and stored for future use. The interviews and the physical assessments were conducted on the day of recruitment while the blood specimens were drawn the following day after the participant had fasted overnight.

2.2.1. Interviews

Socio-demographic data and medical history were obtained using a structured interviewer-administered questionnaire adapted from the World Health Organization's STEPwise approach to Surveillance (STEPS) tool. Self-reported data included duration of being diagnosed HIV infection and CD4 counts, whereas information on HIV treatment was obtained by capturing medications brought to by the participants.

2.2.2. Physical Examination

Anthropometric parameters including height, weight, and waist circumference (WC) were measured using standardized techniques. Height was measured to the nearest millimeter using a Leicester Height Scale (Seca, Liverpool, UK) with the participant barefoot and in the upright position. Weight was measured to the nearest gram using A&D Personal Scale (Model UC-321, Toshima-Ku, Tokyo, Japan) with the participant in light clothes, and without shoes. WC, recorded to the nearest millimeter, was taken at the level of umbilicus. After the participant was seated in a resting position for at least five minutes, blood pressure (BP) was measured in mmHg on the right arm, using a digital automatic BP monitor (Omron, M6 Comfort, Hoofddorp, The Netherland); three measurements were taken three minutes apart.

2.2.3. Laboratory Measurements

Biochemical parameters were analyzed at an ISO 15189 accredited pathology laboratory (PathCare, Reference Laboratory, Cape Town, South Africa) which had no access to participants' clinical information. All analyses were performed on venous blood samples collected after an overnight fast of at least eight hours. Serum cholesterol and triglycerides were measured by enzymatic colorimetric methods; ultrasensitive C-reactive protein was read; plasma glucose was measured by hexokinase method; all implemented using a Beckman Coulter AU 500 spectrophotometer. Insulin concentrations were measured by the Chemiluminesecence Immunoassay method while HbA1c level was determined using high-performance liquid chromatography technique. The homeostatic model assessment of insulin resistance (HOMA-IR) was calculated as the product of insulin (mIU/L) and glucose (mmol/L) by 22.5 [18].

2.3. *Definitions*

2.3.1. Socio-Demographic Characteristics

Education level was distinguished into primary education and secondary education or above. Smoking status was categorized as never-smoker, past-smoker (stopped smoking during the past 12 months), and current-smoker. Alcohol intake behavior was classified as non-heavy drinker (consumed <5 standard alcoholic drinks for men and < 4 standard alcoholic drinks for women in a row during the past 30 days), and heavy-drinker (consumed ⩾5 standard alcoholic drinks for men and ⩾4 standard alcoholic drinks for women in a row during the past 30 days). A standard alcoholic drink was corresponding to one can (340 mL) of beer, one glass (125 mL) wine, or one shot (25 mL) of spirits. Duration of diagnosed HIV infection was the time since being diagnosed with HIV. ARTs were categorized as first line ART, second line ART, and other regimens [19].

2.3.2. Body Size Phenotype

Body mass index (BMI) was calculated as weight (kg)/height × height (m^2). BMI was used to classify participants into three categories: normal weight (BMI < 25 kg/m^2), overweight (BMI ⩾ 25 kg/m^2 and BMI < 30 kg/m^2) and obese (BMI ⩾ 30 kg/m^2). There is no consensus on the definition and number of cardio-metabolic abnormalities to use when characterizing obesity phenotypes [20]. In the current study, we considered the following four abnormalities: (1) elevated BP determined using the average of the second and third BP measurements (systolic BP ⩾ 130 mmHg or diastolic BP ⩾ 85 mmHg or known hypertension on treatment); (2) high triglycerides (⩾1.69 mmol/L); (3) low high-density lipoprotein cholesterol (HDL-C ⩽ 1.0 mmol/L in men; ⩽1.3 mmol/L in women); (4) high blood glucose (fasting plasma glucose (FPG) ⩾ 5.6 mmol/L or known diabetes mellitus). In secondary analysis, in a subset of participants with data available on insulin levels, we included insulin resistance as a fifth metabolic abnormality, by classifying as insulin resistant all participants with HOMA-IR above the data specific 90th percentile. Considering the lack of consensus on waist circumference (or waist-to-hip ratio) threshold to define abdominal obesity in African populations, the criteria of abdominal obesity which has been included in about 30% of studies on obesity phenotype [20] was not included in our panel of metabolic abnormalities.

Participants were then classified for metabolic status as "metabolically healthy" if they had none or one metabolic abnormality, and as "metabolically abnormal" if they had two or more metabolic abnormalities. Cross-classification of participants by BMI and metabolic status led to the following six phenotypes: (1) normal weight and metabolically healthy (NWMH); (2) normal weight and metabolically abnormal (NWMA); (3) overweight and metabolically healthy (OvMH); (4) overweight and metabolically abnormal (OvMA); (5) obese and metabolically healthy (OMH); and (6) obese and metabolically abnormal (OMA).

2.4. Statistical Analysis

Participants' characteristics are summarized as means (standard deviation, SD) and medians (25th to 75th percentiles) for continuous variables, and as count (percentages) for categorical variables. Comparison of baseline characteristics across BMI categories, by metabolic status, and by HIV-related characteristics were done using chi-square tests, fisher-exact test, *t*-tests or Kruskal-wallis tests for non-parametric data or Analysis of Variance test (ANOVA) where appropriate. The linear trends across BMI categories overall and by metabolic status were examined using the Cochrane-Armitage trend tests and Brown-Forsythe Levene procedures. The two-way interactions between BMI categories and metabolic status (B × M), and metabolic status and gender (M × G) were tested using linear and logistic regression models, by incorporating in the same model the main effects of the variables of interest as well as their interaction term.

To assess the association between each continuous metabolic trait and BMI categories, multinomial logistic regressions models (age and sex adjusted) were used to derive the odds ratio (OR) and 95% confidence interval for a unit higher level of each metabolic trait in relation with overweight and obesity risk, always using normal weight are reference category. The McFadden's R^2 [21] was then used as a measure of the overall performance of models containing age, gender, and each metabolic trait of interest. A two-side p-value < 0.05 indicates a statistical significance. All analyses were performed using the R statistical software version 3.0.3 (the R Foundation for Statistical Computing Platform, Vienna, Austria. For a z-value of 1.96 (corresponding to a 95% confidence interval), and an effective sample size of 748 participants, our study had a margin of error of 0.05% to detect a prevalence of normal weight metabolically abnormal phenotype of 1% in the total sample. The acceptable margin of error is 5%, indicating that our study was well-powered for the overall and subgroup analyses.

3. Results

3.1. Socio-Demographic Characteristics

Of the 831 participants who were interviewed and clinically assessed, 754 (91%) returned for biochemical measurements. Blood samples from six participants were inadequate for analyses resulting in 748 (99%) participants being included in the study. This comprised 591 women and 157 men who had complete data on the variables of interest.

The median age (25th–75th percentiles) was 38 (32–44) years overall, 41 (35–47) years in men, and 37 (31–43) years in women ($p < 0.001$). As shown in Table 1, most participants (84.9%) had secondary education or higher with a lower prevalence in men (75.8%) than in women (87.3%) ($p < 0.001$). About half of the participants (54.6%) were employed with similar rates in men and women (49.7% *vs.* 55.9%, $p = 0.162$). Current smoking was more prevalent in men than in women (58.8% *vs.* 16.1%, $p < 0.001$) but heavy alcohol consumption was similar (34.1% *vs.* 34.1%, $p = 0.975$).

Table 1. Characteristics of the HIV/AIDS patients (*n* (%), or median (25th–75th percentiles)).

Characteristics	Overall, ($n = 748$)	Men, ($n = 157$)	Women, ($n = 591$)	p
Age, year	38 (32–44)	41 (35–47)	37 (31–43)	<0.001
Education level, *n* (%)				<0.001
Primary	113/746 (15.1)	38/157 (24.2)	75/589 (12.7)	
Secondary and above	633/746 (84.9)	119/157 (75.8)	514/589 (87.3)	
Employed, *n* (%)	408/747 (54.6)	78/157 (49.7)	330/590 (55.9)	0.162
Smoking habit, *n* (%)				<0.001
Never smoke	461/718 (64.7)	34/156 (22.2)	427/562 (76.4)	
Current smoker	187/718 (25.3)	93/156 (58.8)	90/562 (16.1)	
Past smoker	70/718 (13.3)	29/156 (45.3)	42/562 (9.0)	
Heavy drinker, *n* (%)	64/187 (34.2)	22/64 (34.4)	42/123 (34.1)	0.975
HIV duration, years	5 (2–9)	4 (2–7)	5 (2.5–9)	<0.001
CD4, cells/mm^3	392(240–604)	272(193–448)	410(253–627)	0.001
ART treatment, *n* (%)				0.005
Non-ART	46/699 (6.6)	7/149 (4.7)	39/550 (7.1)	
first line	426/699 (60.9)	78/149 (52.3)	348/550 (63.3)	
second line	79/699 (11.3)	17/149 (11.4)	62/550 (11.3)	
Others	148/699 (21.2)	47/149 (31.5)	101/550 (18.3)	
Body mass index (kg/m^2)				
Median (P25–P75)	26.3 (22.1–32)	21.4 (19.8–22.4)	28.3 (23.8–28.9)	<0.001
<25, *n* (%)	325 (43.4)	126 (80.3)	199 (33.7)	
25.0–29.9, *n* (%)	171 (22.9)	21 (13.4)	150 (25.4)	
⩾30, *n* (%)	252 (33.7)	10 (6.4)	242 (40.9)	
Waist circumference, cm	88 (77.5–98)	78.9 (73.9–88.3)	90 (79.5–100.8)	<0.001
Systolic BP, mmHg	117 (107–129.5)	123.5 (114.5–140)	115 (105.8–127)	<0.001
Diastolic BP, mmHg	82 (75–90.5)	83 (76–94)	81.5 (74.8–89.8)	0.129
Total cholesterol, mmol/L	4.3 (3.7–5.1)	4.2 (3.5–5.0)	4.4 (3.8–5.1)	0.009
HDL-cholesterol, mmol/L	1.27 (1.03–1.5)	1.2 (1.0–1.5)	1.29 (1.08–1.52)	0.010
LDL-cholesterol, mmol/L	2.5 (2.0–3.1)	2.3 (1.7–3.0)	2.5 (2.0–3.1)	0.012
Triglycerides, mmol/L	1.0 (0.74–1.34)	1.12 (0.75–1.27)	0.97 (0.74–1.28)	0.023
Fasting glucose, mmol/L	5.0 (4.6–5.4)	5.1 (4.8–5.5)	4.9 (4.6–5.4)	0.010
HOMA-IR	1.36 (0.84–2.24)	0.94 (0.53–1.64)	1.49 (0.93–2.37)	<0.001
C-reactive protein, mg/L	5.6 (2.4–12)	5.0 (2.1–16.2)	5.6 (2.4–14.2)	0.728
Treated hypertension, *n* (%)	110 (14.7)	11 (7)	99 (16.8)	0.002
Treated diabetes, *n* (%)	28 (3.7)	8 (5.1)	20 (3.4)	0.432

ART, antiretroviral; BP, blood pressure; HDL, high density lipoprotein; HIV, human immunodeficiency virus; AIDS, acquired immunodeficiency syndrome; HOMA-IR, homeostatic model assessment of insulin resistance; LDL, low density lipoprotein.

3.2. Profile of HIV Infection

The median duration of diagnosed HIV infection was five years (25th–75th percentiles: 2–9) with no difference by gender ($p = 0.223$). The median CD4 count was 392 cells/mm^3 (25th–75th percentiles:

240–604) with higher levels in women than in men (410 cells/mm^3 *vs.* 272 cells/mm^3, $p = 0.002$). Most participants were receiving ART (93.4%) with the majority on first line ART (63.9%), while 11.8% received second line ART and 17.4% were on other ART regimens. Interestingly, there were significant differences in the distribution by gender ($p = 0.005$).

3.3. *Profile of Cardio-Metabolic Abnormalities*

The mean BMI was 26.3 kg/m^2 overall with significantly lower levels in men compared with women (21.4 kg/m^2 *vs.* 28.3 kg/m^2, $p < 0.001$). Overall, 43.4% of participants had normal BMI levels while 22.9% were overweight and 33.7% obese with significant differences by gender ($p < 0.001$). Women compared to men had larger WCs (90 cm *vs.* 79 cm, $p < 0.001$), higher HOMA-IR indices (1.49 *vs.* 0.94, $p < 0.001$), and total cholesterol levels (4.4 *vs.* 4.2 mmol/L, $p = 0.009$). However, they had lower levels of triglycerides (0.97 *vs.* 1.12 mmol/L, $p = 0.023$), fasting glucose (4.9 *vs.* 5.1 mmol/L, $p = 0.010$) and systolic BP (115 *vs.* 124 mmHg, $p < 0.001$). Furthermore, HDL-cholesterol levels (1.29 *vs.* 1.2 mmol/L, $p = 0.010$) and prevalent treated hypertension (16.8% *vs.* 7.0%, $p = 0.002$) were higher in women than men. Diastolic BP, hs-CRP, as well as prevalent treated diabetes were similar in both genders (all $p \geqslant 0.129$) (Table 1).

3.4. *Distribution of Body Size Phenotypes*

The proportion of $\geqslant$2 metabolic abnormalities across normal-weight (27.1%), overweight (41.5%), and obese (44.8%) categories increased significantly in a linear trend (p-trend = 0.001). The distribution of body size phenotypes in the overall sample was 31.7% (NWMH), 11.7% (NWMA), 13.4% (OvMH), 9.5% (OvMA), 18.6% (OMH), and 15.1% (OMA), Figure 1.

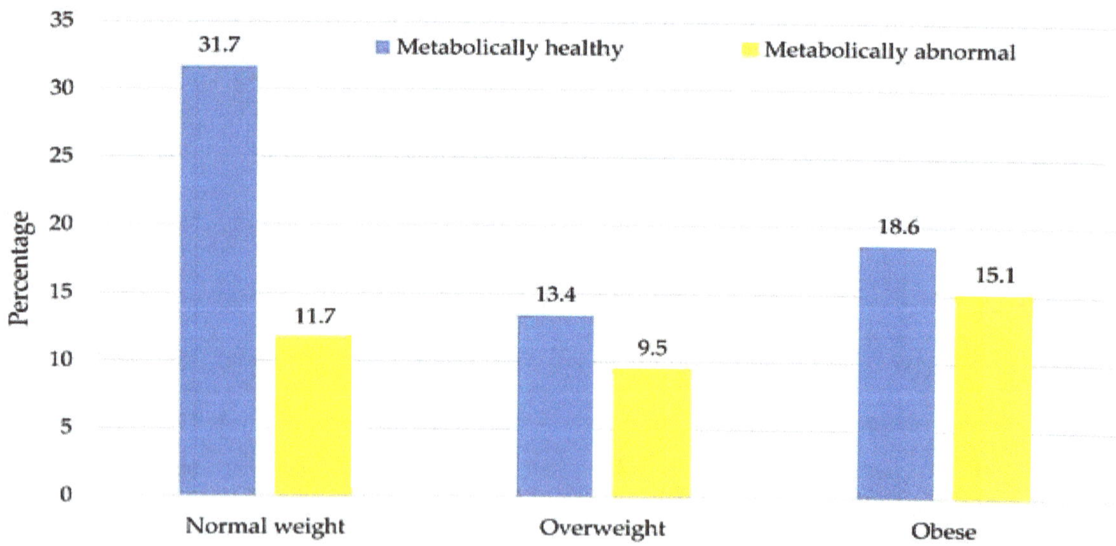

Figure 1. Distribution of metabolic phenotypes across body mass index categories. Each vertical bar represents the proportion of participants in the total sample with the corresponding combination of body size (normal-weight, overweight, or obese) and metabolic phenotype (healthy or abnormal). The accompanying proportions are shown at the tip of each bar.

In men, the majority (54.1%) were NWMH, just over a quarter (26.1%) were NWMA, while few fell into the other categories: 6.4% (OvMH), 7% (OvMA), 0.7% (OMH), and 5.7% (OMA). In contrast, the distribution in women was as follows: 25.7% (NWMH), 8% (NWMA), 15.2% (OvMH), 10.1% (OvMA), 23.4% (OMH), and 17.6% (OMA) (Figure 2). There was no statistically significant interaction by gender in the distribution of body size phenotypes (p-interaction = 0.062).

The distribution of metabolic phenotypes across BMI categories was not significantly different by longer or shorter duration of diagnosed HIV infection (median five years, p-interaction = 0.897)

(Figure 3a), higher or lower CD4 count (median 392 cells/mm^3, p-interaction = 0.447) (Figure 3b) or across the three ART regimens (p-interaction = 0.205) (Figure 3c). The proportion of ⩾2 metabolic abnormalities tended to increase significantly and linearly across BMI categories within most of the latter subgroups except for lower CD4 count and the second line ART regimen.

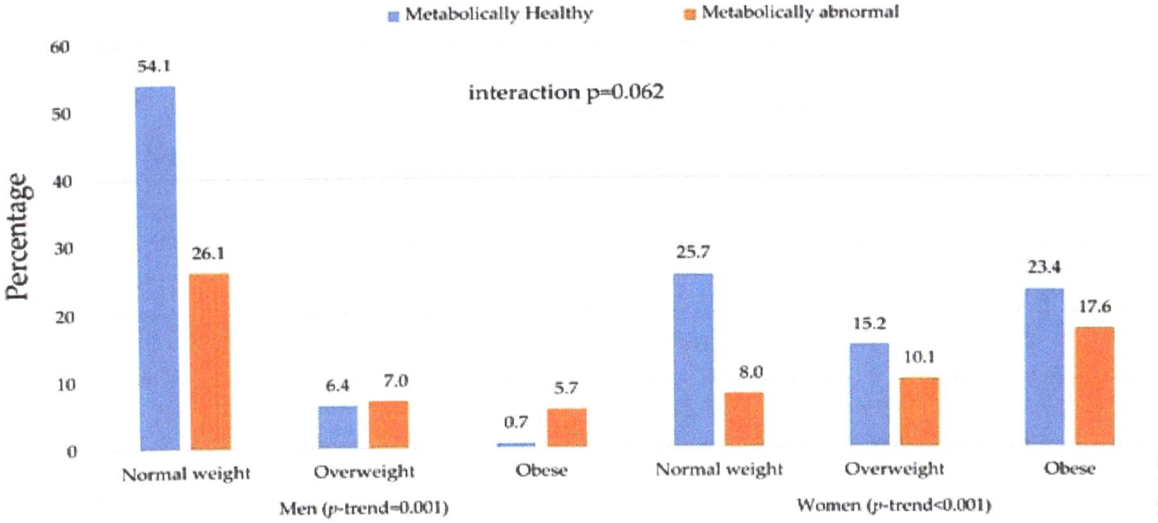

Figure 2. Distribution of metabolic phenotypes across body mass index categories in men and women. Each vertical bar represents the proportion of participants in the total gender-specific sub-sample with the corresponding combination of body size (normal-weight, overweight, or obese) and metabolic phenotype (healthy or abnormal). The accompanying gender-specific proportions are shown at the tip of each bar. The p-value for the interaction by gender in the distribution are shown, together with the p-value for le linear trend (p-trend) in the distribution of metabolic phenotypes across body mass index categories, seperately in men and women.

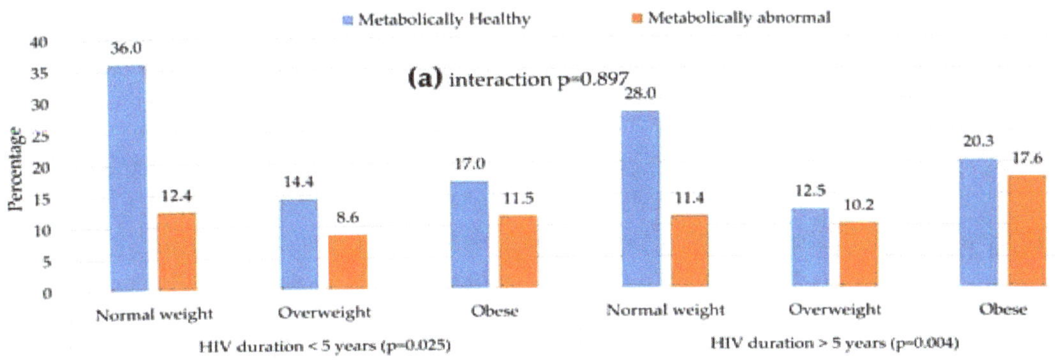

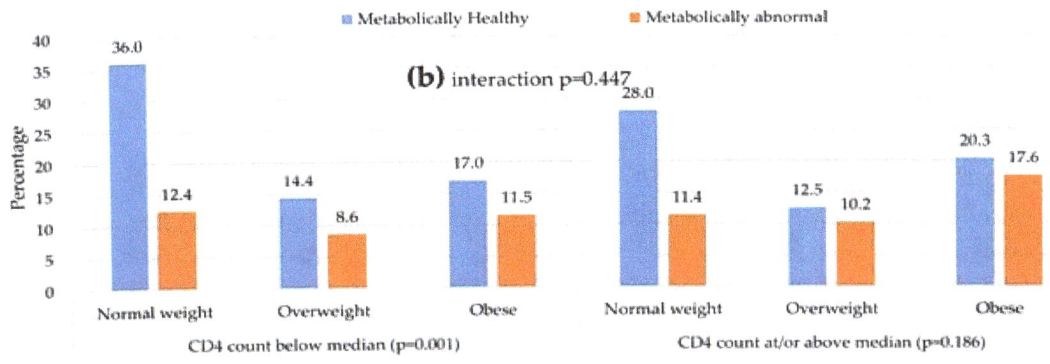

Figure 3. *Cont.*

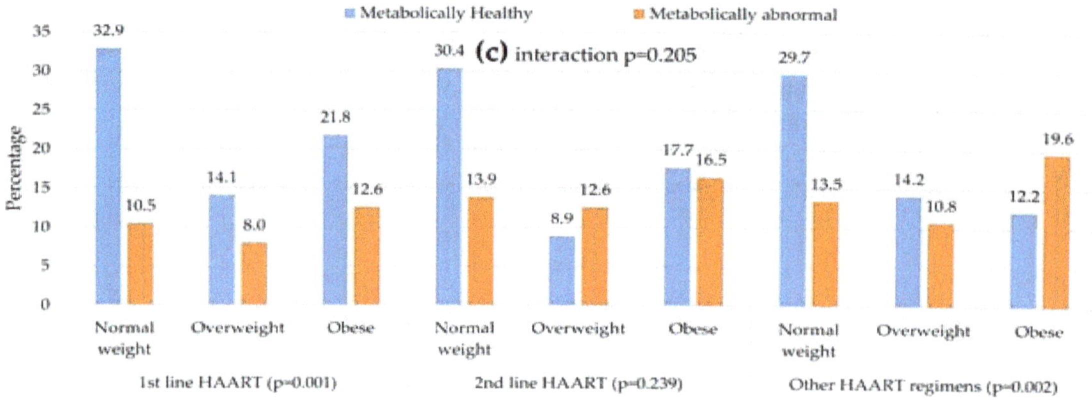

Figure 3. Distribution of body size phenotypes by major HIV predictive characteristics: (**a**) Distribution of metabolic phenotype across body mass index categories in participants below, and those at or above the median of diagnosed duration of HIV infection; (**b**) Distribution of metabolic phenotype across body mass index categories in participants below, and those at or above the median CD4 count; (**c**) Distribution of metabolic phenotype across body mass index categories in participants on different antiretroviral treatment regimens. For each figure panel, the *p*-values for the interactionb (interaction *p*) in the distribution across complementary subgroups are, together with the *p*-value for linear trend in the distribution of metabolic phenotype across body mass index categories within each subgroup (*p*-value attached to the name of the subgroup). Each vertical bar represents the proportion of participants in the subgroup specific sample with the corresponding combination of body size (normal-weight, overweight, or obese) and metabolic phenotype (healthy or abnormal). The accompanying proportions are shown at the tip of each bar.

3.5. Distribution of Metabolic Phenotypes within and Across BMI Categories

Within BMI categories, in addition to the expected differences in the levels of cardio-metabolic risk factors, participants with metabolically abnormal phenotypes tended to be older (all $p \leqslant 0.001$) and unemployed, although differences were significant only among normal weight and overweight (all $p \leqslant 0.002$), but not among obese participants (both $p \geqslant 0.215$). Furthermore, metabolically abnormal obese participants were likely to be men (8.0% *vs.* 0.7%, $p = 0.006$) and included fewer participants on first line ART ($p = 0.009$).

Age and level of education across BMI categories increased linearly overall (both $p \leqslant 0.012$), driven by a significant linear trend in metabolically healthy participants (both $p \leqslant 0.005$) but not in the metabolically abnormal (both $p \geqslant 0.396$), with however no evidence of statistical interaction (both *p*-interaction $\geqslant 0.065$). The proportion of men who were current smokers decreased linearly overall across increasing BMI categories ($p < 0.001$ for linear trend), and within both metabolic phenotype groups (*p*-trend = 0.001), with no evidence of statistical interaction (both interactions $p > 0.759$), Table 2.

Median WC, HOMA-IR, and HDL-C levels across BMI categories increased significantly overall (*p*-trend $\leqslant 0.001$) and within the metabolic phenotype groups (all *p*-trend $\leqslant 0.024$), without evidence of statistical interaction (all *p*-interaction $\geqslant 0.560$). Fasting glucose, triglycerides, and prevalence of hypertension also increase across increasing BMI categories, but only on the total cohort (*p*-trend $\leqslant 0.038$). Interaction analyses found BMI categories and metabolic status interacted to affect the distribution of fasting glucose (*p*-interaction = 0.044) whereas metabolic status interacted with gender to influence triglycerides distributions across BMI categories (*p*-interaction = 0.002).

Moreover, when further analyses in the subgroup of participants with data on insulin level (n = 711) that included insulin resistance (HOMA-IR in 90th) as a fifth metabolic abnormality. The prevalence $\geqslant$2 risk factors was found to increase slightly across BMI categories: NWMA (12.8%), OvMA (9.3%), and OMA (16.6%), but the patterns within and across subgroups were mostly similar (Figure 4).

Table 2. Characteristics of participants across body mass index (BMI) categories and metabolic status [*n* (%), or median (25th–75th percentiles)].

BMI Categories	Normal Weight (n = 325)			Overweight (n = 171)			Obese (n = 252)			*p*-Trend			*p*-Interaction	
Metabolic Status	**Healthy**	**Abnormal**	***p***	**Healthy**	**Abnormal**	***p***	**Healthy**	**Abnormal**	***p***	**Overall**	**Healthy**	**Abnormal**	**B × M**	**M × G**
Prevalence, *n* (%)	237 (31.7)	88 (11.7)		100 (13.4)	71 (9.5)		139 (18.6)	113 (15.1)		<0.001	-	-	-	-
Men, *n* (%)	85 (35.9)	41 (46.6)	0.078	10 (10.0)	11 (15.5)	0.281	1 (0.7)	9 (8.0)	0.006	<0.001	<0.001	<0.001	0.759	-
Age, years	36 (30–44)	42 (34–49)	<0.001	36 (31–42)	43 (36–47.5)	<0.001	37 (31.5–41)	39 (34–47)	0.001	0.002	<0.001	0.396	0.065	0.34
≥7 school-years, *n* (%)	190/236 (80.5)	71/88 (80.7)	0.972	89/100 (89.0)	58/70 (82.9)	0.249	128/139 (92.1)	97/113 (85.8)	0.111	0.012	0.005	0.617	0.532	0.067
Unemployed, *n* (%)	84/236 (35.6)	48/88 (54.5)	0.002	38/100 (38.0)	47/71 (66.2)	<0.001	64/139 (46.0)	58/113 (51.3)	0.404	0.081	0.131	0.132	0.056	0.061
Smoking habit, *n* (%)			0.523			0.327			0.144	<0.001	<0.001	<0.001	0.925	0.238
Never	105/230 (45.7)	33/85 (38.8)		78/96 (81.3)	49/68 (72.0)		111/132 (84.1)	85/107 (79.4)						
Current smoker	99/230 (43.0)	40/85 (47.1)		12/96 (12.5)	11/68 (16.2)		15/132 (11.4)	10/107 (9.3)						
Past smokers	26/230 (11.3)	12/85 (14.1)		6/96 (6.2)	8/68 (11.8)		6/132 (4.5)	12/107 (11.2)						
Heavy drinkers, *n* (%)	26/74 (35.1)	8/27 (29.6)	0.643	7/25 (28.0)	8/19 (42.1)	0.356	7/22 (31.8)	8/20 (40.0)	0.748	0.973	0.801	0.638	0.518	0.766
HIV diagnosed duration, years	4 (2–7.8)	5 (2–8)	0.577	4.3 (2–8)	6 (2–9)	0.149	5 (3–10)	6 (4–10)	0.334	0.413	0.435	0.436	0.820	>0.999
Median CD4 count, /mm^3	311 (172–473)	350 (232–544)	0.288	433 (187–630)	395 (252–626)	0.494	452 (297–677)	434 (267–699)	0.627	0.335	0.213	0.627	0.77	0.430
Antiretroviral regimens, *n* (%)			0.448			0.201			0.009	0.947	0.386	0.963	0.363	0.179
First line	140/208 (67.3)	45/76 (59.2)		60/88 (68.3)	34/60 (56.6)		93/125 (74.4)	54/96 (56.2)						
Second line	24/208 (11.5)	11/76 (14.5)		7/88 (8.0)	10/60 (16.7)		14/125 (11.2)	13/96 (13.5)						
Others	44/208 (21.2)	20/76 (26.3)		21/88 (23.7)	16/60 (26.7)		18/125 (14.4)	29/96 (30.2)						
Waist circumference, cm	77 (72–80)	78 (72–86)	0.016	89 (85–92)	93 (86–95)	0.005	101 (95–108)	104 (99–111)	0.005	<0.001	<0.001	0.016	0.560	0.780
Systolic blood pressure, mmHg	114 (105–125)	128 (116–145)	<0.001	112 (104–124)	125 (117–140)	<0.001	113 (106–119)	124 (114–138)	<0.001	0.230	0.136	0.560	0.620	0.610
Diastolic blood pressure, mmHg	78 (72–85)	88 (81–92)	<0.001	81 (73–85)	88 (82–97)	<0.001	81 (75–85)	88 (80–96)	<0.001	0.954	0.771	0.819	0.230	0.510
Fasting glucose, mmol/L	4.9 (4.6–5.2)	5.3 (4.8–6.3)	<0.001	4.9 (4.6–5.2)	5.2 (4.7–5.7)	0.001	4.9 (4.6–5.2)	5.6 (5.0–6.4)	<0.001	0.010	0.583	0.049	0.044	0.510
Median HOMA-IR	0.85 (0.57–1.27)	1.16 (0.82–1.79)	<0.001	1.31 (0.931.81)	1.76 (1.05–2.49)	0.003	1.9 (1.33–2.44)	2.52 (1.54–4.67)	<0.001	<0.001	0.001	0.006	0.630	0.290
Diabetes [a], *n* (%)	2/227 (0.9)	21/87 (24.1)	<0.001	1/96 (1.0)	10/68 (14.7)	0.001	2/128 (1.6)	27/110 (24.6)	<0.001	0.077	0.839	0.252	0.148	0.752
Hypertension [b], *n* (%)	52 (21.9)	50 (56.8)	<0.001	20 (20.0)	43 (60.6)	<0.001	35 (25.2)	70 (62.0)	<0.001	0.038	0.615	0.757	0.841	0.107

Table 2. *Cont.*

BMI Categories	Normal Weight (n = 325)			Overweight (n = 171)			Obese (n = 252)			*p*-Trend			*p*-Interaction	
Metabolic Status	**Healthy**	**Abnormal**	***p***	**Healthy**	**Abnormal**	***p***	**Healthy**	**Abnormal**	***p***	**Overall**	**Healthy**	**Abnormal**	**B × M**	**M × G**
Triglycerides, mmol/L	0.9 (0.7–1.2)	1.2 (1.0–1.9)	<0.001	0.9 (0.7–1.2)	1.2 (1.0–1.9)	<0.001	0.9 (0.7–1.2)	1.4 (1.0–1.9)	<0.001	0.033	0.647	0.472	0.720	0.002
HDL-cholesterol, mmol/L	1.4 (1.1–1.7)	1.2 (0.9–1.3)	<0.001	1.4 (1.2–1.7)	1.1 (1.0–1.2)	<0.001	1.4 (1.2–1.6)	1.1 (1.0–1.2)	<0.001	0.001	0.021	0.024	0.790	0.640
LDL-cholesterol, mmol/L	2.2 (1.8–2.9)	2.5 (1.9–3.1)	0.181	2.4 (2.0–3.0)	2.5 (2.0–3.3)	0.423	2.6 (2.2–3.1)	2.8 (2.3–3.4)	0.019	0.867	0.769	0.713	0.910	0.330
Total cholesterol, mmol/l	4.2 (3.6–5.0)	4.2 (3.5–4.9)	0.483	4.3 (3.7–5.1)	4.2 (3.6–4.9)	0.665	4.5 (3.9–5.1)	4.5 (4.0–5.2)	0.208	0.126	0.350	0.438	>0.999	0.710
C-reactive protein, mg/L	4.2 (1.5–12.1)	5.2 (2.5–16.1)	0.102	4.4 (2.3–10.4)	4.4 (2.0–8.5)	0.959	7.8 (3.5–15.8)	8.0 (3.8–16.6)	0.590	0.803	0.523	0.236	0.770	0.130

[a] Diabetes as FPG ⩾ 7.0 mmol/L or on treatment; [b] hypertension as blood pressure (BP) ⩾ 140/90 mmHg or on treatment.

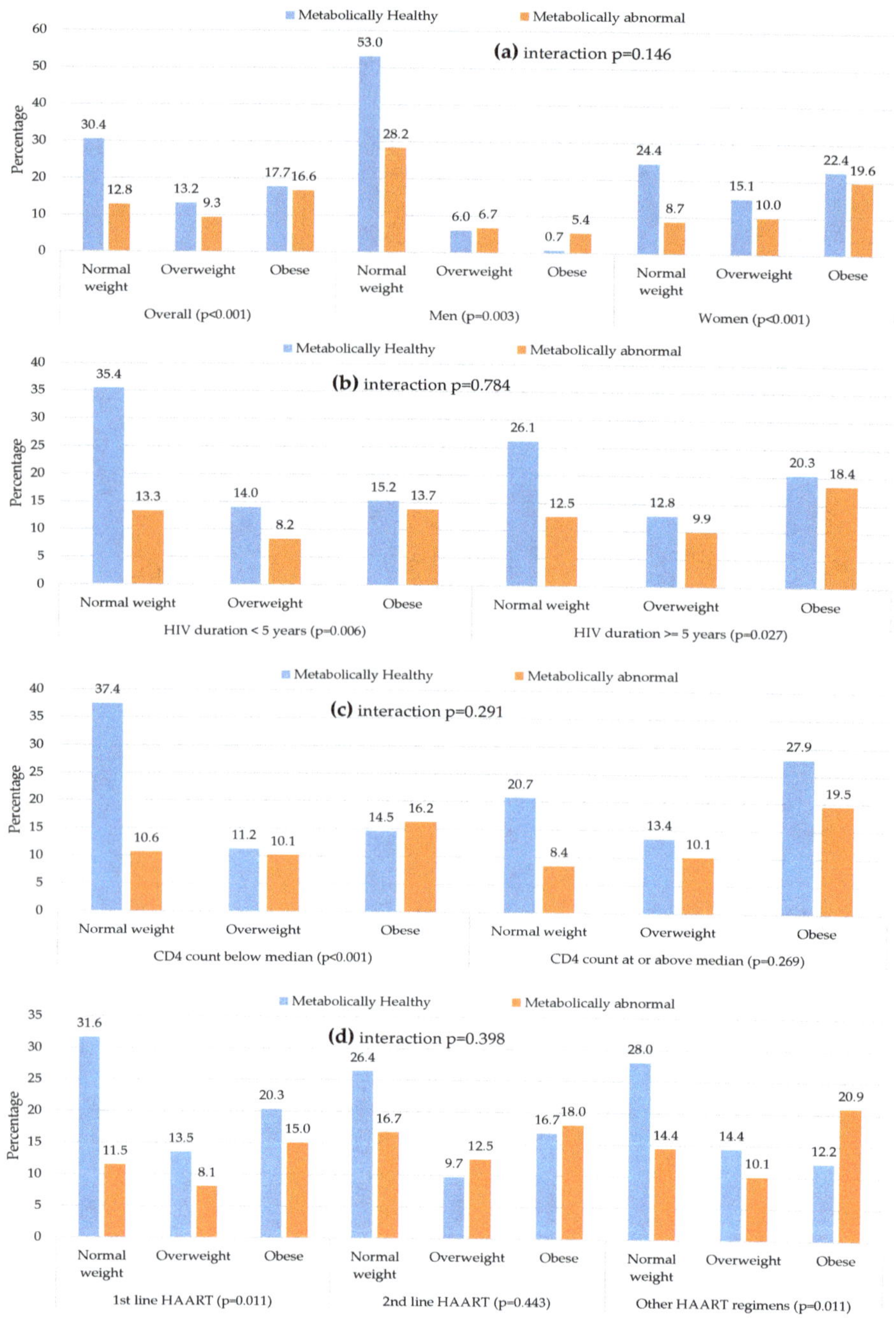

Figure 4. Distribution of metabolic phenotypes across body mass index by major characteristics: (**a**) Overall and in men and women; (**b**) in participants below, and those at or above the median of diagnosed duration of HIV infection; (**c**) in participants below and those at or above the median CD4 count; (**d**) in participants on different antiretroviral treatment regimens. Metabollically abnormal phenotype is based on the presence of any two of the following five abnormalities: elevated blood pressure or known hypertension; high triglycerides; low HDL-cholesterol, high blood glucose, or known diabetes; insulin resistance. For each figure panel, the *p*-values for the interaction (interaction *p*) in the distribution across complementary subgroups are, together with the *p*-value for linear trend in the distribution of metabolic phenotype across body mass index categories within each subgroup (*p*-value attached to the name of the subgroup). Each vertical bar represents the proportion of participants in the subgroup specific sample with the corresponding combination of body size (normal-weight, overweight, or obese) and metabolic phenotype (healthy or abnormal). The accompanying proportions are shown at the tip of each bar.

3.6. Prediction of Body Mass Index Categories by the Continuous Metabolic Traits

In multinomial logistic regression models, mutually adjusted for each other and using normal weight as a reference, male sex was associated with 81% (95% confidence interval: 68%–89%) lower odds of overweight and 94% (89%–97%) lower odds of obesity; while each year of older age was associated with 2% (0%–4%) higher odds of overweight and a non-significant 1% (−1% to 4%) higher odds of obesity. The McFadden R^2 for the overall performance of this basic model was 0.081. In the presence of age and sex, all metabolic trait with the exception of systolic blood pressure (for both overweight and obesity) and fasting plasma glucose (for overweight only) were significantly associated with odds of overweight and obesity (Table 3). The direction of the effect with increasing metabolic traits levels was always positive, except for HDL-cholesterol where increasing levels were associated with decreasing odds of overweight and obesity. The highest R^2 for the overall performance of resulting models was recorded for the model containing HOMA-IR (R^2 = 0.183); and ranged from 0.083 (for the model containing systolic blood pressure) to 0.103 (for the model containing either triglycerides or HDL-cholesterol), Table 3.

Table 3. Odds ratios (OR) and 95% confidence intervals (95% CI) from multinomial age and sex adjusted multinomial logistic regression models, showing the association of metabolic traits with body mass index categories.

Predictors	Normal Weight	Overweight		Obese		R^2
	Reference	OR (95% CI)	p-Value	OR (95% CI)	p-Value	
Age, per year	1.00	1.02 (1.00–1.04)	0.093	1.01 (0.99–1.04)	0.195	0.081
Sex, men	1.00	0.19 (0.11–0.32)	<0.001	0.06 (0.03–0.11)	<0.001	
Systolic blood pressure, per mmHg	1.00	1.01 (1.00–1.02)	0.204	1.01 (1.00–1.02)	0.167	0.083
Diastolic blood pressure, per mmHg	1.00	1.02 (1.00–1.04)	0.012	1.02 (1.01–1.04)	0.005	0.087
Triglycerides, per mmol/L	1.00	2.06 (1.41–3.02)	<0.001	2.70 (1.86–3.92)	<0.001	0.102
HDL-Cholesterol, per mmol/L	1.00	0.40 (0.24–0.66)	<0.001	0.27 (0.16–0.44)	<0.001	0.102
LDL-cholesterol, per mmol/L	1.00	1.15 (0.92–1.45)	<0.001	1.56 (1.26–1.93)	<0.001	0.092
Fasting plasma glucose, per mmol/L	1.00	0.93 (0.79–1.10)	0.417	1.18 (1.04–1.32)	0.007	0.090
HOMA-IR	1.00	1.42 (1.19–1.70)	<0.001	1.77 (1.49–2.10)	<0.001	0.183

R^2 is the McFadden pseudo-R^2 for the overall performance of the model containing age, sex, and the metabolic trait of interest.

4. Discussion

Although there have been rigorous reports on fat distribution and obesity in individuals with HIV infection, to our knowledge, this is one of the first studies to document the distribution of cardio-metabolic abnormalities in relation with body size in an HIV-infected population. Metabolically abnormal phenotypes, defined as the presence of ⩾2 cardio-metabolic risk factors, were high across all BMI categories. Even in normal weight participants, over a quarter (27.1%) had metabolically abnormal phenotypes with this rising to 41.5% and 44.8% in the overweight and the obese, respectively. This suggests the likely influence of multiple factors in the development of cardio-metabolic abnormalities in this population. The high prevalence in normal weight HIV-infected individuals suggests the possible contribution of HIV-related factors and underscores the need to examine for cardio-metabolic abnormalities even in the absence of overweight and obesity.

In contrast, the much higher prevalence demonstrated with increasing adiposity may be attributable to the greater role of this conventional risk factor in the development of cardio-metabolic abnormalities in the HIV-infected population. This highlights the fine balance that needs to be maintained between ensuring adequate nutrition and optimal weight in the HIV-infected while simultaneously monitoring and guarding against excess weight gain. Thus, there is a need for holistic management of these co-morbidities that may indirectly be associated with HIV infection.

The prevalence of overweight and obesity, at 13.4% and 6.4% in men and 25.4% and 40.9% in women in this study approximated the adiposity distribution reported in South African National Health and Nutrition Survey (SANHANES-1) [22]. The overweight and obesity rates in the SANHANES-1 were 20.1% (95% CI: 13.7–26.4) and 11.6% (95% CI: 7.5–15.7) in men and 26.4% (95% CI: 21.7–31.0) and 44.8% (95% CI: 38.8–50.8) in women, respectively. Similar findings have been reported in the United States where obesity levels in HIV-infected men (19%) and women (42%) were comparable to the general population (men: 24.7%, women: 37%) [17]. It is thus important to assess adiposity in HIV-infected individuals and to implement appropriate management strategies for weight reduction, similar to general populations. Notably, that the distribution of overweight and obesity in this study mirrors that of the general population in the country is testimony of the successful implementation of ART strategies in this community.

Although the prevalence of the metabolically abnormal phenotypes by the BMI categories described in this study were significant at 11.7% (NWMA), 9.5% (OvMA), and 15.1% (OMA), a substantial proportion of participants were obese but metabolically healthy (18.6%). This agrees with the 6%–75% estimate of OMH in general populations globally and is likely because BMI is a proxy marker of cardiovascular risk. BMI measures general fat distribution and not visceral adipose tissue specifically, which is linked closely to insulin resistance and cardio-metabolic abnormalities. A better proxy for visceral adipose tissue is WC and, unsurprisingly, within BMI categories, participants with compared to without metabolic abnormalities had greater WC and elevated HOMA-IR index, a proxy measure of insulin resistance. Similar findings have also been reported in other studies [20,23–25]. Recent studies in Caucasians that have included insulin resistance among abnormal metabolic traits, have reported high prevalence of metabolically abnormal phenotypes both in obese and non-obese people [26,27].

The distribution of body size phenotypes in our study is comparable with results of local studies conducted in the general population in South Africa [24,28]. Our previous community-based study in mixed-ancestry adults in Cape Town applying the same definition criteria found OMH and NWMA to be present respectively 16.5% and 5% of the sample [24]. Furthermore, among normal-weight participants (17.1% of the sample), 29.1% were classified as metabolically abnormal, while among obese participants (53.7% of the sample), 30.8% were classified as metabolically healthy [24]. In another study in 103 normal-weight and 122 obese premenopausal urban black South African women, Jennings and co-workers found that 22% of the normal-weight participants were metabolically abnormal (defined by the presence of insulin resistance), while 38% of obese women were metabolically healthy (*i.e.*, did not have insulin resistance) [28]. There are no recent reports available from Africa for comparison of the metabolically abnormal phenotypes that include insulin resistance. Nevertheless, data from a study conducted almost two decades ago in Cameroon revealed a much lower prevalence of metabolic abnormalities with 1.4% (NWMA), 1.6% (OvMA), and 1.7% (OMA) [23]. This highlights the epidemiological transition under way in Sub-Saharan Africa with the majority of this study's participants having normal weight (61%) in the year 1994, unlike more recent reports, and the expected lower prevalence of cardio-metabolic risk factors compared with the present study [23]. Interestingly, there was no significant difference in the distribution of metabolic abnormalities across BMI groups by duration of diagnosed HIV infection, CD4 count levels or ART regimens. There have been diverse reports on the effects of HIV-specific factors on body fat de-arrangement, dyslipidemia, hyperglycemia, and metabolic syndrome. However, results from a recent systematic review and meta-analysis indicated that HIV-related characteristics had minor, if any, influence on the presence of metabolic syndrome [29]. Nevertheless, longitudinal studies are ideally required to pronounce on the absence or presence, if any, of a relationship between specific HIV-related factors and the development of cardio-metabolic abnormalities by body size phenotype.

The relationship of gender, smoking status, and alcohol consumption on the distribution of body size phenotypes remains inconclusive in studies conducted in general populations [10,30,31]. The findings of this study accorded with reports that showed little or no effect of smoking status and alcohol use on the distribution of body size phenotypes [26]. However, a few studies showed a higher prevalence of OMH in women than in men [26,32].

Limitations and Strengths

The cross-sectional design of this study precludes inferences of causal associations between the variables of interest and the development of cardio-metabolic abnormalities. The inclusion of an HIV-uninfected and HIV-infected ART-naïve comparative groups would have strengthened our analyses. Seeing that this was a clinic-based study limits its generalizability since it did not include HIV-infected individuals not attending healthcare facilities. However, these limitations are inevitable because the present project is part of a broad intervention study, which aims to explore the utilization of HIV-care infrastructure as a gateway to detect, manage, and control non-communicable diseases in HIV-infected populations in Africa. The relatively fewer men compared to women in the study, characteristic of epidemiological studies in the country, might overestimate the prevalence of obesity phenotypes. In the absence of detailed information on dietary habits/food consumption and data on ethnicity, we could not explore possible effects of lifestyle factors and ethnicity on the distribution of body size phenotypes among the participants. Nevertheless, differences in MHO prevalence according to ethnicity have been reported, although this recent meta-analysis did not include any studies based on African cohorts [33]. There are reports indicating that overall dietary intake was not associated with healthy obesity in both Europeans and African Americans [27,34]. In addition to lifestyle and ethnicity, data was not available on the pharmacological compounds included in the ART regimens of the participants as well as the duration of treatment with those compounds, precluding detailed analyses by potency of pharmacological compounds and duration of treatments.

Nonetheless, the inclusion of participants from 17 healthcare facilities, including both urban and rural sites strengthens the representativeness in terms of the characteristics assessed. Furthermore, this study is among the first to describe the high prevalence of metabolically abnormal phenotypes across BMI categories in a relatively young HIV-infected population. The study findings underscore the need for further research, particularly longitudinal studies, to understand the development of cardio-metabolic abnormalities in the local HIV-infected population and the differential role played by conventional risk factors as opposed to HIV-related influences.

5. Conclusions

The high prevalence of metabolically abnormal phenotypes across all BMI categories, notably in a relatively young HIV-infected population, highlights the importance of holistic management in HIV-infected individuals. Ideally, cardio-metabolic assessments/screenings should be done at baseline and at regular intervals thereafter, particularly in high-risk groups. Furthermore, considering the high prevalence of overweight and obesity in the HIV-infected, lifestyle measures for weight reduction need to be encouraged. This is a captive audience who present regularly to healthcare facilities and the opportunity should be used to raise greater awareness on cardiovascular disease prevention. Such a strategy, targeting all HIV-infected patients, may contribute to a general improvement in cardiovascular health across the spectrum of BMI distribution. If proven successful, it may possibly have wider applicability in the general population.

Acknowledgments: Grand Challenge Canada, through the Global Alliance on Chronic Diseases initiative. KAN is supported by the NRF Innovation Doctoral Research Scholarship, Doctoral Scholarship, and Yeoman Bequest Bursary through the University of Cape Town. The funding bodies did not make provision for cost of open access publications.

Author Contributions: A.P.K., E.J.M., and B.M. conceived the study and acquired the funding. A.d.V. operationalized and supervised data collection in collaboration with T.E.M. and K.A.N., N.P. analyzed the data and drafted the manuscript. All co-authors substantially revised the manuscript and approved the submission.

Abbreviations

The following abbreviations are used in this manuscript:

ANOVA	analysis of variance
ART	antiretroviral therapy
AIDS	acquired immunodeficiency syndrome
BMI	body mass index
B × M	interaction between BMI and metabolic status
BP	blood pressure
CVD	cardiovascular disease
DBP	diastolic blood pressure
FPG	fasting plasma glucose
HDL-C	high density lipoprotein cholesterol
HIV	human immunodeficiency virus
HOMA-IR	homeostatic model assessment of insulin resistance
Hs-CRP	high sensitivity-C reactive protein
LDL-C	low density lipoprotein cholesterol
M × G	interaction between metabolic status and gender
NWMH	normal-weight metabolically healthy
NWMA	normal weight metabolically abnormal
OvMH	overweight metabolically healthy
OvMA	overweight metabolically abnormal
OMH	obese metabolically healthy
OMA	obese metabolically abnormal
PDA	personal digital assistant
SBP	systolic blood pressure
SD	standard deviation
T2DM	type 2 diabetes mellitus
WC	waist circumference

References

1. Murray, C.J.; Ortblad, K.F.; Guinovart, C.; Lim, S.S.; Wolock, T.M.; Roberts, D.A.; Dansereau, E.A.; Graetz, N.; Barber, R.M.; Brown, J.C.; *et al.* Global, regional, and national incidence and mortality for HIV, tuberculosis, and malaria during 1990–2013: A systematic analysis for the global burden of disease study 2013. *Lancet* **2014**, *384*, 1005–1070. [CrossRef]
2. World Health Organisation. Millennium Development Goals (mdgs) 6: Combat HIV/AIDS, Malaria and Other Diseases. Available online: http://www.who.int/topics/millennium_development_goals/diseases/en/ (accessed on 21 March 2016).
3. Samji, H.; Cescon, A.; Hogg, R.S.; Modur, S.P.; Althoff, K.N.; Buchacz, K.; Burchell, A.N.; Cohen, M.; Gebo, K.A.; Gill, M.J.; *et al.* Closing the gap: Increases in life expectancy among treated HIV-positive individuals in the United States and Canada. *PLoS ONE* **2013**, *8*, e81355. [CrossRef] [PubMed]
4. Boodram, B.; Plankey, M.W.; Cox, C.; Tien, P.C.; Cohen, M.H.; Anastos, K.; Karim, R.; Hyman, C.; Hershow, R.C. Prevalence and correlates of elevated body mass index among HIV-positive and HIV-negative women in the women's interagency HIV study. *AIDS Patient Care STDS* **2009**, *23*, 1009–1016. [CrossRef] [PubMed]
5. Crum-Cianflone, N.; Roediger, M.P.; Eberly, L.; Headd, M.; Marconi, V.; Ganesan, A.; Weintrob, A.; Barthel, R.V.; Fraser, S.; Agan, B.K. Increasing rates of obesity among HIV-infected persons during the HIV epidemic. *PLoS ONE* **2010**, *5*, e10106. [CrossRef] [PubMed]
6. Weber, R.; Ruppik, M.; Rickenbach, M.; Spoerri, A.; Furrer, H.; Battegay, M.; Cavassini, M.; Calmy, A.; Bernasconi, E.; Schmid, P.; *et al.* Decreasing mortality and changing patterns of causes of death in the swiss HIV cohort study. *HIV Med.* **2013**, *14*, 195–207. [CrossRef] [PubMed]

7. Palella, F.J., Jr.; Baker, R.K.; Moorman, A.C.; Chmiel, J.S.; Wood, K.C.; Brooks, J.T.; Holmberg, S.D. Mortality in the highly active antiretroviral therapy era: Changing causes of death and disease in the HIV outpatient study. *J. Acquir. Immune Defic. Syndr.* **2006**, *43*, 27–34. [CrossRef] [PubMed]
8. World Health Organisation. *Global Status Report on Noncommunicable Diseases 2014*; WHO: Geneva, Switzerland, 2014; p. 298.
9. Cornier, M.A. The metabolic syndrome. *Endocr. Rev.* **2008**, *29*, 777–822. [CrossRef] [PubMed]
10. Wildman, R.P.; Muntner, P.; Reynolds, K.; McGinn, A.P.; Rajpathak, S.; Wylie-Rosett, J.; Sowers, M.R. The obese without cardiometabolic risk factor clustering and the normal weight with cardiometabolic risk factor clustering: Prevalence and correlates of 2 phenotypes among the US population (NHANES 1999–2004). *Arch. Intern. Med.* **2008**, *168*, 1617–1624. [CrossRef] [PubMed]
11. Van Wijk, J.P.H.; Cabezas, M.C. Hypertriglyceridemia, metabolic syndrome, and cardiovascular disease in HIV-infected patients: Effects of antiretroviral therapy and adipose tissue distribution. *Int. J. Vasc. Med.* **2012**, *2012*. [CrossRef] [PubMed]
12. Giralt, M.; Domingo, P.; Guallar, J.P.; de la Concepcion, M.L.R.; Alegre, M.; Domingo, J.C.; Villarroya, F. HIV-1 infection alters gene expression in adipose tissue, which contributes to HIV-1/haart-associated lipodystrophy. *Antivir. Ther.* **2006**, *11*, 729–740. [PubMed]
13. Grinspoon, S.; Carr, A. Cardiovascular risk and body-fat abnormalities in HIV-infected adults. *N. Engl. J. Med.* **2005**, *352*, 48–62. [CrossRef] [PubMed]
14. Anuurad, E.; Bremer, A.; Berglund, L. HIV protease inhibitors and obesity. *Curr. Opin. Endocrinol. Diabetes Obes.* **2010**, *17*, 478–485. [CrossRef] [PubMed]
15. Worm, S.W.; Lundgren, J.D. The metabolic syndrome in HIV. *Best Pract. Res. Clin. Endocrinol. Metab.* **2011**, *25*, 479–486. [CrossRef] [PubMed]
16. Stanley, T.L.; Grinspoon, S.K. Body composition and metabolic changes in HIV-infected patients. *J. Infect. Dis.* **2012**, *205*, S383–S390. [CrossRef] [PubMed]
17. Thompson-Paul, A.M.; Wei, S.C.; Mattson, C.L.; Robertson, M.; Hernandez-Romieu, A.C.; Bell, T.K.; Skarbinski, J. Obesity among HIV-infected adults receiving medical care in the United States: Data from the cross-sectional medical monitoring project and national health and nutrition examination survey. *Medicine* **2015**, *94*. [CrossRef] [PubMed]
18. Matthews, D.R.; Hosker, J.P.; Rudenski, A.S.; Naylor, B.A.; Treacher, D.F.; Turner, R.C. Homeostasis model assessment: Insulin resistance and beta-cell function from fasting plasma glucose and insulin concentrations in man. *Diabetologia* **1985**, *28*, 412–419. [CrossRef] [PubMed]
19. South African National Department of Health. *National Consolidated Guidelines for the Prevention of Mother-to-Child Transmission of HIV (Pmtct) and the Management of HIV in Children, Adolescents and Adults*; National Department of Health of Republic of South Africa: Pretoria, South Africa, 2015.
20. Rey-Lopez, J.P.; de Rezende, L.F.; Pastor-Valero, M.; Tess, B.H. The prevalence of metabolically healthy obesity: A systematic review and critical evaluation of the definitions used. *Obes. Rev.* **2014**, *15*, 781–790. [CrossRef] [PubMed]
21. McFadden, D.L. Conditional logit analysis of qualitative choice behavior. In *Frontiers in Econometrics*; Zarembka, P., Ed.; Academic Press: New York, NY, USA, 1973; pp. 105–142.
22. Shisana, O.; Labadarios, D.; Rehle, T.; Simbayi, L. *South African National Health and Nutrition Examination Survey (Sanhanes-1)*; Human Science Research Council (HSRC) Press: Cape Town, South Africa, 2013.
23. Mbanya, V.N.; Echouffo-Tcheugui, J.B.; Akhtar, H.; Mbanya, J.C.; Kengne, A.P. Obesity phenotypes in urban and rural cameroonians: A cross-sectional study. *Diabetol. Metab. Syndr.* **2015**, *7*, 21. [CrossRef] [PubMed]
24. Matsha, T.E.; Hartnick, M.D.; Kisten, Y.; Eramus, R.T.; Kengne, A.P. Obesity phenotypes and subclinical cardiovascular diseases in a mixed-ancestry South African population: A cross-sectional study. *J. Diabetes* **2014**, *6*, 267–270. [CrossRef] [PubMed]
25. Beraldo, R.A.; Meliscki, G.C.; Silva, B.R.; Navarro, A.M.; Bollela, V.R.; Schmidt, A.; Foss-Freitas, M.C. Comparing the ability of anthropometric indicators in identifying metabolic syndrome in HIV patients. *PLoS ONE* **2016**, *11*, e0149905. [CrossRef] [PubMed]
26. Velho, S.; Paccaud, F.; Waeber, G.; Vollenweider, P.; Marques-Vidal, P. Metabolically healthy obesity: Different prevalences using different criteria. *Eur. J. Clin. Nutr.* **2010**, *64*, 1043–1051. [CrossRef] [PubMed]

27. Phillips, C.M.; Dillon, C.; Harrington, J.M.; McCarthy, V.J.; Kearney, P.M.; Fitzgerald, A.P.; Perry, I.J. Defining metabolically healthy obesity: Role of dietary and lifestyle factors. *PLoS ONE* **2013**, *8*, e76188. [CrossRef] [PubMed]
28. Jennings, C.L.; Lambert, E.V.; Collins, M.; Joffe, Y.; Levitt, N.S.; Goedecke, J.H. Determinants of insulin-resistant phenotypes in normal-weight and obese black african women. *Obesity* **2008**, *16*, 1602–1609. [CrossRef] [PubMed]
29. Nguyen, K.A.; Peer, N.; Mills, E.J.; Kengne, A.P. A meta-analysis of the metabolic syndrome prevalence in the global HIV-infected population. *PLoS ONE* **2016**, *11*, e0150970. [CrossRef] [PubMed]
30. Lopez-Garcia, E.; Guallar-Castillon, P.; Leon-Muñoz, L.; Rodriguez-Artalejo, F. Prevalence and determinants of metabolically healthy obesity in Spain. *Atherosclerosis* **2013**, *231*, 152–157. [CrossRef] [PubMed]
31. Lee, K. Metabolically obese but normal weight (MONW) and metabolically healthy but obese (MHO) phenotypes in Koreans: Characteristics and health behaviors. *Asia Pac. J. Clin. Nutr.* **2009**, *18*, 280–284. [PubMed]
32. Hirigo, A.T.; Tesfaye, D.Y. Influences of gender in metabolic syndrome and its components among people living with HIV virus using antiretroviral treatment in Hawassa, Southern Ethiopia. *BMC Res. Notes* **2016**, *9*, 145. [CrossRef] [PubMed]
33. Wang, B.; Zhuang, R.; Luo, X.; Yin, L.; Pang, C.; Feng, T.; You, H.; Zhai, Y.; Ren, Y.; Zhang, L.; *et al.* Prevalence of metabolically healthy obese and metabolically obese but normal weight in adults worldwide: A meta-analysis. *Horm. Metab. Res.* **2015**, *47*, 839–845. [CrossRef] [PubMed]
34. Kimokoti, R.W.; Judd, S.E.; Shikany, J.M.; Newby, P.K. Metabolically healthy obesity is not associated with food intake in white or black men. *J. Nutr.* **2015**, *145*, 2551–2561. [CrossRef] [PubMed]

An Investigation of the Clinical Utility of the Proposed ICD-11 and DSM-5 Diagnostic Schemes for Eating Disorders Characterized by Recurrent Binge Eating in People with a High BMI

Marly Amorim Palavras [1,2], Phillipa Hay [2] and Angélica Claudino [1,*]

1 Eating Disorders Program (PROATA), Department of Psychiatry, Universidade Federal de São Paulo (UNIFESP), São Paulo 04017030, Brazil; marlypalavras@gmail.com
2 Translational Health Research Institute, School of Medicine, Western Sydney University, Sydney 2751, Australia; p.hay@westernsydney.edu.au
* Correspondence: amclaudino@gmail.com

Abstract: The aims of this paper were to compare (1) the proportion of participants diagnosed with threshold or subthreshold Bulimia Nervosa (BN) and Binge Eating Disorder (BED) (clinical utility), and (2) the severity of participants' clinical features and mental Health-Related Quality of Life (HRQoL) (convergent validity), when diagnosed according to either the Diagnostic and Statistical Manual of Mental Disorders—5th edition (DSM-5) or the proposed International Classification of Diseases 11th edition (ICD-11) schemes. One hundred and seven adult men and women, with a high Body Mass Index (BMI) were evaluated by interview to confirm their eating disorder diagnoses. All participants completed self-report assessments of current symptoms and mental HRQoL. The majority of participants in either diagnostic scheme were included in the main categories of BN or BED (102/107, 95% in the ICD-11 and 85/107, 79% in the DSM-5). Fewer individuals received a subthreshold other or unspecified diagnosis with the ICD-11 compared to the DSM-5 scheme (5% vs. 21%). No significant differences in demographic, clinical features or mental HRQoL of participants with complete or partial BN or BED were found between diagnostic categories. Compared to the DSM-5, the proposed ICD-11 was not over inclusive, i.e., it did not appear to include people with less severe and potentially less clinically relevant symptoms. These results support the greater clinical utility of the ICD-11 whilst both schemes showed convergent validity.

Keywords: Bulimia Nervosa; binge-eating disorder; Diagnostic and Statistical Manual of Mental Disorders; International Classification of Diseases

---

1. Introduction

Currently two diagnostic classification systems guide the field of mental disorders, the Diagnostic and Statistical Manual of Mental Disorders in its 5th edition (DSM-5) [1] and the International Classification of Diseases, now in its 10th edition (ICD-10) [2]. The 11th edition of the ICD-is in preparation [3,4]. A World Psychiatric Association Global Survey (WPA-WHO) involving 4887 psychiatrists in 44 countries indicated that 79.2% of the sample often or almost always/always used one of these formal classification systems as part of their day-to-day clinical work [5]. The DSM-5, which covers mental health exclusively, is very commonly used in the United States, United Kingdom, Australasia, and in international research. The ICD-10 is more extensive, as it includes all medical diagnoses, and it is the official government classification scheme in the majority of countries worldwide [2,5]. Further, the two schemes differ substantively in their structure, definitions and diagnostic guidelines, particularly concerning disorders characterized by recurrent binge eating such as Binge Eating Disorder (BED) and Bulimia Nervosa (BN) [6,7].

In both schemes, BED is now included as the third major eating disorder after BN and anorexia nervosa (AN). Both systems also became more inclusive aiming to reduce the formerly very high number of cases (around 60%) diagnosed within the residual poorly specified categories. DSM-5 now has two such categories—Other Specified Feeding or Eating Disorder (OSFED) and Unspecified Feeding or Eating Disorder (UFED), respectively. OSFED has five diagnostic groups: (1) atypical anorexia nervosa; (2) BN of low frequency and/or limited duration; (3) BED of low frequency and/or duration; (4) purging disorder; and (5) night eating syndrome. UFED is the residual category with no specific criteria [1]. The proposed ICD-11 guidelines [8,9] have such category—Other Feeding or Eating Disorder (OFED). The proposed OFED is closer to the DSM-5 UFED, in being a more general, nonspecific category of people who fall outside diagnostic criteria for a main eating disorder. The main features of OFED are the inclusion of atypical eating behaviors; symptoms that do not fulfill criteria for other Feeding and Eating Disorder (FED), for another mental and behavioral disorder, for another health condition, or that are not secondary to the use of substance or medication interfering on the central nervous system; symptoms and behaviors that are not sanctioned by cultural aspects; and finally, symptoms that impact on the person's personal, social, or work life.

In the DSM-5 [1] and the provisional ICD-11 guidelines [9], the essential features of binge eating are: (1) frequency of once weekly or more; (2) loss of control over the binge eating episode; and (3) marked distress. ICD-11 differs in the inclusion of subjective binge eating episodes (SBEs), where the amount consumed is normal or small although subjectively considered as large by the individual. This is supported by a large body of research [10–13]. A second point of difference between the DSM-5 and proposed ICD-11 criteria for BN and BED is the duration of binge eating episodes. In the DSM-5 this is at least 3 months for both disorders. In the proposed ICD-11 the recommendation is at least one month for BN and three months for BED except where the binge eating episodes are very frequent and the diagnosis of BED may be made for shorter period, such as one month. Third, the presence of diagnostic specifiers are required as diagnostic criteria for BED in DSM-5, while these are not essential in the provisional ICD-11.

In the DSM-5, a mental disorder is defined as "associated with significant distress or disability in social, occupational, or other important activities" (p. 20, [1]) and the proposed ICD-11 states the same [2]. Whilst functional disability is not further specified for either BN or BED, many studies do attest to the poor mental Health-Related Quality of Life (HRQoL) and role impairment, defined as "days in which the person was unable to perform the usual work or other activities, e.g., caring for children in the home" [14]. As the ICD-11 proposes broader symptomatic criteria, it is important to know if these define a syndrome of individuals with less impairment or poorer HRQoL than would be found using the DSM-5 scheme, and who may not meet the over-arching requirement for social or functional impairment as suggested in recent epidemiological studies [15,16].

Thus, the aims of this study were to compare (1) the proportion of participants diagnosed with threshold or subthreshold BN and BED (clinical utility); and (2) the severity of clinical features and mental HRQoL of these categories (convergent validity), in either scheme. We hypothesized that the broader criteria proposed in the ICD-11 would decrease the number of diagnoses of unspecified or not otherwise specified categories to a greater degree than in the DSM-5.

2. Materials and Methods

2.1. Procedures

Data were collected in a sample of 107 individuals of both genders, with threshold and subthreshold BN or BED, who attended the second phase of assessment for eligibility to participate in a randomized controlled trial (RCT) testing the efficacy of a new psychological intervention to treat overweight or obese people with BN or BED [17]. Participants were recruited from the waiting list of a Brazilian university center specialized in the treatment of eating disorders and advertisements in printed, internet and oral media. Assessment started with a brief screening interview by telephone. Volunteers were then assessed in person with the Mini International Neuropsychiatric Interview (MINI) [18,19], administered by psychiatrists, and height and weight measured with calibrated scales and a stadiometer.

A third assessment phase involved the administration of a semi-structured interview named the Eating Disorder Examination Edition 17.0 D (EDE) [20]. This interview was used both to confirm the eating disorder diagnoses of participants and to collect detailed data on overall eating disorder symptoms and behaviors. One author (MAP), who had been trained at the Centre for Research on Eating Disorders at Oxford, administered the EDE and made the diagnoses of each patient based on DSM-5 criteria [1] and the provisional ICD-11 diagnostic guidelines [8,9]. For the purpose of this secondary study, inclusion criteria were: participants that met DSM-5 diagnostic criteria for BN, BED, OSFED–BN, OSFED-BED, or UFED, were aged ≥18 years and had a Body Mass Index (BMI) between 27 and 39.9 kg/m^2. Thus, in this secondary study, 107 participants were selected, including 98 people who enrolled in the RCT and 9 participants who participated in all selection and recruitment assessments, but declined to enter the treatment intervention. Figure 1 shows the participant flow and reasons for exclusion during recruitment phases.

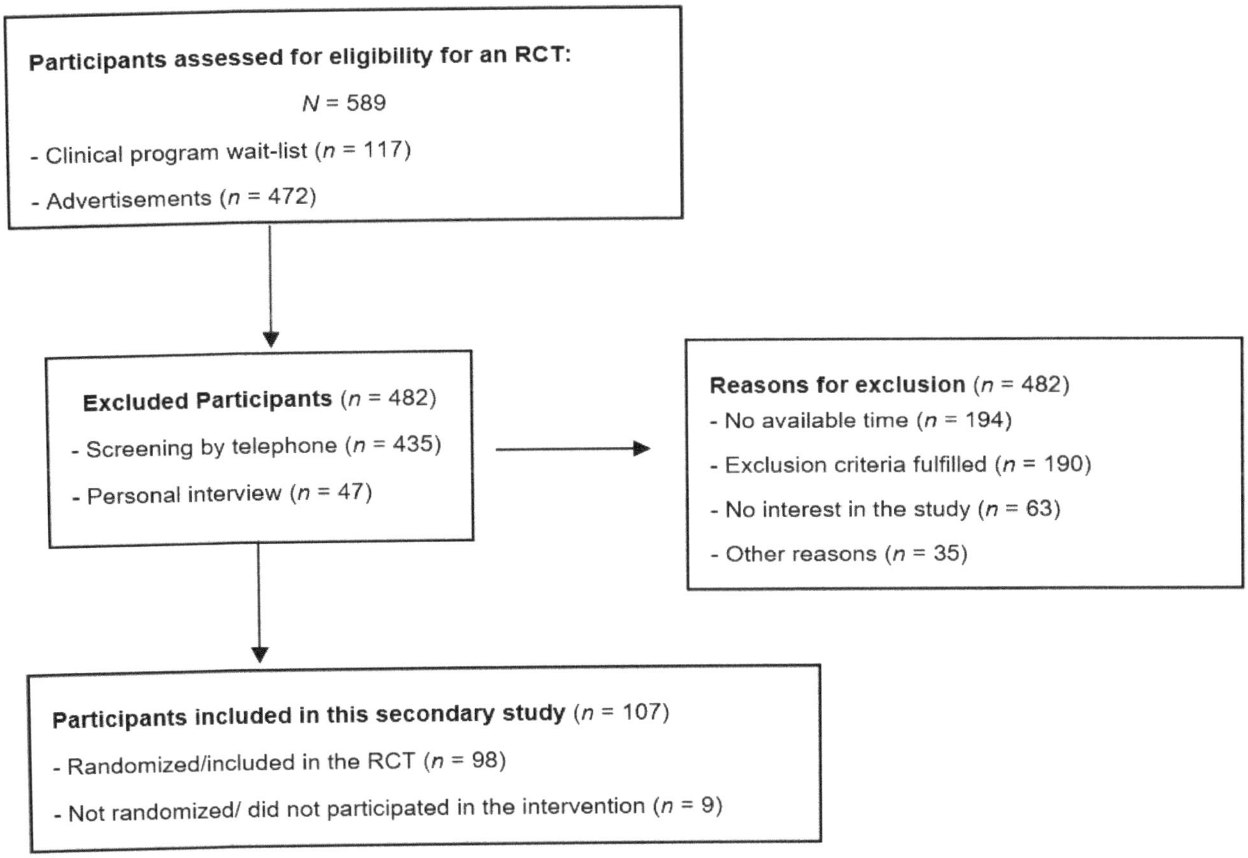

Figure 1. Flow chart of patient selection.

2.2. Measures

The assessment measures used for the study are detailed below:

1. Mini International Neuropsychiatric Interview (MINI) [18,19]: this structured interview is reliable and validated for diagnoses according to the DSM-5 [1]. The MINI version 5 [21] assessing DSM-IV diagnoses [22] has been translated into Portuguese. Thus, the MINI-5 was used in this study, with modifications to coding according to DSM-5 criteria, as in the MINI-7 [19].

2. Eating Disorder Examination (EDE) Edition 17.0D [20]: the EDE is a semi-structured interview. It assesses eating disorder features. It has four subscales measuring levels of dietary restraint, eating, shape and weight concerns. The global score is a mean of subscale scores. In this study, the new Version 17.0D item scoring, that included "being in control" as a reason for the behavior or cognition, was used. EDE version 16.0 [23] has been translated to Brazilian/Portuguese by researchers from the Universidade Federal do Rio de Janeiro (Silvia Freitas, José Carlos Appolinario), by authors of this paper (MAP, AC) and by an eating disorder specialist and member of the Eating Disorder Program (Christina Morgan—CM). A certified translator then back translated it into English. An author of the EDE (O'Connor, M) approved the final version. The translated EDE interrater reliability and concurrent validity were tested and found to be satisfactory. In the validity study, the diagnoses were made according to the eating disorder module of the SCID-I/P interview [24] (Portuguese version) [25]. Diagnostic agreement between the Portuguese EDE version 16.0 and the SCID I/P (both testing DSM-IV diagnoses) was found to be moderate (Kappa = 0.66; n = 149), with a Cronbach α of 0.91 (95% CI: 0.88 0.92) (unpublished data provided by AC). For the purpose of the present study, small adjustments were made by MAP, so that the Portuguese version used was consistent with the 17th version of the EDE [20], in order to derive DSM-5 categories. Cronbach α in this sample was 0.66, n = 107.
3. Binge Eating Scale (BES) [26]: the BES is a 16-item self-report instrument that was translated and validated in a Brazilian sample [27]. The BES measures frequency and severity of binge eating. The Brazilian version has undergone psychometric assessment and has a cut-off point for normality of 17 for the screening of eating disorders in obese individuals seeking treatment for weight loss. Cronbach α in this sample was 0.83, n = 106.
4. Loss of Control over Eating Scale (LOCES) [28]. This 24-item self-report scale measures loss of control during binge eating episodes in the last 4 weeks, with a mean score of 1.70 (SD = 5.72). It has been translated into Brazilian/Portuguese. This translated version has adequate psychometric properties (factor analysis and convergent validity) [29]. Cronbach α in this sample was 0.91, n = 107.
5. Depression, Anxiety and Stress Scale (DASS-21) [30,31] was used in its translated and validated Brazilian/Portuguese version [32]. The DASS is a 21-item self-report instrument that measures the presence and severity of depressive symptoms, anxiety and stress with a cut-off point for normality of 9 for depression, 7 for anxiety and 14 for stress. Cronbach α in this sample was 0.92, and for each subscale was: stress 0.85, depression 0.89, and anxiety 0.77, n = 107.
6. Health-related quality of life was assessed with the 12-item Short Form Health Survey (SF-12) [33]: a self-report questionnaire. It has two scales, the Physical Health Component Summary scale (PCS) and Mental Health Component Summary scale (MCS). The English language version has sound psychometric properties and it has been translated into Brazilian/Portuguese [34]. Cronbach α in this sample was 0.79, n = 106.
7. Disability was asked with a question closely similar to the 'days out of role' questions employed in the Australian National Survey of Mental Health and Well-Being [35]. Participants were asked to write for the past 4 weeks a response to, *"on how many days, if any, were you unable to complete your work, study or household responsibilities because of any problem with your (physical or emotional) health"*? An author (MAP) translated this text.

2.3. *Statistical Analyses*

Frequency and percentage statistics were used to report the distribution of diagnoses including OSFED, UFED and OFED categories for each scheme. Chi square statistic (χ^2) and Fisher's Exact Test were used to compare the frequency distributions of BN, BED, and OSFED/UFED or OFED for each scheme. The t-test or the Mann-Whitney U test were employed for parametric or non-parametric data and/or very small group sizes respectively, with correction of p to < 0.01 for multiple testing. SPSS v.23 was used for analyses [36].

2.4. *Ethics*

The RCT study was approved by the Human Research Ethics Committee of the Universidade Federal de São Paulo (UNIFESP), Brazil (CAAE 43874315.4.0000.5505). All participants provided written informed consent. Access to the data was limited to investigators and authorized researchers. The trial was formally registered in the U.S. National Institutes of Health Clinical, trial registration number NCT02464345, on 1 June 2015.

3. Results

One hundred and seven participants were included in this study. The majority of the participants were women (96%), and white (75%). A large minority were married (44%), and completed an under-graduate level of education (43%). The mean age was 40.07 years (SD 11.67), and mean BMI was 33.69 (SD 3.32). The sample included 50 (47%) participants with twice weekly Objective Binge Eating Episodes (OBEs) and 36 (34%) with weekly OBEs in the past 3 months. The remainder had a mix of OBEs and SBEs with the exception of one participant who had only SBEs.

Diagnostic evaluation using DSM-5 criteria resulted in 15/107 (14%) participants with BN, 70/107 (65.4%) with BED, 8/107 (7.5%) with OSFED-BN, 5/107 (4.7%) with OSFED-BED, and 9/107 (8.4%) participants with UFED. Applying the proposed ICD-11 criteria, there were 20/107 (18.7%) with BN, 82/107 (76.6%) with BED and 5/107 (4.7%) participants with OFED. The provisional ICD-11 diagnostic guidelines included 102/107 participants (95%) in the main categories of BN or BED compared to DSM-5 with 85/107 (79%), and 5/107 (5%) versus 22/107 (21%) with other or unspecified diagnosis ($\chi^2 = 20.265$, df = 1, $p < 0.001$, Fisher's Exact Test).

Comparative clinical features of the participants diagnosed according to either scheme are reported in Table 1. There were no significant differences in eating disorder or other psychiatric symptom severity, HRQoL, days out of role or BMI between participants with BN, BED or OSFED/UFED/OFED diagnosed according to DSM-5 or the proposed ICD-11.

Table 1. Comparative clinical features of the study participants ($N = 107$).

Clinical Features	Bulimia Nervosa			Binge Eating Disorder			# Osfed/Ufed/Ofed			All
	DSM-5 ($n = 15$)	ICD-11 ($n = 20$)		DSM-5 ($n = 70$)	ICD-11 ($n = 82$)		DSM-5 ($n = 22$)	ICD-11 ($n = 5$)		$N = 107$
	Median (IQR)		Z (p) †	Median (IQR)		Z (p)	Median (IQR)		MWU Z (p)	
EDE global	3.59 (3.27–3.83)	3.80 (2.35–3.83)	−0.044 (0.965)	2.48 (1.95–2.88)	2.27 (1.93–2.41)	−1.233 (0.217)	2.23 (1.98–2.74)	2.60 (2.01–2.77)	−0.196 (0.845)	2.57 (2.03–3.23)
EDE restriction	3.00 (2.70–3.60)	2.20 (1.00–3.80)	−0.394 (0.694)	1.60 (0.08–2.40)	1.40 (0.50–2.20)	−0.994 (0.320)	1.60 (0.60–2.20)	1.40 (1.00–1.60)	−0.157 (0.875)	1.80 (0.80–2.40)
EDE eating concern	2.00 (1.90–2.70)	3.00 (2.60–3.20)	−1.228 (0.220)	1.20 (0.60–2.20)	0.90 (0.20–1.40)	−1.605 (0.108)	1.20 (0.20–2.40)	0.60 (0.40–2.40)	−0.197 (0.844)	1.40 (0.60–2.40)
EDE shape concern	5.00 (4.25–5.37)	4.62 (2.62–4.75)	−0.961 (0.336)	3.62 (2.62–4.50)	3.44 (3.06–4.20)	−0.230 (0.818)	3.50 (3.00–4.62)	3.62 (2.88–3.88)	−0.118 (0.906)	3.75 (2.87–4.62)
EDE weight concern	4.20 (3.30–4.70)	3.20 (3.20–3.80)	−1.488 (0.137)	3.20 (2.40–4.20)	3.20 (2.70–3.67)	−0.263 (0.793)	3.20 (2.80–3.75)	2.80 (2.60–3.60)	−0.472 (0.637)	3.20 (2.60–4.20)
Binge Eating Scale	35.00 (30.50–41.00)	32.00 (31.00–33.00)	−0.963 (0.335)	29.00 (22.00–33.00)	28.00 (21.00–32.50)	−0.677 (0.498)	28.00 (24.00–33.00)	25.00 (25.00–25.00)	−1.061 (0.289)	30.00 (23.00–35.00)
LOCES	3.67 (3.29–4.18)	3.50 (3.08–3.62)	−0.917 (0.359)	3.21 (2.79–3.50)	3.12 (2.62–3.43)	−0.564 (0.573)	3.33 (2.70–3.54)	3.45 (3.41–3.50)	−0.746 (0.456)	3.33 (2.83–3.58)
DASS depression	22.00 (16.50–33.00)	24.00 (24.00–28.00)	−0.044 (0.965)	12.00 (6.00–20.00)	14.00 (7.00–17.00)	−0.066 (0.948)	16.00 (10.00–24.00)	10.00 (8.00–12.00)	−1.178 (0.239)	14.00 (8.00–24.00)
DASS anxiety	12.00 (5.00–14.00)	22.00 (4.00–26.00)	−0.615 (0.539)	8.00 (4.00–14.00)	17.00 (2.00–20.00)	−0.896 (0.370)	18.00 (2.00–22.00)	18.00 (6.00–18.00)	−0.277 (0.782)	10.00 (4.00–16.00)
DASS stress	28.00 (20.00–34.00)	30.00 (26.00–32.00)	−0.307 (0.799)	18.00 (12.00–28.00)	21.00 (14.00–27.00)	−0.059 (0.953)	26.00 (16.00–28.00)	20.00 (18.00–22.00)	−0.511 (0.609)	20.00 (14.00–28.00)
SFMCS	30.12 (26.63–38.70)	34.35 (34.32–40.81)	−1.702 (0.089)	36.34 (26.60–42.70)	37.14 (31.24–42.94)	−0.499 (0.618)	36.70 (32.61–42.74)	42.03 (35.74–44.78)	−1.136 (0.256)	36.02 (27.42–42.71)
SFPCS	46.27 (43.51–52.98)	47.00 (46.50–55.90)	−0.567 (0.570)	50.24 (41.97–56.36)	48.77 (40.64–56.60)	−0.273 (0.785)	47.00 (41.14–55.90)	50.39 (47.13–53.58)	−0.431 (0.667)	49.82 (41.52–56.20)
Body Mass Index (kg/m^2)	32.60 (29.72–34.31)	32.70 (31.30–34.60)	−0.655 (0.513)	33.60 (31.12–35.85)	34.65 (32.63–37.02)	−0.964 (0.335)	33.80 (32.37–36.90)	33.89 (30.70–35.29)	−0.823 (0.411)	33.64 (31.08–35.90)
Days out of role/28 days	10.00 (1.00–15.00)	4.00 (2.00–10.00)	−0.482 (0.630)	5.00 (2.00–12.00)	1.00 (0–11.00)	−1.341 (0.180)	2.00 (0–10.00)	0 (0–0)	−1.466 (0.143)	5.00 (0–12.00)

Note ICD-11 has OFED as the only subthreshold category. † MWU Z = Mann Whitney U Z statistic. BED = binge eating disorder; BN = bulimia nervosa; DASS = Depression, Anxiety and Stress Scale; DSM-5 = Diagnostic and Statistical Manual of Mental Disorders 5th ed; EDE = Eating Disorder Examination; ICD-11 = International Classification of Diseases 11th ed.; IQR = Interquartile Range; LOCES = Loss of Control Over Eating Scale; OFED = Other Feeding or Eating Disorder; OSFED = Other Specified Feeding or Eating Disorder; SFMCS = Short Form Health Survey Mental Health Component Summary score; SFPCS = Short Form Health Survey Physical Health Component Summary score; UFED = Unspecified Feeding or Eating Disorder.

4. Discussion

This study compared the clinical utility and convergent validity of the two main classification systems for psychiatric disorders—the DSM-5 [1] and the provisional ICD-11 [8,9]. Threshold and subthreshold diagnoses of BN and BED were derived using the "gold standard" semi-structured interview for eating disorders—the EDE-17.0D [20]. In both systems, a majority of participants met full BN or BED criteria. This supports the improved clinical utility of both schemes over the former DSM-IV [22] and ICD-10 [2] where a larger proportion of people did not meet full criteria [6,37].

In the present study, a greater number of participants received a main diagnosis of BN or BED with the provisional ICD-11 scheme compared to the DSM-5. Despite the inclusion of some less severe cases in those diagnosed according to ICD-11, overall there were no significant differences in levels of eating disorder or general psychopathology, BMI, mental or physical HRQoL, or role impairment between diagnoses defined by either classificatory system. These data do not support the findings reported by Mitchison et al. [16] where there was less impairment in people with less severe recurrent binge eating. A possible explanation is that the Mitchison study was based on the results of a community sample and this study used a clinical sample of people with high BMIs and an eating disorder who were seeking treatment, i.e., people potentially with more severe illness. Indeed, the present study included a higher proportion of people with twice-weekly OBEs, 58.1% (50/86) compared to 40.5% (158/390) in the Mitchison sample; and in the latter study those with twice weekly binge eating had poorer mental HRQoL, whether associated or not with marked distress.

Thus, the results of this study demonstrated that regardless of the classificatory system used, significant levels of associated general psychopathology and impact on mental HRQoL were observed in people with disorders characterized by recurrent binge eating. Our findings support those of Hudson's et al. [38], in which a high association between lifetime comorbid psychiatric disorders and role impairment in people with BED and BN was reported.

Different approaches guide these two classificatory systems, in particular the fact that the proposed ICD-11 diagnostic guidelines do not provide a "check-list" for diagnostic criteria. The diagnosis is based on a description of the essential features of the conditions, i.e., symptoms and characteristics that clinicians expect to find in all cases of the disorder. Reed [37] highlights that a large number of people with mental disorders around the globe may not receive treatment as a consequence of diagnoses being restricted by over rigid criteria. We anticipate that clinicians will likely find the ICD-11 scheme more user friendly, as it allows for greater clinician judgement [3] and is more flexible than the DSM-5. More of their patients may thereby receive definitive diagnosis and also, be eligible for care that is contingent on having a main diagnosis. On the other hand, the strict criteria of the DSM-5 are more applicable to the research setting where there is a need for tight criteria for reproducibility of studies.

A strength of this study was the use of an interview considered the gold standard (the EDE) for providing eating disorders diagnoses. Limitations include the small numbers of participants with ICD-11 BN and OSFED/UFED/OFED, with a subsequent risk of TYPE II error; a sample characterized by individuals who are overweight or obese; no participants with AN or other eating disorders; and the moderate alpha level of the EDE. Further, the BES has been validated in people with obesity and this sample included a small number (13.1%) with BMI 27.5–29.9. A final limitation is that the present study reports on a secondary analysis of data from a RCT testing the efficacy of psychological interventions for overweight people with bulimic disorders and used an EDE version, which does not collect the distress criterion across both OBEs and SBEs. However, the vast majority, 77 of 82 participants, had distress associated with OBEs.

5. Conclusions

The present article found that both the DSM-5 and ICD-11 diagnostic schemes had a low proportion of participants with a poorly specified (OSFED/UFED) diagnosis. Further, those included as BN or BED in the ICD-11 were not less severe than the ones with BN or BED in the DSM-5 groupings. The increased flexibility of the proposed ICD-11 may extend the clinical utility of this scheme compared to the DSM-5. However, further research is needed in larger samples of people with BN, people who are not overweight, and in people with other eating disorders diagnoses.

Author Contributions: M.A.P. was responsible for writing the original draft and P.H. and A.C. were responsible for writing, review and editing.

Acknowledgments: We thank Alexandre Giffoni, Ana Maria Roma, Bruna Boaretto, Denise Claudino, Elson Asevedo, Juliana Carvalho, Mara Maranhão, Mireille Coelho, Nara Estella, Ruth Grigolon, Sérgio Garnes, and Veruska Amigo for the valuable assistance with participant assessments.

References

1. American Psychiatric Association (APA). *Diagnostic and Statistical Manual of Mental Disorders*, 5th ed.; American Psychiatric Publishing: Arlington, VA, USA, 2013.
2. World Health Organization (WHO). *The ICD-10 Classification of Mental and Behavioural Disorders: Clinical Descriptions and Diagnostic Guidelines*; World Health Organization: Geneva, Switzerland, 1992.
3. First, M.B.; Reed, G.M.; Hyman, S.E.; Saxena, S. The development of the ICD-11 clinical descriptions and diagnostic guidelines for mental and behavioural disorders. *World Psychiatry* **2015**, *14*, 82–90. [CrossRef] [PubMed]
4. Reed, G.M.; First, M.B.; Medina-Mora, M.E.; Gureje, O.; Pike, K.M.; Saxena, S. Draft diagnostic guidelines for ICD-11 mental and behavioural disorders available for review and comment. *World Psychiatry* **2016**, *15*, 112–113. [CrossRef] [PubMed]
5. Reed, G.M.; Correia, J.M.; Esparza, P.; Saxena, S.; Maj, M. The WPA-WHO global survey of psychiatrists' attitudes towards mental disorders classification. *World Psychiatry* **2011**, *10*, 118–131. [CrossRef] [PubMed]
6. Al-Adawi, S.; Bax, B.; Bryant-Waugh, R.; Claudino, A.M.; Hay, P.; Monteleone, P.; Norring, C.; Pike, K.M.; Pilon, D.J.; Herscovici, C.R.; et al. Revision of ICD—Status update on feeding and eating disorders. *Adv. Eat. Disord. Theory Res. Pract.* **2013**, *1*, 10–20. [CrossRef]
7. Uher, R.; Rutter, M. Classification of feeding and eating disorders: Review of evidence and proposals for ICD-11. *World Psychiatry* **2012**, *11*, 80–92. [CrossRef] [PubMed]
8. World Health Organization (WHO). *ICD-11 Diagnostic Guidelines for Internet-Based Field Study—Feeding and Eating Disorders (D), Version 6*, Unpublished work. 2015.
9. Global Clinical Practice Network WHO. ICD-11 Diagnostic Guidelines for Internet Based Field Studies. 2015. Available online: https://gcp.network/en/icd-11-guidelines (accessed on 12 October 2017).
10. Brownstone, L.M.; Bardone-Cone, A.M.; Fitzsimmons-Craft, E.E.; Printz, K.S.; Le Grange, D.; Mitchell, J.E.; Crow, S.J.; Peterson, C.B.; Crosby, R.D.; Klein, M.H.; et al. Subjective and objective binge eating in relation to eating disorder symptomatology, negative affect, and personality dimensions. *Int. J. Eat. Disord.* **2013**, *46*, 66–76. [CrossRef] [PubMed]
11. Forney, K.J.; Bodell, L.P.; Haedt-Matt, A.A.; Keel, P.K. The incremental validity of the episode size criterion in binge-eating definitions: An examination in women with purging syndromes. *Int. J. Eat. Disord.* **2016**, *49*, 651–662. [CrossRef] [PubMed]
12. Jenkins, P.E.; Conley, C.S.; Rienecke Hoste, R.; Meyer, C.; Blissett, J.M. Perception of control during episodes of eating: Relationships with quality of life and eating psychopathology. *Int. J. Eat. Disord.* **2012**, *45*, 115–119. [CrossRef] [PubMed]
13. Palavras, M.A.; Hay, P.J.; Lujic, S.; Claudino, A.M. Comparing symptomatic and functional outcomes over 5 years in two nonclinical cohorts characterized by binge eating with and without objectively large episodes. *Int. J. Eat. Disord.* **2015**, *48*, 1158–1165. [CrossRef] [PubMed]

14. Agh, T.; Kovács, G.; Supina, D.; Pawaskar, M.; Herman, B.K.; Vokó, Z.; Sheehan, D.V. A systematic review of the health-related quality of life and economic burdens of anorexia nervosa, bulimia nervosa, and binge eating disorder. *Eat. Weight Disord.* **2016**, *21*, 353–364. [CrossRef] [PubMed]
15. Hay, P.; Mitchison, D.; Collado, A.E.L.; González-Chica, D.A.; Stocks, N.; Touyz, S. Burden and health-related quality of life of eating disorders, including Avoidant/Restrictive Food Intake Disorder (ARFID), in the Australian population. *J. Eat. Disord.* **2017**, *5*, 21. [CrossRef] [PubMed]
16. Mitchison, D.; Touyz, S.; González-Chica, D.A.; Stocks, N.; Hay, P. How abnormal is binge eating? 18-Year time trends in population prevalence and burden. *Acta Psychiatry Scand.* **2017**, *136*, 147–155. [CrossRef] [PubMed]
17. Palavras, M.A.; Hay, P.; Touyz, S.; Sainsbury, A.; da Luz, F.; Swinbourne, J.; Estella, N.M.; Claudino, A. Comparing cognitive behavioural therapy for eating disorders integrated with behavioural weight loss therapy to cognitive behavioural therapy-enhanced alone in overweight or obese people with bulimia nervosa or binge eating disorder: Study protocol for a randomised controlled trial. *Trials* **2015**, *16*, 578. [CrossRef] [PubMed]
18. Lecrubier, Y.; Weiller, E.; Hergueta, T.; Amorim, P.; Bonora, L.I.; Lépine, J.P. Mini International Neuropsychiatric Interview—Brazilian Version 5.0.0. DSM-IV, 2002. Available online: www.bibliotecadigital.ufmg.br (accessed on 2 July 2015).
19. Sheehan, D.; Janavs, J.; Baker, R.; Sheehan, K.H.; Knapp, E.; Sheehan, M. Mini International Neuropsychiatric Interview—Version 7.0.0 DSM-5 2014. Available online: http://www.medical-outcomes.com (accessed on 2 July 2015).
20. Fairburn, C.G.; Cooper, Z.; O'Connor, M. *The Eating Disorder Examination*, 17th ed.; The Centre for Research on Eating Disorders at Oxford: Oxford, UK, 2014; Available online: www.credo-oxford.com/pdfs/EDE170D.pdf (accessed on 3 July 2015).
21. Sheehan, D.V.; Lecrubier, Y.; Sheehan, K.H.; Amorim, P.; Janavs, J.; Weiller, E.; Hergueta, T.; Baker, R.; Dunbar, G.C. The Mini-International Neuropsychiatric Interview (M.I.N.I.): The development and validation of a structured diagnostic psychiatric interview for DSM-IV and ICD-10. *J. Clin. Psychiatry* **1998**, *59* (Suppl. 20), 22–33. [PubMed]
22. American Psychiatric Association (APA). *Diagnostic and Statistical Manual of Mental Disorders*, 4th ed.; American Psychiatric Association: Washington, DC, USA, 1994.
23. Fairburn, C.G. Eating Disorder Examination (Edition 16.0D). In *Cognitive Behavior Therapy and Eating Disorders*; The Guilford Press: New York, NY, USA, 2008; pp. 270–308.
24. First, M.B.; Spitzer, R.L.; Gibbon, M.; Williams, J.B.W. *Structured Clinical Interview for DSM-IV Axis I Disorders-Patient Edition (SCID-I/P, Version 2.0)*; Biometric Research, New York State Psychiatric Institute: New York, NY, USA, 1996.
25. Versiani, M. *Entrevista Clínica Estruturada—DSM-IV Transtornos do Eixo I. Tradução da Structured Clinical Interview for DSM-IV Axis I/Patient*; Versão 2.1; Programa de Ansiedade e Depressão, Instituto de Psiquiatria IPUB, UFRJ: Rio de Janeiro, Brazil, 1996.
26. Gormally, J.; Black, S.; Daston, S.; Rardin, D. The assessment of binge eating severity among obese persons. *Addict. Behav.* **1982**, *7*, 47–55. [CrossRef]
27. Freitas, S.; Lopes, C.S.; Coutinho, W.; Appolinario, J.C. Tradução e adaptação para o português da escala de compulsão alimentar periódica. *Rev. Bras. Psiquiatr.* **2001**, *23*, 215–220. [CrossRef]
28. Latner, J.D.; Mond, J.M.; Kelly, M.C.; Haynes, S.N.; Hay, P.J. The Loss of Control Over Eating Scale: Development and psychometric evaluation. *Int. J. Eat. Disord.* **2014**, *47*, 647–659. [CrossRef] [PubMed]
29. Luz, F.Q.; Sainsbury, A.; Estella, N.M.; Cogo, H.; Touyz, S.W.; Palavras, M.A.; Latner, J.D.; Claudino, A.; Hay, P. An empirical evaluation of the translation to Brazilian Portuguese of the Loss of Control Over Eating Scale (LOCES). *Arch. Clin. Psychiatry* **2016**, *43*, 1–5. [CrossRef]
30. Henry, J.D.; Crawford, J.R. The short-form version of the Depression Anxiety Stress Scales (DASS-21): Construct validity and normative data in a large non-clinical sample. *Br. J. Clin. Psychol.* **2005**, *44*, 227–239. [CrossRef] [PubMed]
31. Lovibond, P.F.; Lovibond, S.H. The structure of negative emotional states: Comparison of the Depression Anxiety Stress Scales (DASS) with the Beck Depression and Anxiety Inventories. *Behav. Res. Ther.* **1995**, *33*, 335–343. [CrossRef]

32. Vignola, R.C.; Tucci, A.M. Adaptation and validation of the depression, anxiety and stress scale (DASS) to Brazilian Portuguese. *J. Affect. Disord.* **2014**, *155*, 104–109. [CrossRef] [PubMed]
33. Ware, J., Jr.; Kosinski, M.; Keller, S.D. A 12-item short-form health survey: Construction of scales and preliminary tests of reliability and validity. *Med. Care* **1996**, *34*, 220–233. [CrossRef] [PubMed]
34. Silveira, M.F.; Almeida, J.C.; Freire, R.S.; Haikal, D.S.; Martins, A.E.B.L. Propriedades psicométricas do instrumento de avaliação da qualidade de vida: 12-item health survey (SF-12). *Ciência Saúde Coletiva* **2013**, *18*, 1923–1931. [CrossRef] [PubMed]
35. Slade, T.; Johnston, A.; Oakley Browne, M.A.; Andrew, G.; Whiteford, H. 2007 National Survey of Mental Health and Wellbeing: Methods and key findings. *Aust. N. Z. J. Psychiatry* **2009**, *43*, 594–605. [CrossRef] [PubMed]
36. IBM Corp. *Released 2015. IBM SPSS Statistics for Windows*; Version 23.0; IBM Corp: Armonk, NY, USA, 2015.
37. Reed, G.M. Toward ICD-11: Improving the clinical utility of WHO's international classification of mental disorders. *Prof. Psychol. Res.* **2010**, *41*, 457–464. [CrossRef]
38. Hudson, J.I.; Hirpi, E.; Pope, H.G., Jr.; Kessler, R.C. The prevalence and correlates of eating disorders in the National Comorbidity Survey Replication. *Biol. Psychiatry* **2007**, *61*, 348–358. [CrossRef] [PubMed]

12

Cognitive Remediation Therapy for Adolescents with Anorexia Nervosa—Treatment Satisfaction and the Perception of Change

Camilla Lindvall Dahlgren * **and Kristin Stedal**

Regional Department for Eating Disorders, Division of Mental Health and Addiction, Oslo University Hospital, Ullevål HF, Postboks 4950 Nydalen, 0424 Oslo, Norway; post.psykiskhelse@oslo-universitetssykehus.no

* Correspondence: camilla.lindvall@dahlgren.no

Academic Editors: Amanda Sainsbury and Felipe Luz

Abstract: Cognitive remediation therapy (CRT) has recently been developed for children and adolescents with anorexia nervosa (AN). It focuses on decreasing rigid cognitions and behaviors, as well as increasing central coherence. Overall, CRT has been proven feasible for young individuals with AN, but little is known regarding the specifics of its feasibility, and the perception of change associated with the intervention. Consequently, the aim of the current study was to explore service users' perspective on CRT with a specific focus on treatment delivery, treatment content, and perceived change. Twenty adolescents (age 13–18) with AN participated in a 10-session course of CRT. A 20-item treatment evaluation questionnaire was administered at the end of treatment, focusing on four aspects of the intervention: (1) general attitudes towards treatment, (2) treatment specifics, (3) the perception of change and (4) the patient-therapist relation. The main findings suggest high levels of treatment satisfaction, but somewhat limited perceptions of change. The current study is one of the most detailed accounts of adolescents' perspective on CRT published on eating disorders, and highlights several important aspects of the treatment viewed through the eye of the receiver.

Keywords: anorexia nervosa; cognitive remediation therapy; eating disorders; treatment satisfaction; neuropsychology; rigidity; cognitive flexibility; central coherence

---

1. Introduction

Anorexia nervosa (AN) is an eating disorder (ED) characterized by a persistent restriction of energy intake which leads to significant low body weight, an intense fear of gaining weight or becoming fat, a distorted experience of one's own body and an amplified sense of the body's influence on self-worth [1]. Individuals with AN often display rigid behaviors and cognitions characterized by preoccupation with details [2]. Such behaviors and cognitions are predominantly linked to core ED symptoms such as food restriction and preoccupancy with weight and shape, but are also commonly seen in the individual's approach to exercise routines, work or school, or in relation to family and friends [3]. Inflexibility and preoccupation with details are often explained in terms of neuropsychological dysfunction. Studies in adults with AN have yielded consistent evidence of suboptimal executive functioning, especially in cognitive flexibility [4,5], and in information processing which is often characterized by weak central coherence [6]. Cognitive function in children and adolescents with AN has received less attention, and the extant literature report mixed findings with a number of studies failing to find evidence of poor neuropsychological functioning, whereas others have replicated results similar to those reported in adults [7].

Following the introduction of cognitive remediation therapy (CRT) for EDs in 2005 [8], a number of case and feasibility studies have supported its utility in adults with AN [9], and four randomized controlled trials (RCTs) [10–13] have sought to investigate the effect of the intervention. For individuals with AN, CRT aims to decrease rigidity and increase the balance between local and global information processing [14–16]. It is hypothesized that by alleviating some of these cognitive difficulties, ambivalence towards engaging in other psychological interventions might decrease, rendering the individual more open to the prospect of change [8]. In 2010, the original, adult CRT manual [17] was adapted for children and adolescents [18], and although a number of studies have established its feasibility for this younger group [14,19–22], there are no published RCT. There is also a paucity in studies evaluating the treatment from the receiver's perspective. This is in contrast with the increased focus on assessment of client satisfaction in ED health services [23,24]. Additionally, it is well known that that treatment dissatisfaction may lead to treatment delay, failure to engage and, ultimately, to treatment withdrawal [25,26]. The aim of this study is to present post-intervention feedback from a feasibility study of CRT for adolescents with AN, and to examine the results through the aspects of treatment satisfaction and perception of change.

2. Materials and Methods

2.1. Participants

A total of 20 inpatients (N = 10) and outpatients (N = 10) aged 13–18 (mean = 15.9, SD = 1.6) were recruited from Oslo University Hospital HF, Ullevål, and took part in a CRT feasibility trial [14]. All participants were female and in treatment for AN at the time of inclusion. Based on self-reports of binge eating and compensatory behaviors, 18 participants were classified as having a restricting subtype of AN (AN-R). The two remaining participants fitted the description for a binge-purge subtype (AN-BP). Intelligence was assessed using the Wechsler Adult Intelligence Scale—Third Edition (WAIS-III) [27], the Wechsler Abbreviated Scale of Intelligence (WASI) [28] or the Wechsler Intelligence Scale for Children-Third Edition (WISC-III) [29]. All participants scored within the normal range. There were no significant differences between in- and out-patients in any of the baseline assessment variables. Descriptive data at baseline is presented in Table 1.

Table 1. Descriptive data for the sample (N = 20) at baseline.

	N	Mean (SD)	Range
Age (years)	20	15.9 (1.6)	13.1–18.7
BMI Percentile	20	10.2 (17.2)	0.0–28.0
Duration of illness [1]	19	2.7 (2.1)	1–7
Global EDE-Q [2]	20	3.4 (1.4)	0.6–5.4
BDI	20	32.2 (15.1)	7–58
STAI	20	58.6 (9.7)	43–78

Note. SD = Standard Deviation; BMI = Body Mass Index; [1] = Years, self-reported; [2] = Eating Disorder Examination Questionnaire Global Score [30]; BDI = Beck Depression Inventory [31]; STAI = State Trait Anxiety Inventory [32].

2.2. Procedure

Participants were assessed using an extensive neuropsychological and psychiatric test battery both before and after receiving CRT. The neuropsychological assessment battery included tests focusing primarily on set-shifting and central coherence, whereas the psychiatric assessment included self-reported measures of depression, anxiety and ED psychopathology. A more detailed account of the assessment procedure and content have been presented elsewhere [3,14,33]. After the initial assessment, participants received, on average, 10 once- or twice-weekly individually delivered sessions, and were then re-tested using the same measures as before the treatment started. In addition, participants were asked to fill out a treatment evaluation questionnaire, allowing for exploration of treatment acceptability and the perception of change after treatment. The study was conducted at the Regional Department for Eating Disorders at Oslo University Hospital, Ullevål, HF. All necessary ethical procedures were followed; the data protection service approved the project, and the Regional Committees for Medical and Health Research Ethics granted us ethical approval. Informed consent was sought from all participants as well as from their parents when below the age of 16.

2.3. *The Intervention—Cognitive Remediation Therapy*

All CRT sessions were delivered face-to-face, and followed the structure and content outlined in a CRT manual specifically developed for children and adolescents with AN [34]. In accordance with previous CRT studies [14,35], no efforts were made to explore themes normally addressed in ED treatment such as food, weight or shape. One to two tasks were administered each session followed by discussion. The selection of tasks was based on the therapist's clinical judgment, and chosen to address particular cognitive styles or difficulties specific to each individual. To help participants to engage in the meta-cognitive process, all tasks were accompanied or followed by questions encouraging the patients to reflect on their thinking processes. As an important part of CRT is to explore how experiences acquired in therapy can be transferred to real-life settings, homework tasks were introduced around session three or four. The aim of these tasks was for participants to use the knowledge acquired during CRT sessions, and to experiment with this knowledge outside the therapy context (e.g., in social settings, at school, or at work). Examples of these homework tasks can be found in the CRT Resource Pack [34,36].

2.4. *Assessment—The CRT Treatment Evaluation Questionnaire*

A treatment evaluation questionnaire was developed to investigate various aspects of treatment satisfaction and the participants' perspective of change (see Table 2). The questionnaire combines CRT-specific items generated by clinicians and researchers at the unit where CRT was delivered, and items derived from treatment satisfaction questionnaires published by Kunnskapssenteret (the Knowledge Center for Health Services) [37] and RIKSÄT (a Swedish national register for ED treatment) [38]. The 20-item questionnaire was divided into four sections each exploring different aspects of treatment: (1) general attitudes towards CRT (items 1–5), (2) treatment-specific items (items 7–10), (3) the perception of change (items 6, 11–16c), and (4) the relationship to the CRT therapist (items 17–20). Aspects 1, 2 and 4 were labelled *treatment satisfaction* and aspect 3 was labelled *perceived change*. All but one item (item 13) were closed questions, and with one exception (item 9), response options were rated on a 5-point Likert scale. Response options differed depending on the wording of each item, i.e. where the response options to the question "*How do you feel about the number of sessions*" (item 8) were "Way too few", "A little few", "Just enough", "A little too many" or "Way too many", the corresponding response options to the question "How did you experience the collaboration between you and your CRT therapist?" were "Very poor", Quite poor", "Both", "Quite good" or "Very good".

Table 2. The CRT Treatment Evaluation Questionnaire.

Item No.	Question
1.	Overall, how satisfied or dissatisfied are you with the course of CRT you have received? [1]
2.	Before you initiated CRT, you were informed about the treatment. Was this information useful? [1]
3.	How did your CRT experiences match the expectations you had prior to treatment initiation? [1]
4.	To what extent did you feel that the CRT sessions were useful to you? [1]
5.	Did you experience CRT as being relevant to your situation? [1]
6.	Did you acquire any skills during CRT that might be useful in your everyday life? [3]
7.	How do you feel about the length of the sessions? [2]
8.	How do you feel about the number of sessions? [2]
9.	How did you experience the division between practical exercises and discussion during the session (you can check as many boxes as you like)? [2]

Table 2. *Cont.*

Item No.	Question
10.	What is your opinion on the tasks used during the sessions? [2]
11.	How has the way you reflect on your own thinking changed during the course of CRT? [3]
12.	To what extent do you experience distress in relation to your eating disorder now, compared to before you started the CRT treatment program? [3]
13.	Are there other areas in your life which have become more or less difficult now, compared to before you started the CRT program? a) Example no. 1, b) Example no. 2
14.	What is your relationship to your family like now compared to before you started the CRT program? [3]
15.	How are things working out in your everyday life now, compared to before you entered the CRT treatment program? a) School/work? b) Leisure time/friends? [3]
16.	Do you think the CRT sessions have had an impact on your ability to change with regards to: a) Your eating disorder? b) School/work? c) Leisure time/friends? [3]
17.	How did you experience the collaboration between you and your CRT therapist? [4]
18.	Did you feel that you were treated with respect during the course of CRT? [4]
19.	Did the CRT therapist listen to you? [4]
20.	Did your therapist explain the tasks in a way that was easy to understand? [4]

Note: [1] = Items assessing general aspects of treatment; [2] = Items assessing treatment-specific aspects; [3] = Items assessing the perception of change; [4] = items assessing the participants' view of the CRT therapist. Items 1–5, 7–10 and 17–20 represent items specific *to treatment satisfaction*. Items 6, 11–15, and 16a,b represent items specific to *perceived change*. CRT = cognitive remediation therapy.

2.5. Analyses

Results are presented using bar graphs (see Appendix A), with the response option being presented on the x axis, and number of responses on the y axis. As response options differed depending on the wording of each item, it was not possible to create bar graphs reporting collated results. Items were therefore divided into the following four categories: (1) General attitudes towards treatment (items 1–5), (2) Treatment-specific items (items 7–10), (3) The perception of change (items 6 and 11–16c) and (4) The relationship to the CRT therapist (items 17–20) and presented as individual item graphs. Item 13a-b was excluded due to the low response rate ($N^{13a} = 5$, $N^{13b} = 9$), and large variations in examples of areas that had become more or less difficult after the course of CRT.

3. Results

A detailed overview of the results from the CRT treatment evaluation questionnaire is presented in Appendix A. There were no voluntary drop-outs, and 19 out of 20 participants completed the entire course of treatment. Eighteen out of the 20 participants completed the treatment evaluation questionnaire post-CRT.

3.1. Treatment Satisfaction

In terms of the general assessment, 16 participants (89%) were either "very satisfied" or "satisfied" with the course of CRT they had received. Seventeen participants (94%) reported that the course of treatment had matched their expectations, and the same number of participants also reported having acquired skills that could be useful in their everyday life (with answers ranging from "very few" to "many"). All participants (N = 18) reported that the CRT sessions had been useful. As for treatment-specific items, 100% of the participants (N = 18) were either "very satisfied" or "extremely satisfied" with the tasks used during the sessions. Thirteen participants (72%) felt that the session length and the division between practical exercises and discussion were "just right". Ten participants (56%) reported the total number of sessions to be "a little few", whereas seven participants (39%) reported that the number of sessions were "just enough". Overall, participants responded highly affirmative with regards to the therapist-specific items (items 17–20). For example, 15 (83%) participants reported that the collaboration between the patient and therapist was "very good", and an equal number felt they had been treated with respect during the intervention and that the therapist had listened to them. Seventy-eight percent of the participants (N = 14) reported that the therapist had explained the tasks in a way that was easy to understand (item 20).

3.2. *The Perception of Change*

The perception of change was evaluated in relation to ED-specific items, but also in terms of other aspects of life, such as school or work, leisure time, friends and family. Eleven out of 18 participants (61%) reported that they were either slightly, or much more aware of their thinking style post CRT. Fifty-nine percent of the participants (N = 10) reported that ED-related distress was "more or less the same as before" CRT, and seven participants (41%) chose the same response when probed to appraise their relationship to their family post-CRT. Eight participants (47%) reported a "slightly better" relationship to their family after the intervention. As for items related to everyday functioning (item 15a-b), the majority of participants (61%, N = 11) reported that school/work was "more or less the same as before" CRT. Corresponding numbers for leisure time/friends was N = 8 (44%). Whereas 10 participants (56%) reported that the CRT sessions had had "a little" (N = 7), "quite a lot" (N = 2) or "a lot" (N = 1) of impact on their ability to change with regards to the ED, 44% of the patients (N = 8) reported that CRT had had either "very little" (N = 5) or "none not at all" (N = 3) impact on ED-related change. Results were almost identical with regards to perceived change in relation to school and/or work. The intervention appeared to have had limited impact on the participants' perceived change with regards to leisure and/or social activities with six participants (40%) choosing the response option "very little", five participants (33%) "little", three participants (20%) quite a lot and one patient (7%) "a lot".

4. Discussion

The aim of the current study was to investigate post-intervention feedback from a feasibility study on CRT for adolescents, and to delineate the individuals' perspective in terms of general and specific attitudes towards treatment, and the relationship to the CRT therapist. Perceived change post-CRT was also investigated using ED-specific and non-ED-specific items. Overall, results indicate high levels of treatment satisfaction, both in terms of general attitudes towards treatment, treatment specifics (e.g., treatment length, content, tasks, etc.), and the relationship to the therapist, but somewhat limited perceptions of change.

4.1. *Treatment Satisfaction*

Tasks used in CRT are based on their potential playful capacity, and it is hypothesized that their simple, non-threatening nature help engage patients in treatment, and encourage curiosity rather than resistance [14,39,40]. This was supported in the current study where the majority of patients reported being either slightly or very satisfied with the tasks used to identify and challenge cognitive styles. Our results regarding task specifics are also in line with those recently published by Giombini et al. [20] supporting the use of board games and puzzles presented in the CRT Resource Pack [36]. Ten sessions is the length of treatment most commonly provided in both adult, child and adolescent CRT delivery. However, the results presented here call into question whether ten sessions are enough. More than half of the patients in our study reported that the number of sessions was "a little few", and similar to the study by van Noort et al. [22], some of the patients actually requested additional sessions, an underreported phenomenon in patients with AN. In contrast to patient feedback in Wood et al.'s study from 2011 [40] where sessions exceeding 30 minutes were felt as being too long, the majority of patients in the current study reported the session length to be "just right", and a few patients actually thought the sessions were a little short. In addition, the majority of patients in the current study communicated that they were satisfied with the treatment that they had received, and on an overall level, patients reported that the CRT sessions were both useful and relevant to their situation. Thus, in stark contrast to other treatment studies in EDs where adolescents with AN often report negative recollections of their treatment [41], CRT appears to provide a positive framework for this particular patient group.

High levels of dropout is a recurrent issue in treatment of AN, suggesting that a number of patients are either unwilling or unable to engage in treatment. Dropout rates for adolescents with AN who are hospitalized are reported as high as 24% [42], and even though dropout rates are less frequent in adolescents than in adults, a 95% completion rate, as reported in the current study, is unusual—and highly promising—for this group of patients. As treatment compliance has been shown to be a facilitator for recovery and a predictor of a successful outcome [43], it is paramount that we identify therapies that increase compliance and therapy adherence.

CRT for adolescents has been administered in a variety of modes including individual delivery [19,22,35], family-CRT [44], CRT delivered in collaboration with carers [45] and in groups [39,40]. In the current study, CRT was provided individually with one therapist delivering all treatment. One major advantage of individually delivered CRT is the possibility to tailor the treatment to each specific patient. In our case, CRT sessions were dedicated exclusively to the specific needs and circumstances of each individual, and it is not unlikely that such exclusivity could have had a positive effect in strengthening the therapist–patient bond. A good therapeutic alliance is known to predict treatment adherence and better outcomes in patients with EDs [46], especially young patients [47], and previous research in eating disorders suggests that treatment satisfaction is closely related to the way in which care is delivered [48]. In the current study, the vast majority of patients chose the most favorable response outcome ("very good") when asked about the collaboration between the patient and the therapist, and the remaining therapist-specific items were answered equally, positively affirmative. Favourable outcomes, such as these, might reflect a number of aspects specific to CRT. Firstly, it is likely that the very nature of the intervention plays an important role in this type of feedback. In contrast to traditional ED treatment, CRT does not focus on core ED psychopathology such as weight, shape or eating. The lack of focus on ED symptomatology, which is often emotionally charged, might have rendered patients curious, rather than reluctant, and motivated rather than discouraged to engage and remain in treatment.

4.2. Perception of Change

In line with a recently published study by Giombini et al. [20], individuals in the current study experienced limited transferability of skills from the therapy context to their everyday lives. In Giombini et al.'s study [20], patients were asked to provide feedback on the CRT sessions as a way of evaluating the program. Although CRT was positively received by the majority of patients, a group of patients reported difficulties in understanding how CRT might be helpful in their everyday life, and what impact it would have on their recovery. In an adult CRT study by Easter and Tchanturia [49], similar findings are reported. This study used therapists' feedback letter to investigate the implementation of CRT in the patients' day-to-day life. Comparable to the current study, these patients also found it challenging when attempting to relate skills acquired in CRT to their everyday lives. A similar methodological approach, with comparable findings, was presented in a recently published study by Giombini et al. [50]. In their qualitative appraisal of young peoples' experience of individual CRT, only 13% (N = 9) of the patients were able to describe how they could use knowledge acquired during CRT sessions in their daily life. In the current study, more than half of the patients reported that they had acquired either quite a few or many skills during CRT sessions that could be useful in their everyday life. However, when probed more specifically on whether CRT had impacted the ability to change—either with regards to the eating disorder or their everyday life—the majority of patients reported "Not at all", "Very little" or "Little". These results call into question the direct transferability of in-session learning, suggesting that more work needs to be done in order to help patients to channel new insights and behaviors from the inside to the outside of the therapy room.

To the authors' knowledge, this is one of two [51] existing studies to explicitly investigate how individuals perceive everyday life and ED-related changes post CRT. Despite the majority of participants reporting being slightly more, or more, aware of how they reflect on their own thinking after CRT, our results indicate that they find the impact of CRT on the ability to change to be fairly limited. It could be argued that this is due to difficulties in evaluating one's own change. In a previous study investigating self-reported executive functioning before and after CRT, Dahlgren and colleagues [3] showed that parents reported a greater extent of change in their child's everyday behaviors, in comparison to the patients' own reports. This could be due to biased post-intervention ratings based on anticipation or wishful thinking, or it could be because adolescents have difficulties in evaluating their own behavior and potential changes in behavior and attitudes. Another explanation is that changes in cognitions and behaviors require far more than ten CRT sessions to appear, or in our case, perceived by patients themselves.

5. Strengths and Limitations

Altogether, the participants in the current study appeared to find CRT useful and relevant, and the vast majority of patients reported being very satisfied with the relationship to the CRT therapist. However, since it is well documented that a good alliance between the patient and the therapist is central to engaging patients and motivating them to stay in treatment [46,47], it is possible that the role of the therapist played an important part in treatment adherence. For example, it is difficult to differentiate "treatment satisfaction" from "therapist satisfaction". It is unknown whether the results would have changed if more than one therapist had delivered the CRT, and that such changes had been independent of the treatment per se. Further, we cannot exclude a therapist-specific contribution to the observed low dropout rate. Thus, it remains to be investigated if the results from the current study can be reproduced in other contexts with a number of therapists delivering the intervention remains. The study is also limited in terms of its sample size and the age range. It is likely that the perspective of change more easily can be reflected on and self-assessed by an individual at age 18 compared to someone at age 13. Further, as response options differed between items, it was not possible to report summary scores or merged data from the four different sections of the questionnaire. In-depth interviews could have served as an important adjunct to our questionnaire, allowing for qualitative analyses of the service user's perspective.

Finally, the study is limited by not providing anonymous feedback forms. This is a limitation not just for the current study, but for all studies that have so far been published on patients' perception of CRT. Patients' reports are likely to be biased as all patients knew that the therapist would read their feedback forms. In addition, as AN patients often have a tendency of seeking social approval [52,53], this is especially important to take into consideration when evaluating patient feedback.

6. Conclusions

The current study provides one of the most detailed accounts of the patient's perspective on CRT published for adolescent patients with AN. The findings highlight several important intervention aspects viewed through the eye of the receiver. On an overall level, patients reported CRT sessions as being both useful and relevant to their situation, and the majority of patients communicated that they were satisfied with the treatment they had received. On the other hand, and in line with a number of previous studies, the findings also indicate that patients perceived limited impact of CRT in terms of changes in their everyday-life functioning and their eating disorder. Such results warrant further investigation and a critical evaluation of treatment content, as well as of outcome measures used. Future studies might want to place an emphasis on crystalizing the primary purpose of CRT for adolescents with AN, and choose outcome measures appropriate to assess expected outcomes. If, as pointed out by Dahlgren and Rø [9], the main aim of CRT is to prepare the patients for subsequent treatment, future CRT studies should place further emphasis on motivational aspects of treatment and its likelihood of preventing drop-out, rather than focusing on the direct effect of CRT on measurable cognitive or behavioral changes.

Acknowledgments: This work was funded, in its entirety, by the Regional Department for Eating Disorders (RASP), Oslo University Hospital HF, Ullevål. Costs associated with open access publishing were also funded by RASP.

Author Contributions: Dahlgren, C.L. conceived and designed the experiments; Dahlgren, C.L. performed the experiments; Dahlgren, C.L. and Stedal, K. analyzed the data; Oslo University Hospital contributed materials/analysis tools; Dahlgren, C.L. and Stedal, K. wrote the paper.

Appendix A

Item-Specific Results from the Treatment Evaluation Questionnaire (N = 18). *Note.* Response options are presented on the *x* axis, and number of responses are presented on the *y* axis. Items with an asterisk (*) indicate fewer than N = 18 responses.

Appendix A.1 General Attitudes towards Treatment (Item 1–5)

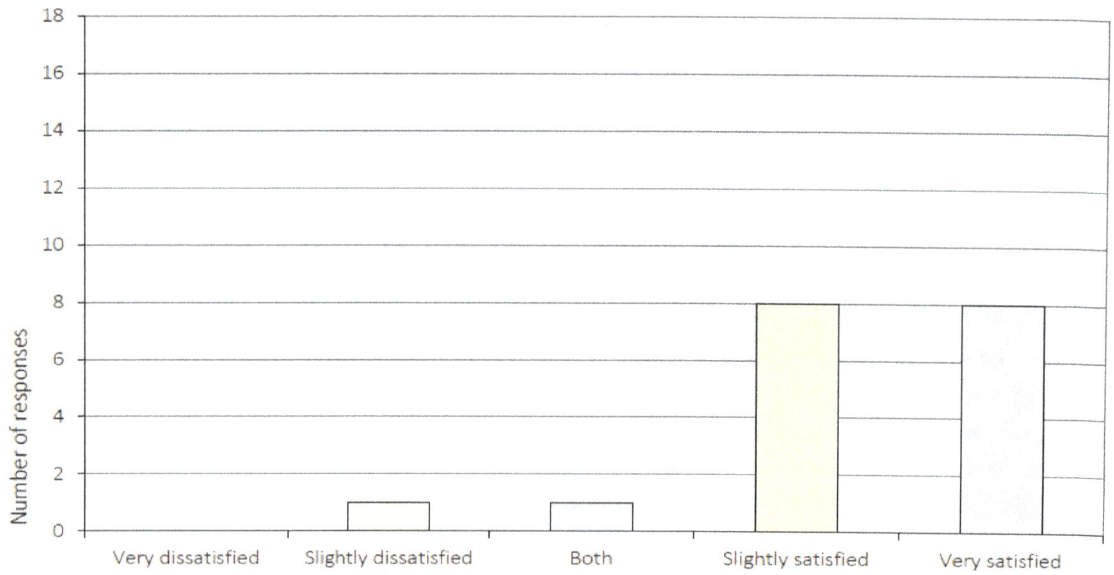

Figure A1. Overall, how satisfied or dissatisfied are you with the course of CRT that you have received?

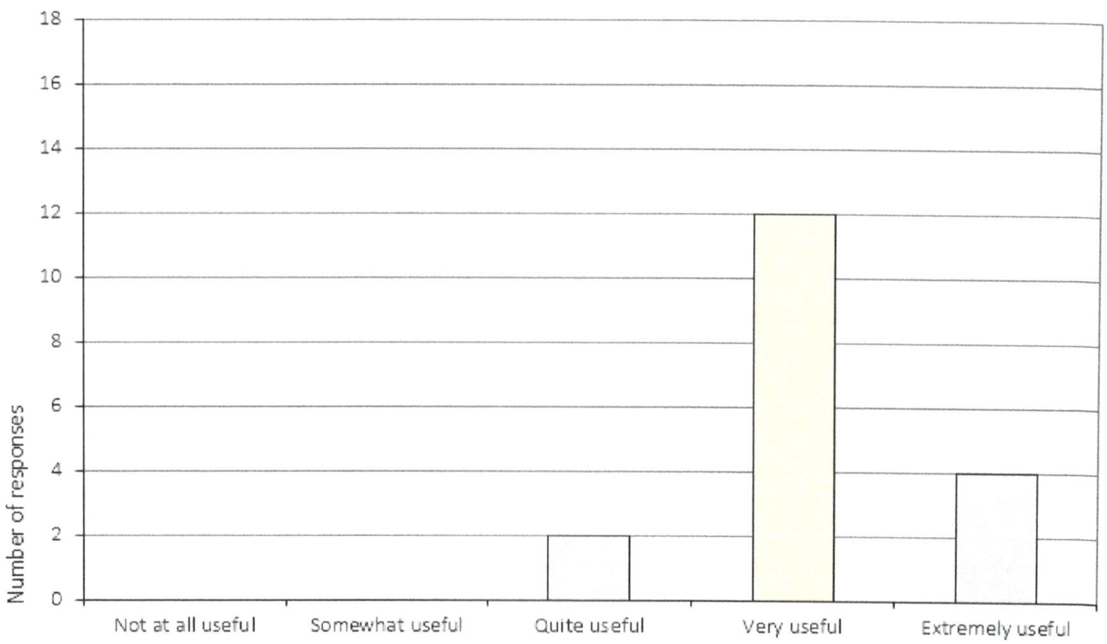

Figure A2. Before initiating CRT you were informed about the treatment. Was this information useful?

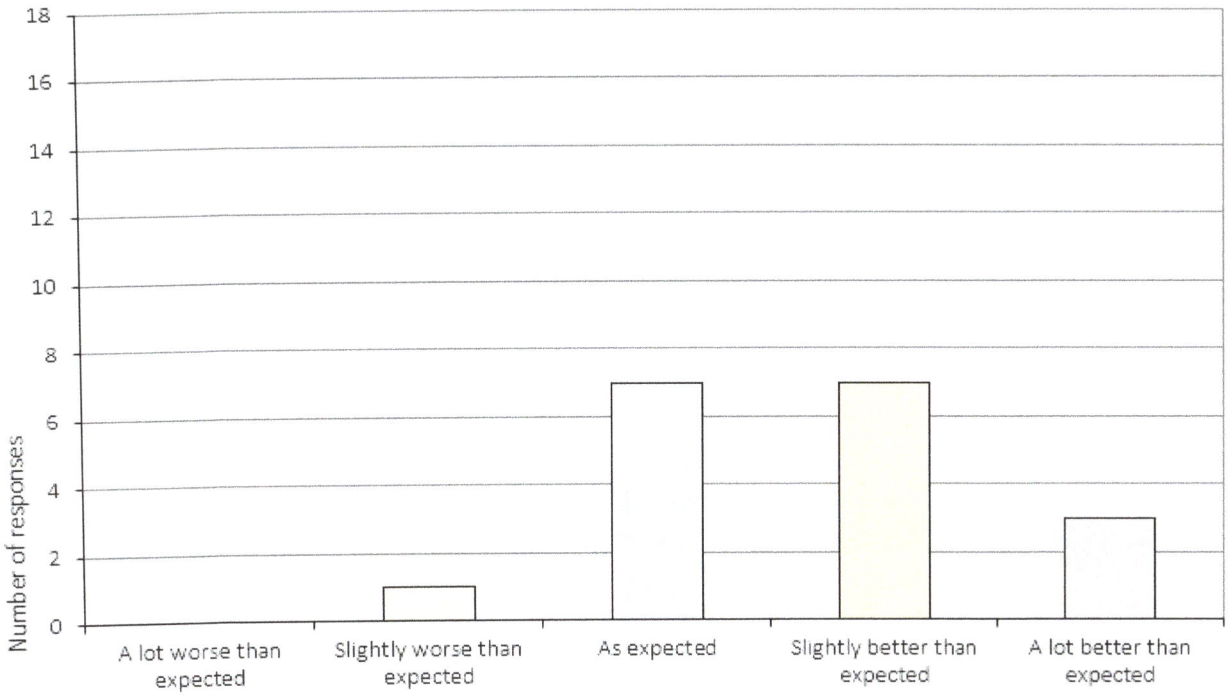

Figure A3. How did your CRT experience match the expectancies you had prior to treatment initiation?

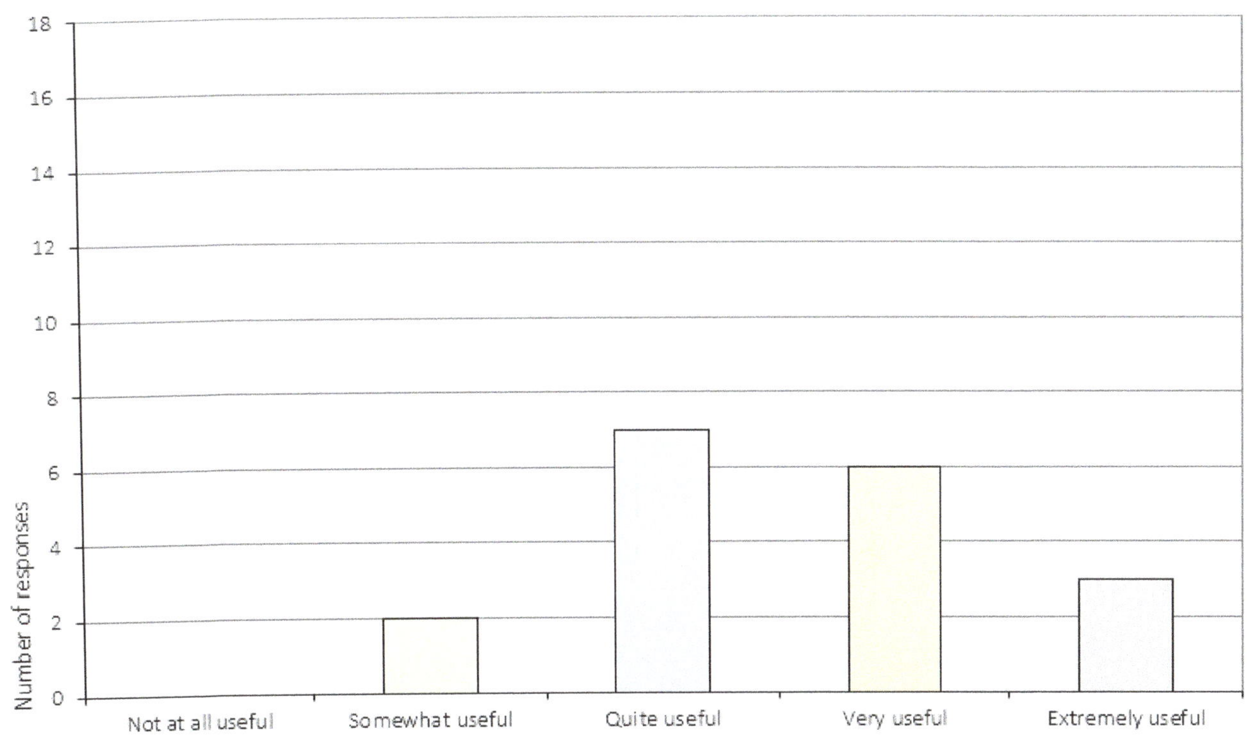

Figure A4. To what extent did you feel that the CRT sessions were useful to you?

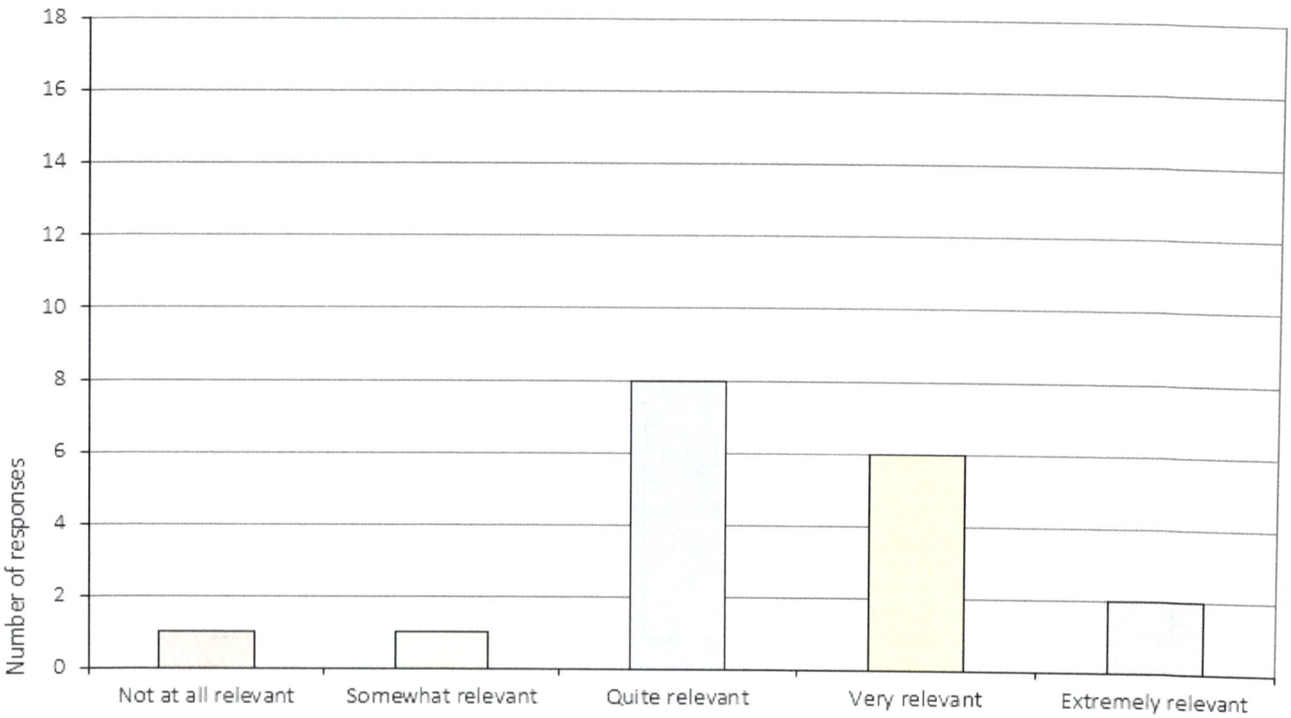

Figure A5. Did you experience CRT as being relevant to your situation?

Appendix A.2 Treatment Specific Items (Item 7–10)

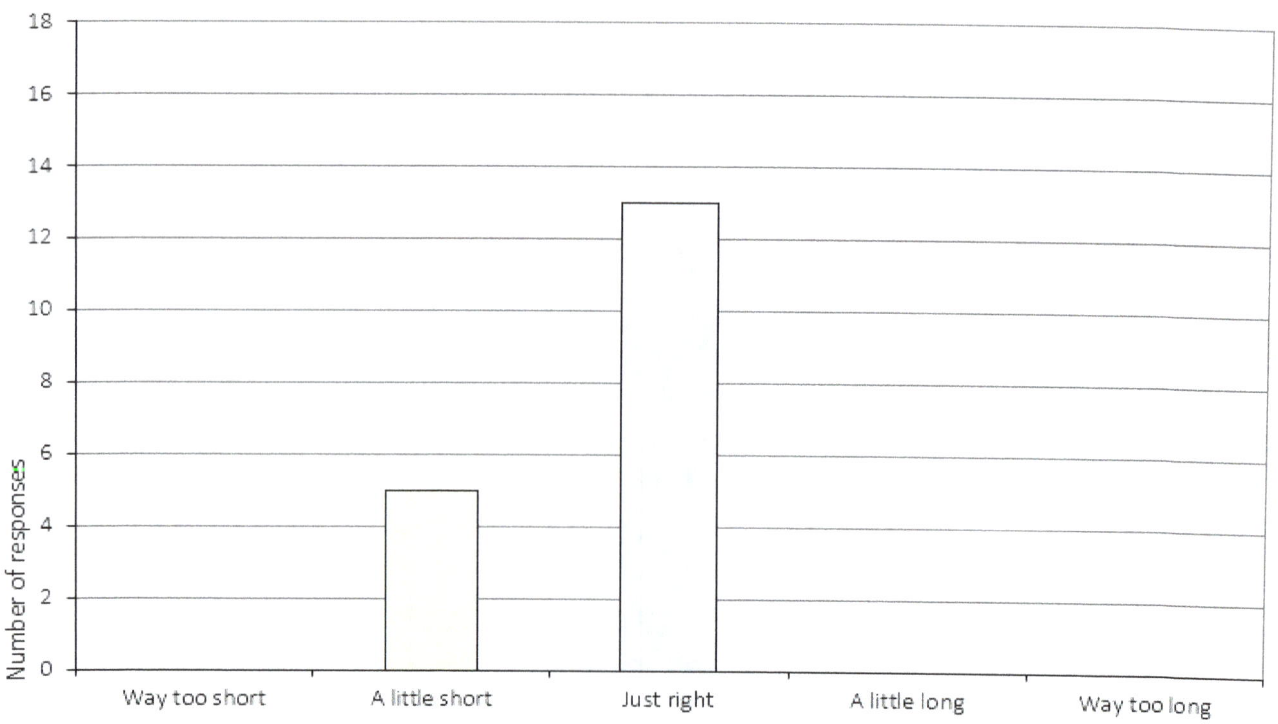

Figure A7. How did you feel about the the length of the sessions?

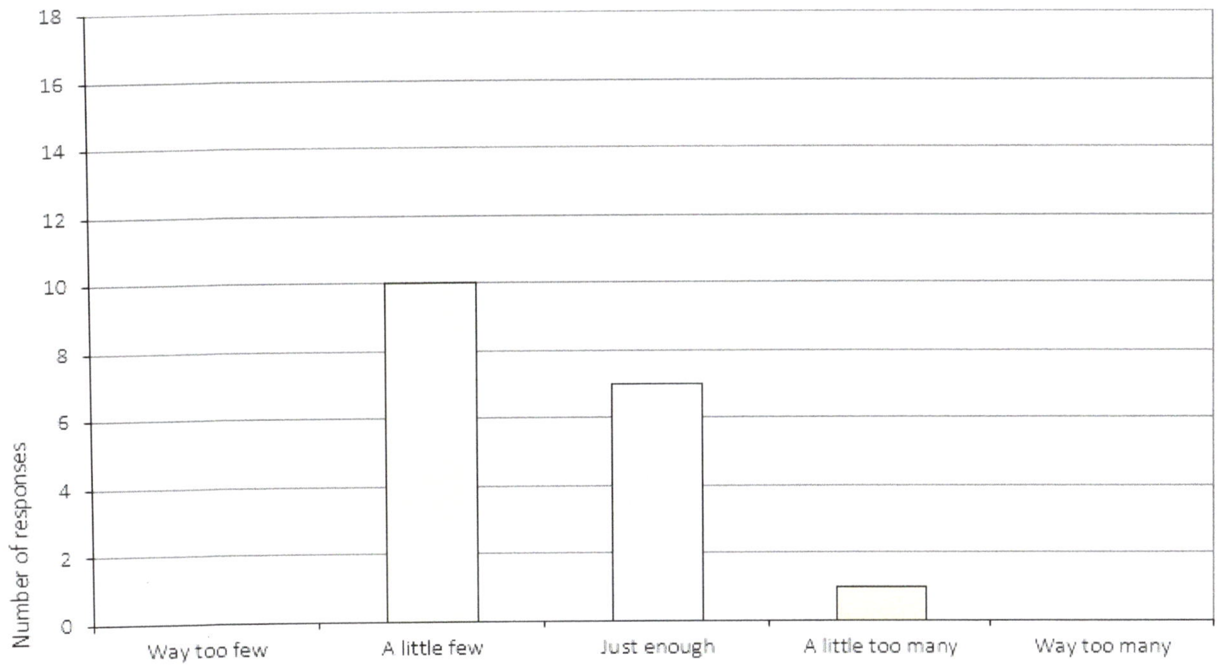

Figure A8. How did you feel about the number of session?

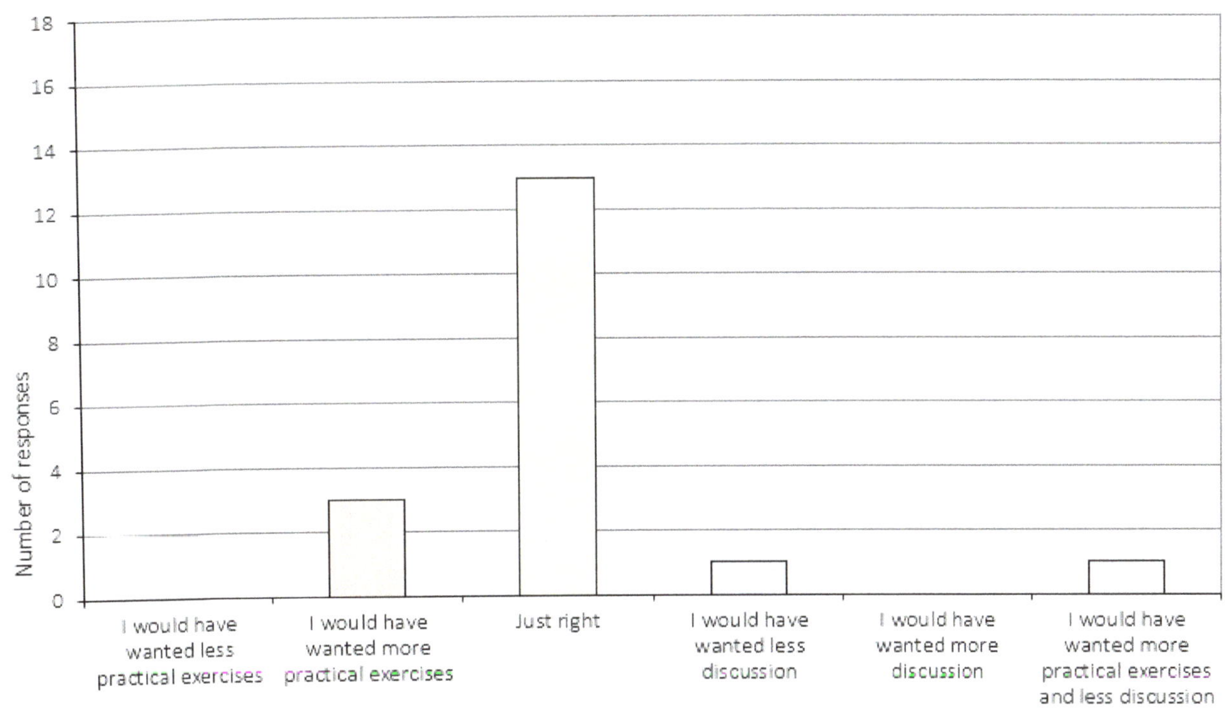

Figure A9. How did you experience the division between practical exercises and discussion during the sessions?

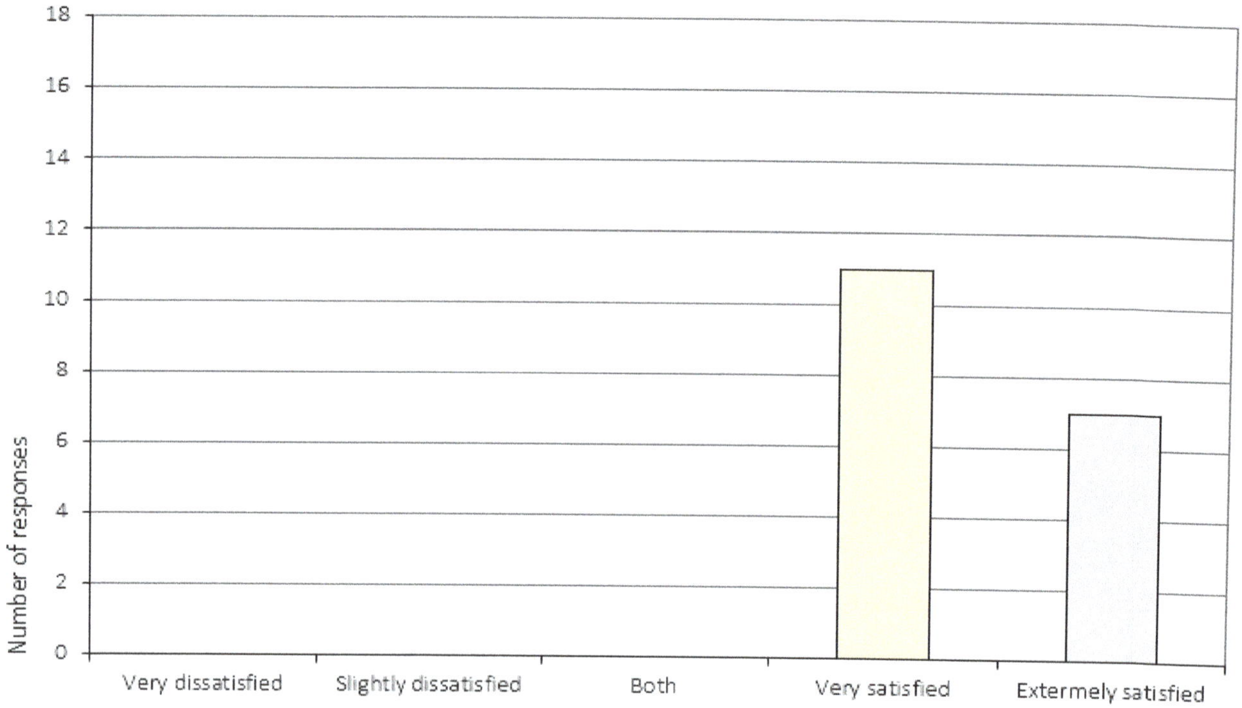

Figure A10. All in all, how satisfied or dissatisfied are you with the course of CRT that you have received?

Appendix A.3 The Perception of Change (Item 6 and 11–16c)

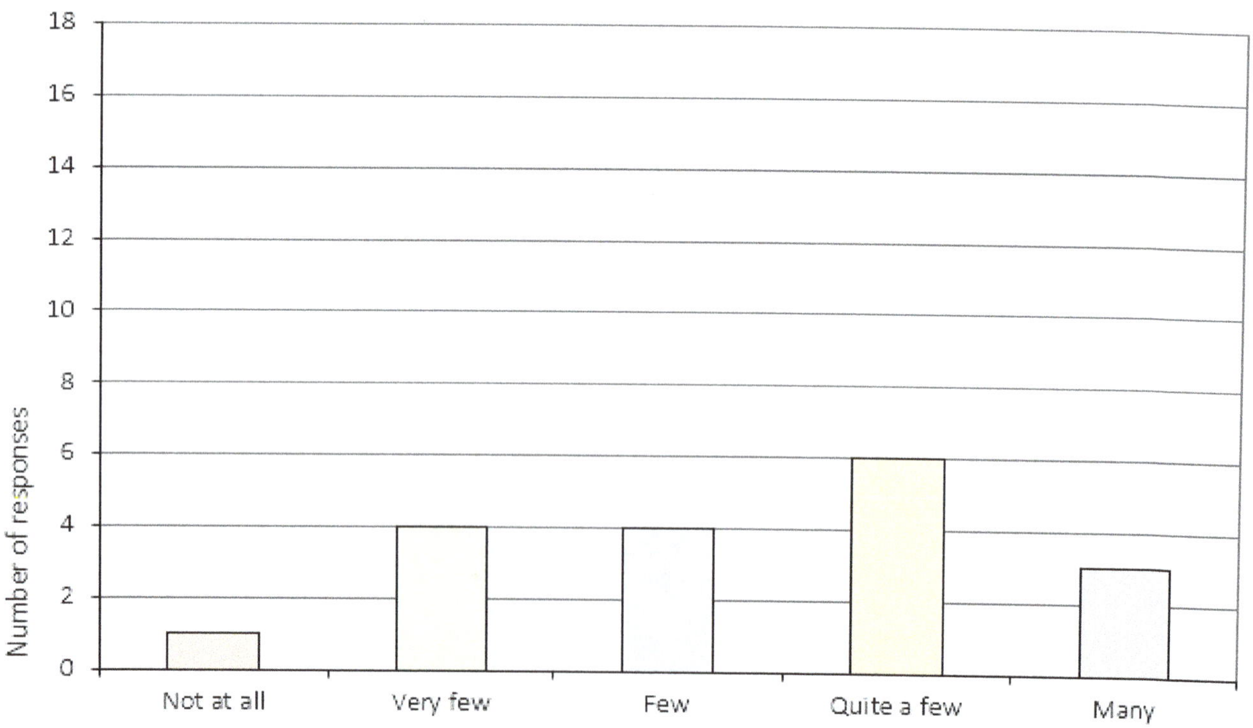

Figure A6. Did you acquire any skills during the CRT sessions that might be useful in your everyday life?

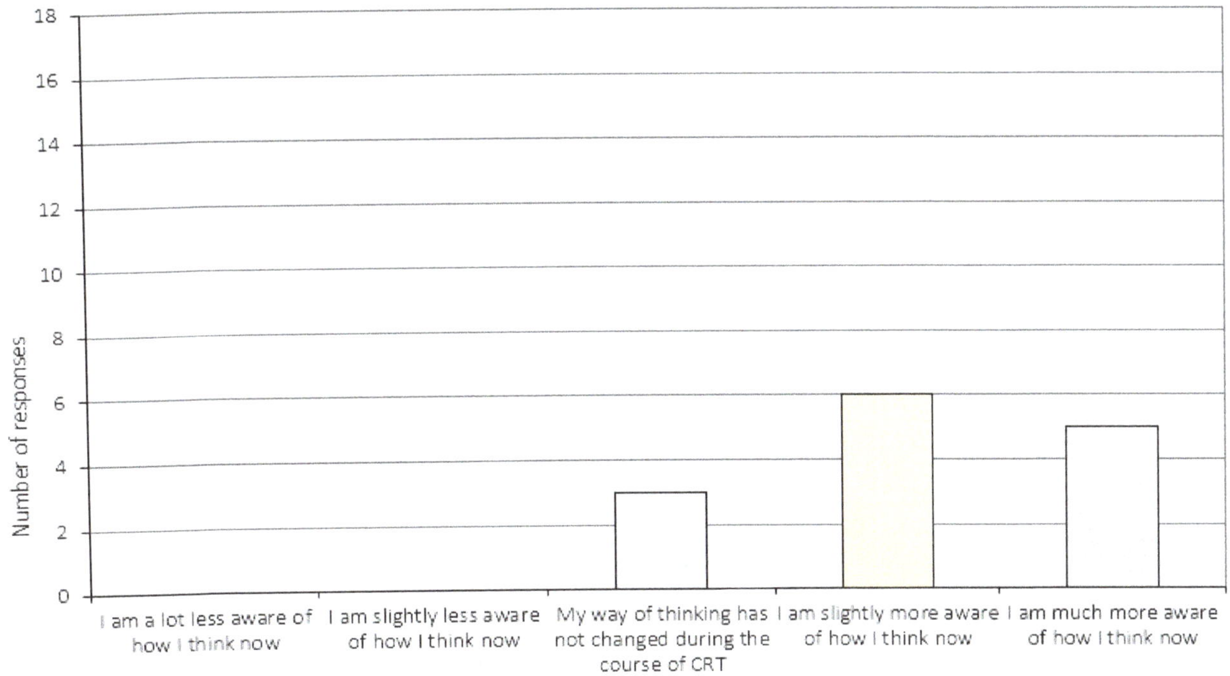

Figure A11. How has the way you reflect on your own thinking changed during the course of CRT? (*N = 14).

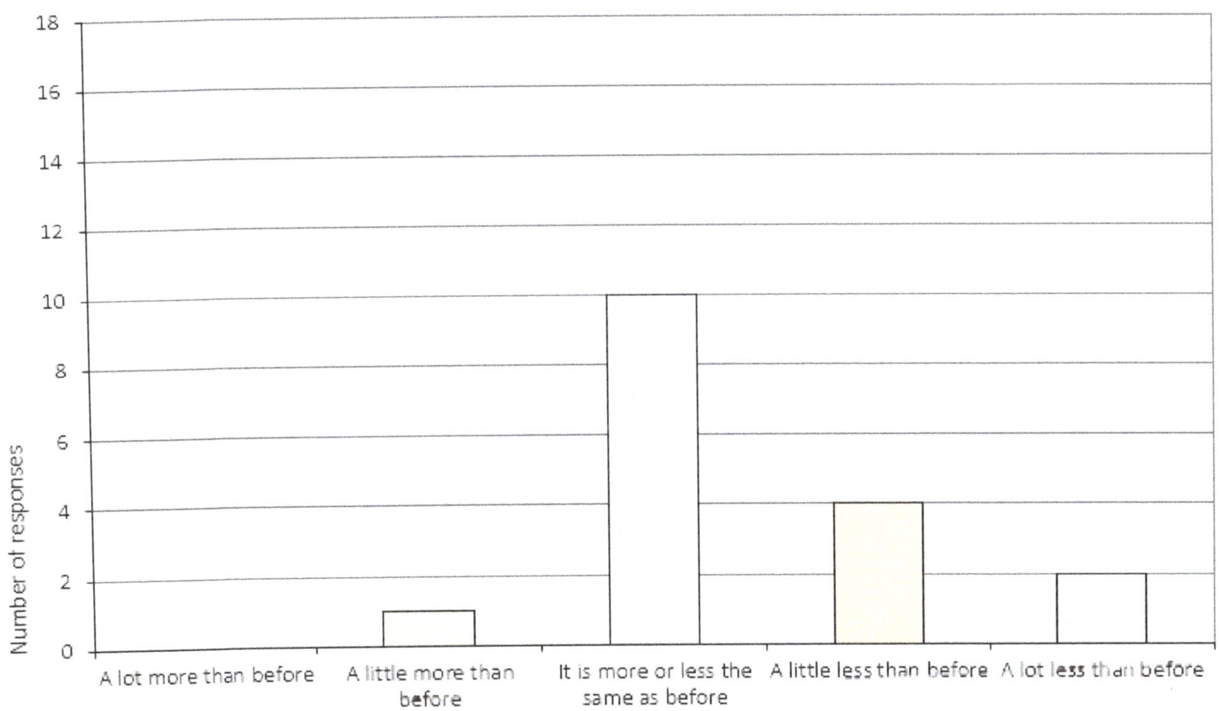

Figure A12. To what extent do you experience distress in relation to your eating disorder now, compared to before you started the CRT treatment program? (*N = 17).

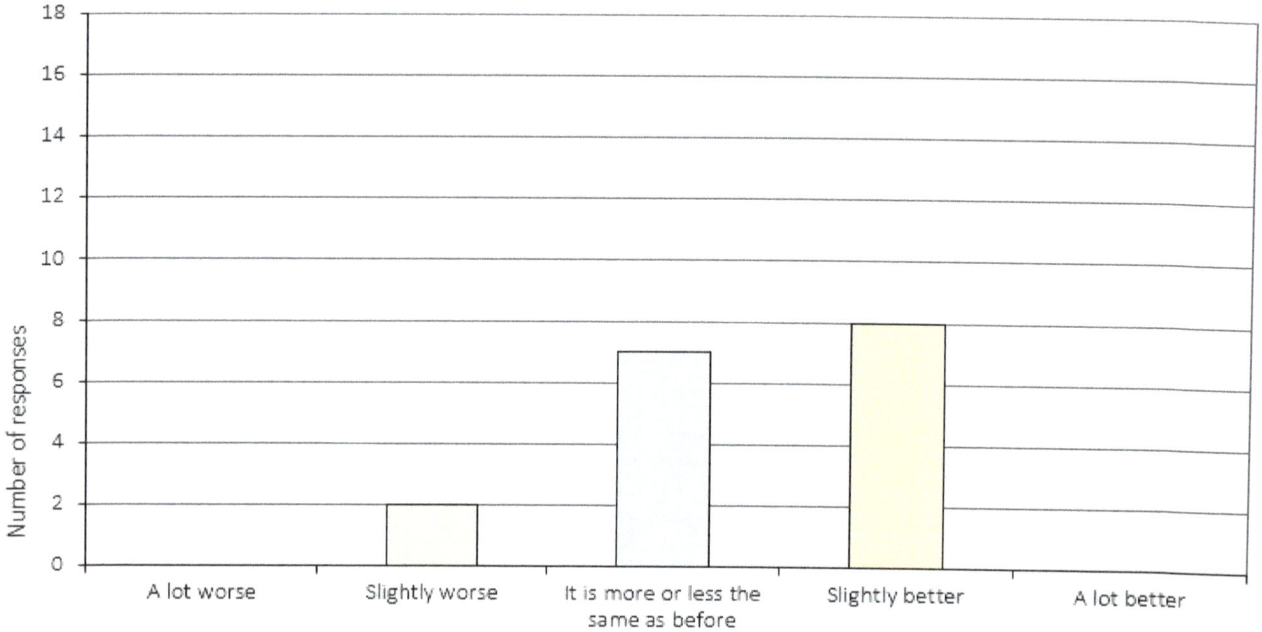

Figure A14. How is your relationship to your family now, compared to before you started the CRT treatment program? (*N = 17).

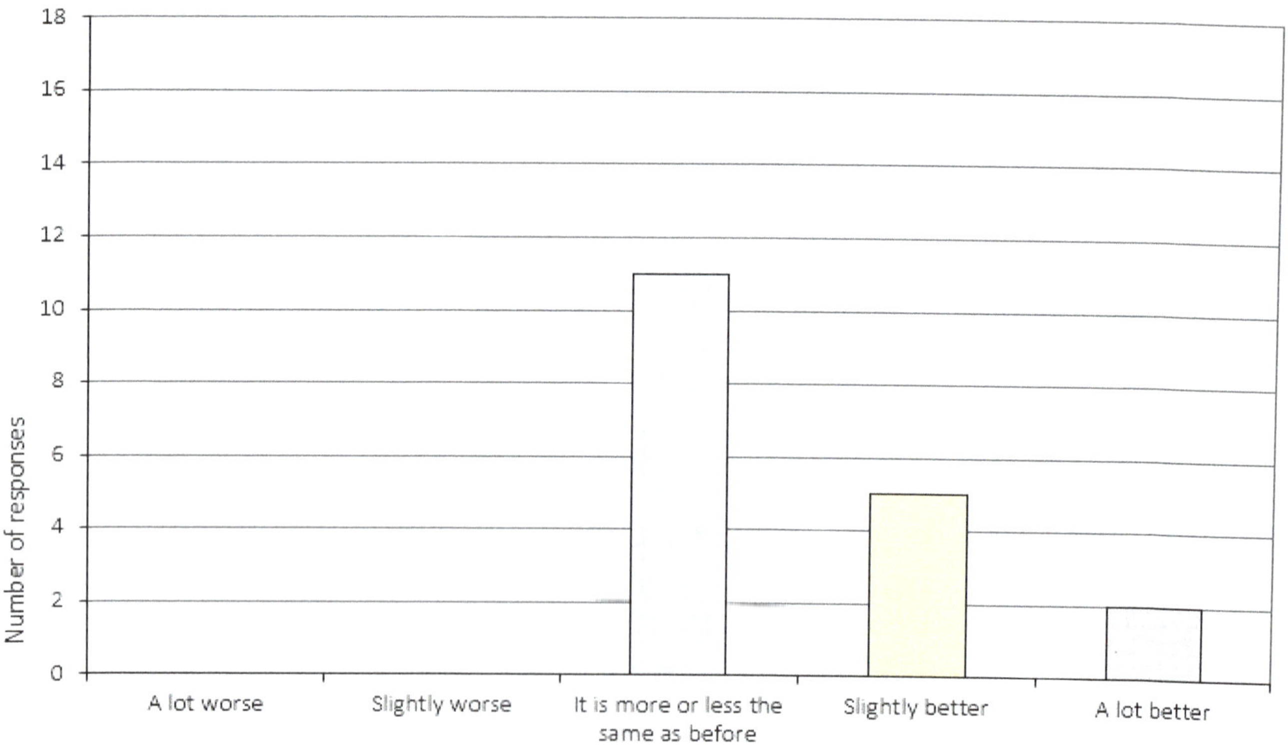

Figure A15a. How are things working out in your daily life now, compared to before you started the CRT treatment program? (**a**) School/Work.

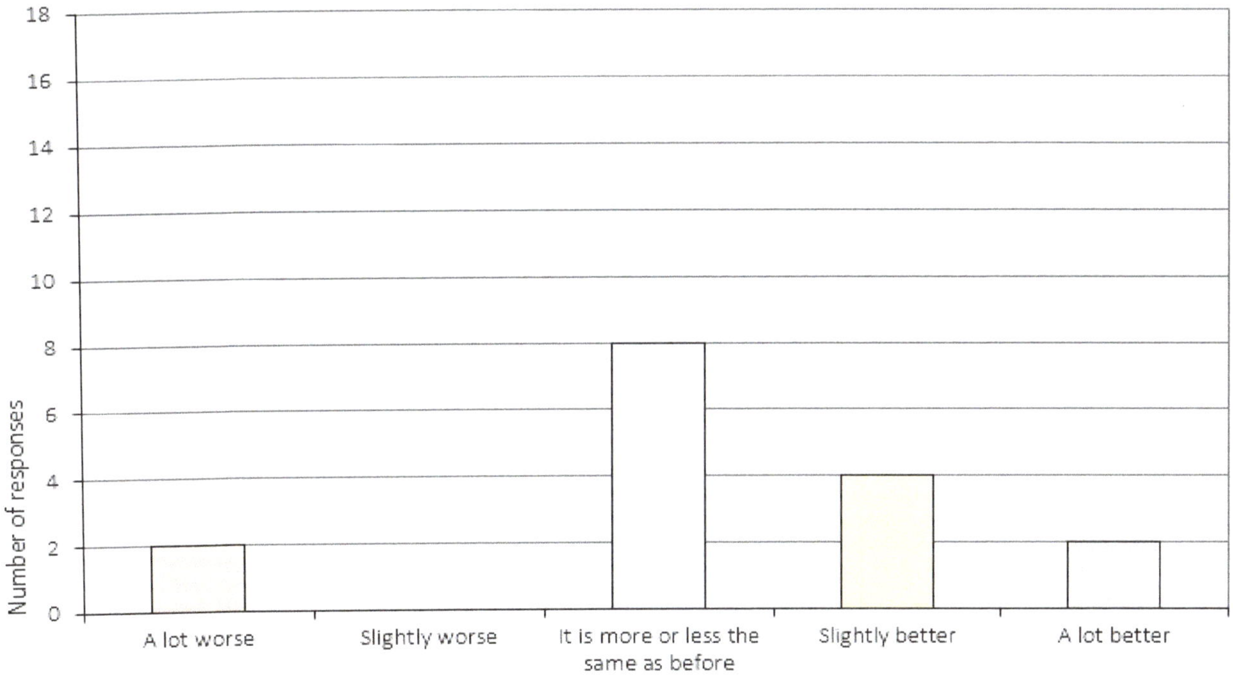

Figure A15b. How are things working out in your daily life now, compared to before you started the CRT treatment program? (b)Leisure time/friends (*N = 16).

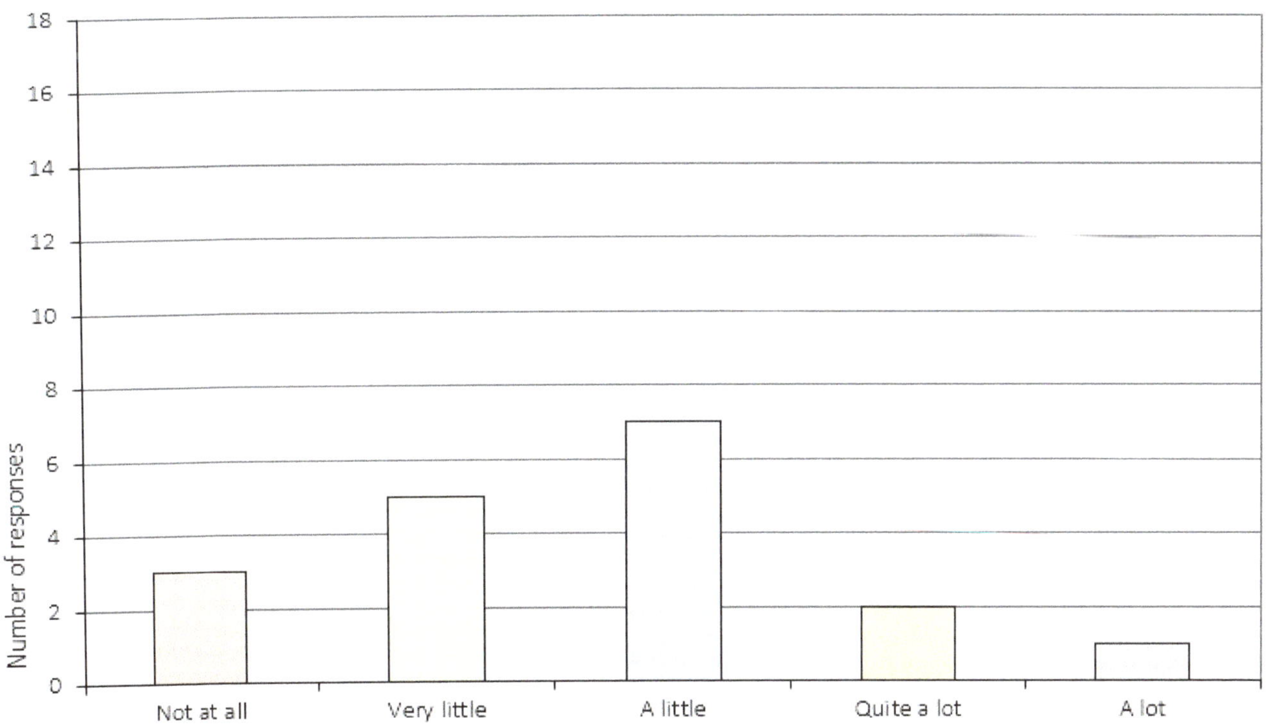

Figure A16a. Do you think the CRT sessions have had an impact on your ability to change with regards to your eating disorder?

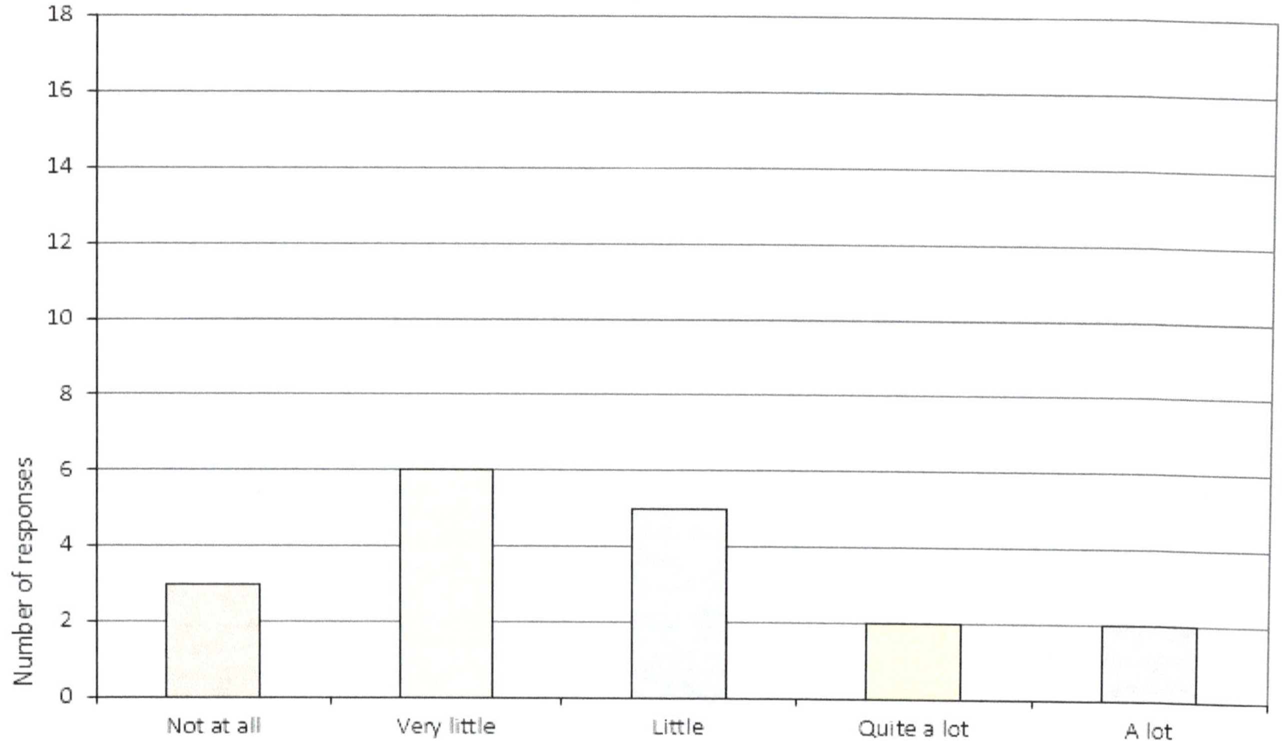

Figure A16b. Do you think the CRT sessions have had an impact on your ability to change with regards to school/work?

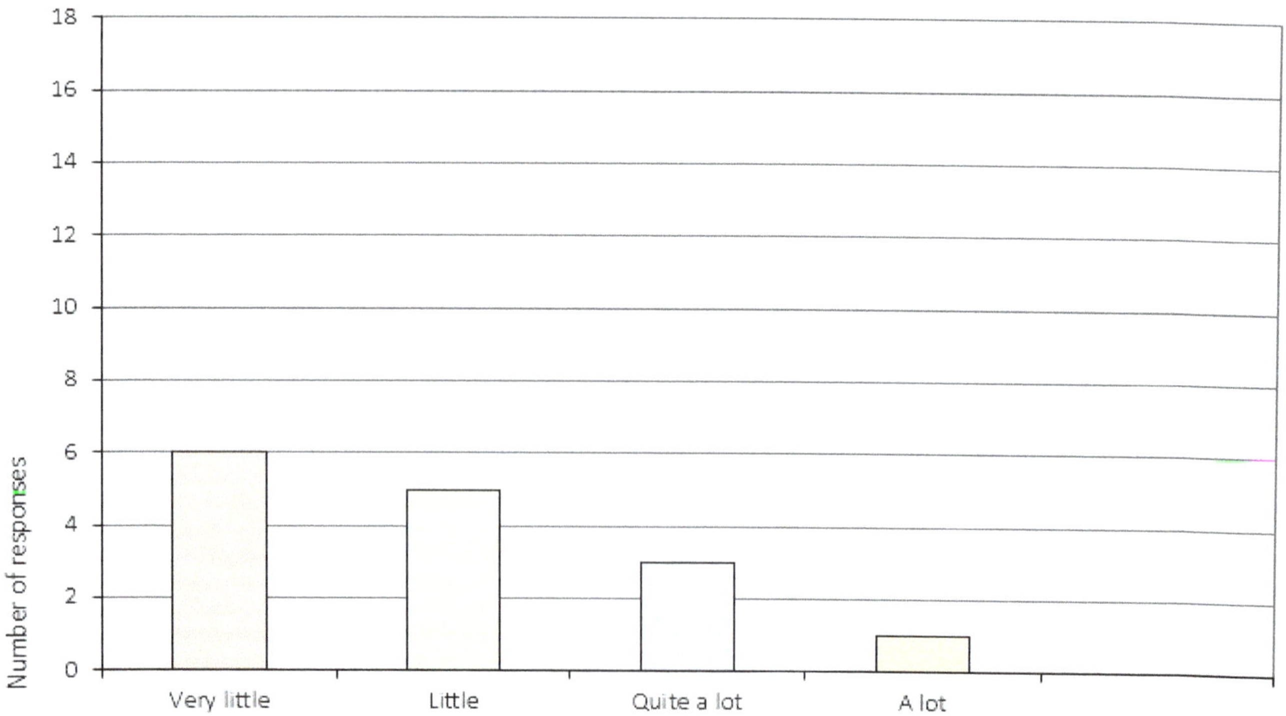

Figure A16c. Do you think the CRT sessions have had an impact on your ability to change with regards to leisure time/friends? (*N = 15).

Appendix A.4 The Relationship to the CRT Therapist (Item 17–20)

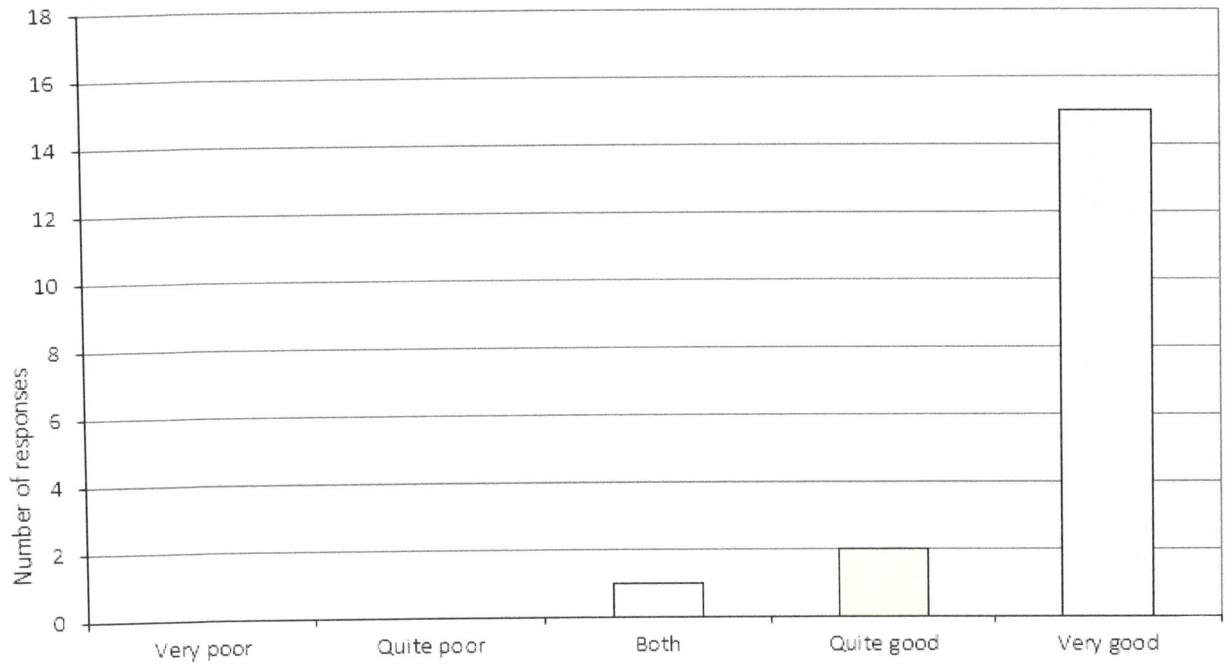

Figure A17. How did you experience the collaboration between you and your CRT therapist?

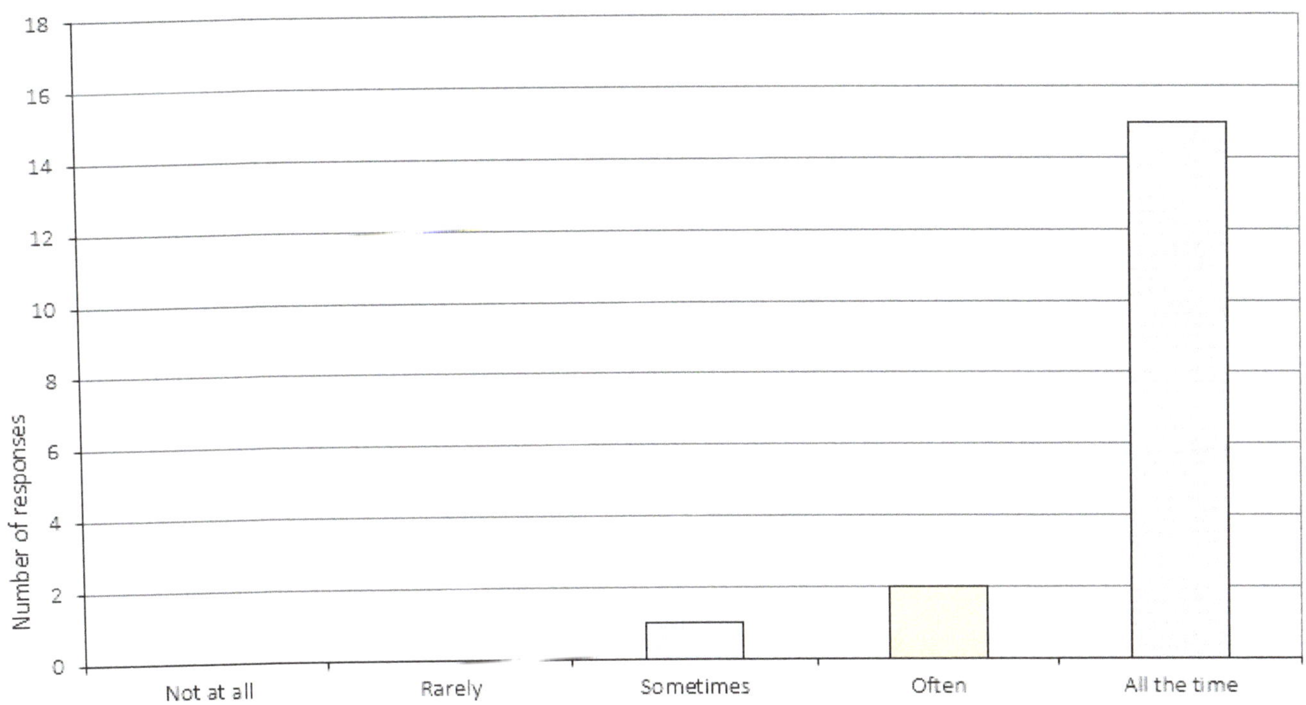

Figure A18. Were you treated with respect during the course of CRT?

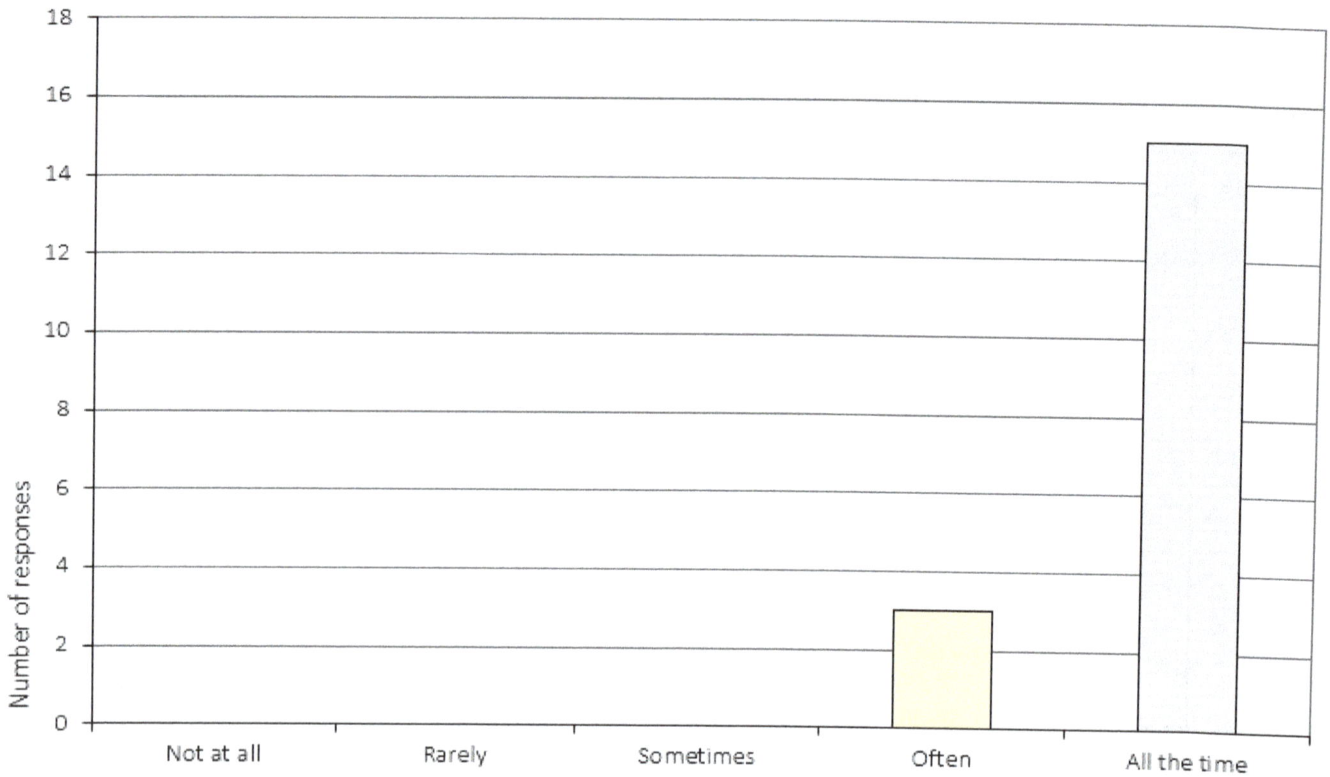

Figure A19. Did the CRT therapist listen to you?

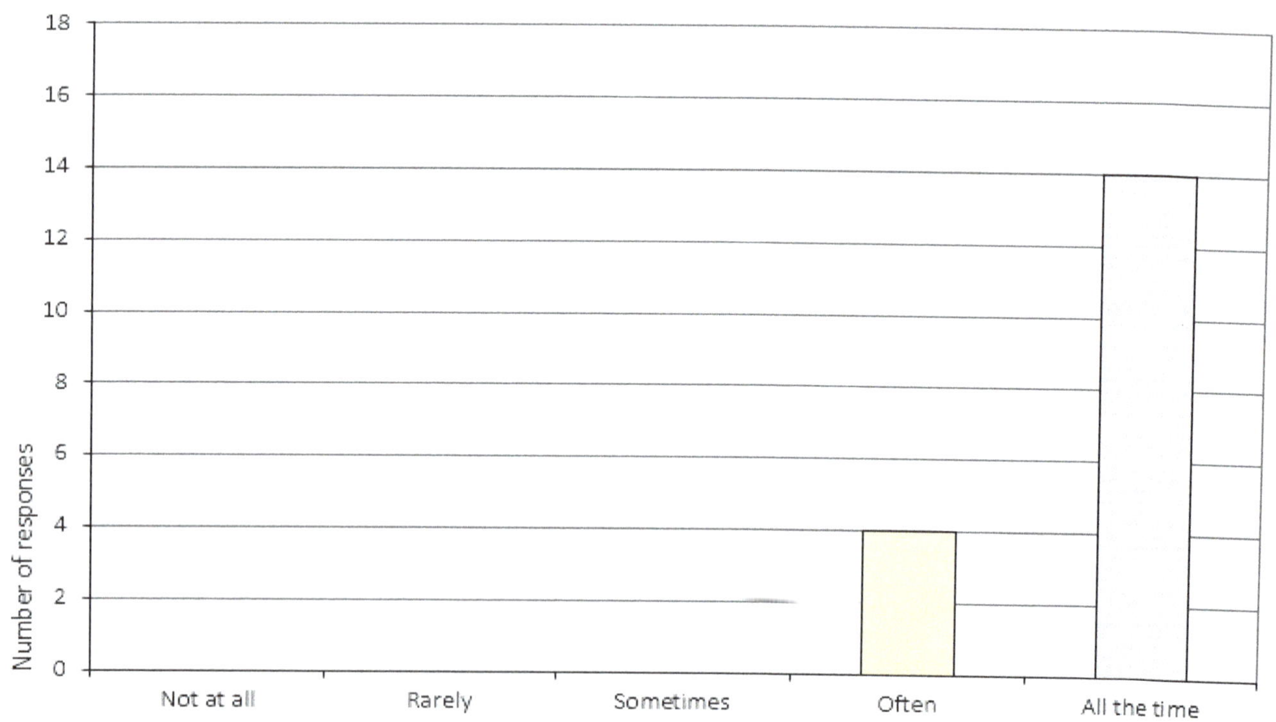

Figure A20. Did your therapist explain the tasks in a way that was easy to understand?

References

1. American Psychological Association. *Diagnostic and Statistical Manual of Mental Disorders*, 5th ed.; American Psychiatric Association: Washington, DC, USA, 2013.

2. Stedal, K.; Frampton, I.; Landrø, N.I.; Lask, B. An Examination of the Ravello Profile—A Neuropsychological Test Battery for Anorexia Nervosa. *Eur. Eat. Disord. Rev.* **2012**, *20*, 175–181.
3. Dahlgren, C.L.; Lask, B.; Landrø, N.I.; Rø, Ø. Patient and Parental Self-reports of Executive Functioning in a Sample of Young Female Adolescents with Anorexia Nervosa Before and After Cognitive Remediation Therapy. *Eur. Eat. Disord. Rev.* **2014**, *22*, 45–52. [CrossRef] [PubMed]
4. Perpina, C.; Segura, M.; Sanchez-Reales, S. Cognitive flexibility and decision-making in eating disorders and obesity. *Eat Weight Disord.* **2016**. [CrossRef]
5. Aloi, M.; Rania, M.; Caroleo, M.; Bruni, A.; Cauteruccio, M.A.; De Fazio, P.; Segura-Garcia, C. Decision making, central coherence and set-shifting: a comparison between Binge Eating Disorder, Anorexia Nervosa and Healthy Controls. *BMC Psychiatr.* **2015**, *15*, 6. [CrossRef]
6. Lang, K.; Lopez, C.; Stahl, D.; Tchanturia, K.; Treasure, J. Central Coherence in Eating Disorders: A Synthesis of Studies Using the Rey Osterrieth Complex Figure Test. *PLoS ONE* **2016**, *11*, e0165467. [CrossRef] [PubMed]
7. Lang, K.; Tchanturia, K. A systematic review of central coherence in children and adolescents with anorexia nervosa. *J. Child. Adolesc. Behav.* **2014**, *2*, 140. [CrossRef]
8. Davies, H.; Tchanturia, K. Cognitive Remediation Therapy as an Intervention for Acute Anorexia Nervosa: A Case Report. *Eur. Eat. Disord. Rev.* **2005**, *13*, 311–316. [CrossRef]
9. Dahlgren, C.; Rø, Ø. A systematic review of cognitive remediation therapy for anorexia nervosa-development, current state and implications for future research and clinical practice. *J. Eat. Disord.* **2014**, *2*, 26.
10. Brockmeyer, T.; Ingenerf, K.; Walther, S.; Wild, B.; Hartmann, M.; Herzog, W.; Bents, H.; Friederich, H.C. Training cognitive flexibility in patients with anorexia nervosa: A pilot randomized controlled trial of cognitive remediation therapy. *Int. J. Eat. Disord.* **2013**, *47*, 24–31. [CrossRef] [PubMed]
11. Lock, J.; Agras, W.S.; Fitzpatrick, K.K.; Bryson, S.W.; Jo, B.; Tchanturia, K. Is outpatient cognitive remediation therapy feasible to use in randomized clinical trials for anorexia nervosa? *Int. J. Eat. Disord.* **2013**, *46*, 567–575. [CrossRef] [PubMed]
12. Brockmeyer, T.; Ingenerf, K.; Walther, S.; Wild, B.; Hartmann, M.; Herzog, W.; Bents, H.; Friederich, H.C. Training cognitive flexibility in patients with anorexia nervosa: A pilot randomized controlled trial of cognitive remediation therapy. *Int. J. Eat. Disord.* **2014**, *47*, 24–31. [CrossRef] [PubMed]
13. Dingemans, A.E.; Danner, U.N.; Donker, J.M.; aardoom, J.J.; van Meer, F.; Tobias, K.; van Elburg, A.A.; van Furth, E.F. The effectiveness of cognitive remediation therapy in patients with a severe or enduring eating disorder: A randomized controlled trial. *Psychother. Psychosom.* **2014**, *83*, 29–36. [CrossRef] [PubMed]
14. Dahlgren, C.L.; Lask, B.; Landrø, N.I.; Rø, Ø. Developing and evaluating cognitive remediation therapy (CRT) for adolescents with anorexia nervosa: a feasibility study. *Clin. Child. Psychol. Psychiatry* **2014**, *19*, 476–487. [CrossRef] [PubMed]
15. Tchanturia, K.; Lounes, N.; Holttum, S. Cognitive remediation in anorexia nervosa and related conditions: A systematic review. *Eur. Eat. Disord. Rev.* **2014**, *22*, 454–462. [CrossRef] [PubMed]
16. van Noort, B.M.; Kraus, M.K.A.; Pfeiffer, E.; Lehmkuhl, U.; Kappel, V. Neuropsychological and Behavioural Short-Term Effects of Cognitive Remediation Therapy in Adolescent Anorexia Nervosa: A Pilot Study. *Eur. Eat. Disord. Rev.* **2016**, *24*, 69–74. [CrossRef] [PubMed]
17. Tchanturia, K.; Davies, H.; Reeder, C.; Wykes, T. Cognitive Remediation Therapy for Anorexia Nervosa. 2010. Available online: www.katetchanturia.com (accessed on 2 March 2017).
18. Owen, I.; Lindvall, C.L.; Lask, B. Cognitive Remediation Therapy. In *Eating Disorders in Childhood and Adolescence*; Lask, B., Bryant-Waugh, R., Eds.; Routledge: New York, NY, USA, 2013; pp. 301–318.
19. Giombini, L.; Moynihan, J.; Turco, M.; Nesbitt, S. Evaluation of individual cognitive remediation therapy (CRT) for the treatment of young people with anorexia nervosa. *Eat. Weight. Disord.* **2016**. [CrossRef] [PubMed]
20. Giombini, L.; Turton, R.; Turco, M.; Nesbitt, S.; Lask, B. The use of cognitive remediation therapy on a child adolescent eating disorder unit: Patients and therapist perspectives. *Clin. Child. Psychol. Psychiatry* **2017**, *22*, 288–300. [CrossRef] [PubMed]
21. van Noort, B.M.; Pfeiffer, E.; Ehrlich, S.; Lehmkuhl, U.; Kappel, V. Cognitive performance in children with acute early-onset anorexia nervosa. *Eur. Child. Adolesc. Psychiatry.* **2016**, *25*, 1233–1244. [CrossRef] [PubMed]
22. van Noort, B.M.; Pfeiffer, E.; Lehmkuhl, U.; Kappel, V. Cognitive Remediation Therapy for Children with Anorexia Nervosa. *Z. Kinder. Jugendpsychiatr. Psychother.* **2015**, *43*, 351–355. [CrossRef] [PubMed]

23. Doran, D.; Smith, P. Measuring service quality provision within an eating disorders context. *Int. J. Health. Care Qual. Assur. Inc. Leadersh. Health Serv.* **2004**, *17*, 377–388. [CrossRef] [PubMed]
24. Newton, T. Consumer involvement in the appraisal of treatment for people with eating disorders: A neglected area of research? *Eur. Eat. Disord. Rev.* **2001**, *9*, 301–308. [CrossRef]
25. Bell, L. What can we learn from consumer studies and qualitative research in the treatment of eating disorders? *Eat. Weight Disord.* **2003**, *8*, 181–187. [CrossRef] [PubMed]
26. de la Rie, S.; Noordenbos, G.; Donker, M.; van Furth, E. Evaluating the treatment of eating disorders from the patient's perspective. *Int. J. Eat. Disord.* **2006**, *39*, 667–676. [CrossRef] [PubMed]
27. Wechsler, D. *Wechsler Adult Intelligence Scale-Third Edition (WAIS-III)*; Harcourt Assessment: London, UK, 1997.
28. Wechsler, D. *Wechsler Abbreviated Scale of Intelligence (WASI)*; NCS Pearson Inc.: San Antonio, TX, USA, 1999.
29. Wechsler, D. *Wechsler Intelligence Scale for Children-Third Edition (WISC-III)*; The Psychological Corporation Europe: London, UK, 1992.
30. Fairburn, C.G.; Beglin, S.J. Assessment of Eating Disorders, Interview or Self-Report Questionnaire. *Int. J. Eat. Disord.* **1994**, *16*, 363–370. [PubMed]
31. Beck, A.T.; Steer, R.A.; Brown, G.K. *Manual for the Beck Depression Inventory-II*; Psychological Corporation: San Antonio, TX, USA, 1996.
32. Spielberger, C.D.; Goursuch, R.; Lushene, R. *Manual for the State Trait Anxiety Inventory*; Consulting Psychologists Press: Mountain View, CA, USA, 1983.
33. Dahlgren, C.L. *Cognitive Remediation Therapy for Young Female Adolescents with Anorexia Nervosa—Assessing the Feasibility of a Novel Eating Disorder Intervention*; Oslo University Hospital: Oslo, Norway, 2014.
34. Lindvall, C.; Owen, I.; Lask, B. *The CRT Resource Pack for Children and Adolescents with Anorexia Nervosa*; Oslo University Hospital: Ullevål HF, Oslo, Norway, 2010; Available online: http://www.researchgate.com (accessed on 1 April 2016).
35. Dahlgren, C.L.; Lask, B.; Landrø, N.I.; Rø, Ø. Neuropsychological functioning in adolescents with anorexia nervosa before and after cognitive remediation therapy: A feasibility trial. *Int. J. Eat. Disord* **2013**, *46*, 576–581.
36. Dahlgren, C.L.; van Noort, B.M.; Lask, B. *The Cognitive Remediation Therapy (CRT) Resource Pack for Children and Adolescents with Feeding and Eating Disorders*, 2nd ed.; Oslo University Hospital: Oslo, Norway, 2015; Available online: http://www.rasp.no/ (accessed on 1 January 2017).
37. Holmboe, O.; Groven, G.; Olsen, R.V. *Brukererfaringer med poliklinikker for voksne i det psykiske helsevernet 2007*; PasOpp-rapport nr 6-2008 fra Kunnskapssenteret; Norwegian Knowledge Centre for the Health Services: Olso, Norway, 2008.
38. Lago, C.; Norring, C.; Engström, I. Enkät om behandlingstillfredsställelse: RIKSÄT: Nationellt Kvalitetsregister för Ätstörningsbehandling. Available online: http://kcp.se/kvalitetsregister/riksat/arbetsmaterial-dokument/ (accessed on 15 January 2010).
39. Pretorius, N.; Dimmer, M.; Power, E.; Eisler, I.; Simic, M.; Tcanturia, K. Evaluation of a cognitive remediation therapy group for adolescents with anorexia nervosa: Pilot study. *Eur. Eat. Disord. Rev.* **2012**, *20*, 321–325. [CrossRef] [PubMed]
40. Wood, L.; Al-Khairulla, H.; Lask, B. Group cognitive remediation therapy for adolescents with anorexia nervosa. *Clin. Child Psychol. Psychiatry* **2011**, *16*, 225–231. [CrossRef] [PubMed]
41. Halvorsen, I.; Heyerdahl, S. Treatment perception in adolescent onset anorexia nervosa: Retrospective views of patients and parents. *Int. J. Eat. Disord.* **2007**, *40*, 629–639. [CrossRef] [PubMed]
42. Roux, H.; Ali, A.; Lambert, S.; Radon, L.; Huas, C.; Curt, F.; Berthoz, S.; Godart, N. Predictive factors of dropout from inpatient treatment for anorexia nervosa. *BMC Psychiatr.* **2016**, *16*, 339. [CrossRef] [PubMed]
43. Towell, D.B.; Woodford, S.; Reid, S.; Rooney, B.; Towell, A. Compliance and outcome in treatment-resistant anorexia and bulimia: A retrospective study. *Br. J. Clin. Psychol.* **2001**, *40*, 189–195. [CrossRef] [PubMed]
44. Lask, B.; Roberts, A. Family cognitive remediation therapy for anorexia nervosa. *Clin. Child Psychol. Psychiatr.* **2015**, *20*, 207–217. [CrossRef] [PubMed]
45. Lang, K.; Treasure, J.; Tchanturia, K. Acceptability and feasibility of self-help Cognitive Remediation Therapy for anorexia nervosa delivered in collaboration with carers: A qualitative preliminary evaluation study. *Psychiatry Res.* **2015**, *225*, 387–394. [CrossRef] [PubMed]

46. Graves, T.A.; Tabri, N.; Thompson-Brenner, H.; Franko, D.L.; Eddy, K.T.; Bourion-Bedes, S.; Brown, A.; Constantino, M.J.; Fluckiger, C.; Forsberg, S.; et al. A meta-analysis of the relation between therapeutic alliance and treatment outcome in eating disorders. *Int. J. Eat. Disord.* **2017**, *50*, 323–340. [CrossRef] [PubMed]
47. Zaitsoff, S.; Pullmer, R.; Cyr, M.; Aime, H. The role of the therapeutic alliance in eating disorder treatment outcomes: A systematic review. *Eat. Disord.* **2015**, *23*, 99–114. [CrossRef] [PubMed]
48. Gulliksen, K.S.; Espeset, E.M.; Nordbø, R.H.; Skårderud, F.; Geller, J.; Holte, A. Preferred therapist characteristics in treatment of anorexia nervosa: The patient's perspective. *Int. J. Eat. Disord.* **2012**, *45*, 932–941. [CrossRef] [PubMed]
49. Easter, A.; Tchanturia, K. Therapists' experiences of cognitive remediation therapy for anorexia nervosa: Implications for working with adolescents. *Clin. Child Psychol. Psychiatr.* **2011**, *16*, 233–246. [CrossRef] [PubMed]
50. Giombini, L.; Nesbitt, S.; Waples, L.; Finazzi, E.; Easter, A.; Tchanturia, K. Young people's experience of individual cognitive remediation therapy (CRT) in an inpatient eating disorder service: A qualitative study. *Eat. Weight Disord.* **2017**. [CrossRef]
51. Whitney, J.; Easter, A.; Tchanturia, K. Service users' feedback on cognitive training in the treatment of anorexia nervosa: A qualitative study. *Int. J. Eat. Disord.* **2008**, *41*, 542–550. [CrossRef] [PubMed]
52. Strober, M. Personality and symptomatological features in young, nonchronic anorexia nervosa patients. *J. Psychosom. Res.* **1980**, *24*, 353–359. [CrossRef]
53. Amianto, F.; Abbate-Daga, G.; Morando, S.; Sobrero, C.; Fassino, S. Personality development characteristics of women with anorexia nervosa, their healthy siblings and healthy controls: What prevents and what relates to psychopathology? *Psychiatr. Res.* **2011**, *187*, 401–408. [CrossRef] [PubMed]

13

Association between Body Mass Index and All-Cause Mortality in Hypertensive Adults: Results from the China Stroke Primary Prevention Trial (CSPPT)

Wei Yang [1], Jian-Ping Li [1], Yan Zhang [1], Fang-Fang Fan [1], Xi-Ping Xu [2], Bin-Yan Wang [2], Xin Xu [2], Xian-Hui Qin [2], Hou-Xun Xing [3], Gen-Fu Tang [3], Zi-Yi Zhou [3], Dong-Feng Gu [4], Dong Zhao [5] and Yong Huo [1,*]

1. Department of Cardiology, Peking University First Hospital, Beijing 100034, China; ywyy2008@163.com (W.Y.); lijianping@medmail.com.cn (J.-P.L.); drzhy1108@163.com (Y.Z.); fang9020@126.com (F.-F.F.)
2. National Clinical Research Center for Kidney Disease, State Key Laboratory for Organ Failure Research, Renal Division, Nanfang Hospital, Southern Medical University, Guangzhou 510515, China; xipingxu126@126.com (X.-P.X.); binyanwang126@126.com (B.-Y.W.); xux007@163.com (X.X.); xianhuiqin@126.com (X.-H.Q.)
3. Institute for Biomedicine, Anhui Medical University, Hefei 230032, China; ausachina@163.com (H.-X.X.); tanggenfu@163.com (G.-F.T.); zhouziyi19920319@126.com (Z.-Y.Z.)
4. State Key Laboratory of Cardiovascular Disease, Fuwai Hospital, National Center for Cardiovascular Diseases, Chinese Academy of Medical Sciences and Peking Union Medical College, Beijing 100037, China; gudongfeng@vip.sina.com
5. Department of Epidemiology, Beijing Anzhen Hospital, Capital Medical University, Beijing Institute of Heart, Lung and Blood Vessel Diseases, Beijing 100029, China; deezhao@vip.sina.com

* Correspondence: huoyong@263.net.cn

Abstract: The association between elevated body mass index (BMI) and risk of death has been reported in many studies. However, the association between BMI and all-cause mortality for hypertensive Chinese adults remains unclear. We conducted a post-hoc analysis using data from the China Stroke Primary Prevention Trial (CSPPT). Cox regression analysis was performed to determine the significance of the association of BMI with all-cause mortality. During a mean follow-up duration of 4.5 years, 622 deaths (3.0%) occurred among the 20,694 participants aged 45–75 years. A reversed J-shaped relationship was observed between BMI and all-cause mortality. The hazard ratios (HRs) for underweight (<18.5 kg/m^2), overweight (24.0–27.9 kg/m^2), and obesity (≥28.0 kg/m^2) were calculated relative to normal weight (18.5–23.9 kg/m^2). The summary HRs were 1.56 (95% CI, 1.11–2.18) for underweight, 0.78 (95% CI 0.64–0.95) for overweight and 0.64 (95% CI, 0.48–0.85) for obesity. In sex-age-specific analyses, participants over 60 years of age had optimal BMI in the obesity classification and the results were consistent in both males and females. Relative to normal weight, underweight was associated with significantly higher mortality. Excessive weight was not associated with increased risk of mortality. Chinese hypertensive adults had the lowest mortality in grade 1 obesity.

Keywords: obesity; body mass index; mortality; hypertension; China

---

1. Introduction

Obesity is a global epidemic issue that is highly prevalent in both developed and developing countries; it affects people of both sexes and all ages, has adverse health consequences, accrues large economic costs, and has negative social implications [1]. Body mass index (BMI), defined as weight in kilograms divided by the square of the height in meters, is commonly used in clinical practice to screen for overweight and obesity and to guide weight loss recommendations. In China, an increasingly large proportion of the population has a BMI $\geqslant$ 25 kg/m^2, the standard definition of overweight [2]. Although obesity has been demonstrated to be associated with multiple non-communicable diseases, including hypertension, type 2 diabetes, coronary heart disease, stroke and several cancers [3], the association between BMI and all-cause mortality remains controversial: a direct association, a J-shaped, a U-shaped, or a reversed J-shaped relationship have all been recently reported [4–8].

The World Health Organization (WHO) defines the following six categories based on BMI values: <18.5 kg/m^2 = underweight; 18.5 to 24.9 kg/m^2 = normal weight; 25.0 to 29.9 kg/m^2 = overweight; 30.0 to 34.9 kg/m^2 = grade 1 obesity; 35.0 to 39.9 kg/m^2 = grade 2 obesity; and $\geqslant$40 kg/m^2 = grade 3 obesity [9]. These definitions of overweight and obesity are mainly based on criteria derived from studies that involved populations of European origin. It has been suggested that the associations of BMI with body composition and health outcomes may differ between Asian and European populations [10]. The BMI cut-off points for overweight and obesity should be lower for Asian populations than they are for European populations (suggested cut-off points for Asians are $\geqslant$23.0 kg/m^2 for overweight and $\geqslant$27.5 kg/m^2 for obesity) [10]. However, a consensus statement from the WHO concluded that the available data were not sufficient to support Asian-specific cut-off points [10]. The Ministry of Health of the People's Republic of China determined a reclassification of BMI for Chinese adults that differs from the WHO classification: underweight (<18.5 kg/m^2), normal weight (18.5–23.9 kg/m^2), overweight (24.0–27.9 kg/m^2) and obesity ($\geqslant$28.0 kg/m^2) [11].

For decades, the prevalence of hypertension has been increasing in China, and by the year 2010 it reached 20% [12]. During the period of 2005–2009, about 42% of Chinese adults aged 35–70 years were hypertensive [12]. Although obesity is clearly regarded as a risk factor for developing hypertension, the optimal BMI for middle-aged or elderly hypertensive Chinese remains unclear. Therefore, the objective of this study was to evaluate the relationship between BMI and all-cause mortality in hypertensive Chinese adults.

2. Materials and Methods

2.1. Data Sources

This post-hoc analysis utilizes data from the China Stroke Primary Prevention Trial (CSPPT), which enrolled 20,702 subjects with primary hypertension in a multi-community, randomized, double-blind, controlled trial to assess whether enalapril maleate and folic acid supplementation was more effective in reducing risk of stroke than enalapril maleate supplementation alone. This study was conducted in accordance with the principles of the Declaration of Helsinki. The Human Subjects Committee at the Biomedical Institute of Anhui Medical University approved the study protocol. All patients provided written informed consent prior to data collection.

2.2. Participants and Treatment

The methods and primary results of the CSPPT trial have been reported elsewhere [13]. Briefly, the CSPPT was conducted from 19 May 2008 to 24 August 2013 in 32 communities in Jiangsu and Anhui Provinces in China. Eligible participants were men and women aged 45–75 years old who had hypertension, defined as seated resting systolic blood pressure (SBP) $\geqslant$140 mmHg or diastolic blood pressure (DBP) $\geqslant$90 mmHg at both the screening and recruitment visit, or who were on anti-hypertensive medication. The major exclusion criteria included history of physician-diagnosed stroke, myocardial infarction (MI), heart failure, post-coronary revascularization, or congenital heart disease.

The current analysis was designed to investigate the relationship between BMI and all-cause mortality in this cohort. All-cause mortality included death due to any reason. After excluding eight subjects with missing information on weight and height, the final analysis included 20,694 subjects.

Participants contributed person-years from the date of recruitment until date of death or end of follow-up (24 August 2013). BMI classifications as set according to the guidelines from the Ministry of Health of the People's Republic of China were used and included: underweight (<18.5 kg/m^2), normal weight (18.5–23.9 kg/m^2), overweight (24.0–27.9 kg/m^2) and obesity (⩾28.0 kg/m^2). At the initial study visit trained research staff measured and recorded height (to the nearest 0.1 cm) and weight (to the nearest 0.1 kg) for each participant. In addition, trained staff collected baseline demographic data, medical history, and medication use. Cigarette smoking was classified into never, former, and current smoker (defined as smoke at least one cigarette per day for more than one year). Alcohol drinking was stratified into never, former and current drinker (defined as drink alcohol at least twice weekly for more than one year). Education was categorized into illiterate (0 years of education), primary school (1–6 years), and secondary school (>6 years) or above. Stress was defined as mild, moderate or severe according to the participant's personal evaluation.

2.3. *Follow-Up and Outcomes*

Patients were evaluated every three months for an average of five years to assess blood pressure (BP), adherence to medication, and adverse outcomes including stroke, composite major cardiovascular (CV) events and resultant death, and all-cause death. The study outcomes were adjudicated according to standard criteria by a clinical end points committee.

2.4. *Statistical Analysis*

All participants were divided into four groups according to the Chinese classification for BMI (<18.5, 18.5–23.9, 24.0–27.9, ⩾28.0 kg/m^2). Baseline characteristics of all participants were compared using the analysis of variance (ANOVA) for continuous variables and the χ^2 test for categorical variables. All-cause mortality was first assessed using the Kalpan-Meier method and log-rank tests, and then multivariable Cox proportional-hazards regression models were applied to calculate hazard ratios (HR) and 95% confidence intervals (CI) for the risk of all-cause mortality in each of the BMI groups. Potential confounders were adjusted including sex, age, center, baseline and on-treatment BP, smoking status, alcohol drinking, education, stress, fasting blood glucose (FBG), total cholesterol (TC), triglycerides (TG), serum creatinine (SCr), homocysteine (Hcy) and albumin. Further stratified analyses by subgroups including sex, age, center, smoking and alcohol drinking status, education, stress and albumin levels were also explored by Cox proportional-hazards regression models to test for consistency of results. All tests were two-sided, and p-values less than 0.05 were considered statistically significant. All analyses were performed by EmpowerStats [14] and the statistical package R [15].

3. Results

3.1. *Patient Characteristics*

Baseline characteristics of all patients are presented in Table 1. Of the 20,694 participants, 59.0% were female, and the mean age was 60.0 years (SD, 7.5 years), with a range from 45 to 75 years. The mean BMI was 25.0 kg/m^2 (SD, 3.4 kg/m^2). Men had a lower of BMI 24.2 kg/m^2 (SD, 3.7 kg/m^2) than women, who had a BMI of 25.4 kg/m^2 (SD, 3.4 kg/m^2). The percentages of underweight, normal weight, overweight and obese were 2.5%, 39.1%, 38.9% and 19.5%, respectively. Higher BMI categories were associated with younger age, female gender, better education, and higher levels of FBG, TC, TG, albumin, and baseline and on-treatment blood pressure measurements. Lower BMI categories were associated with higher HDL-C levels and current smoking status.

Table 1. Baseline characteristics of the study participants by BMI categories [1].

Variables	BMI Categories, kg/m^2					
	All Subjects	<18.5	18.5–23.9	24.0–27.9	⩾28.0	p-Value
Number (%)	20,694	526(2.5)	8083 (39.1)	8043 (38.9)	4042 (19.5)	
Age, mean (SD), years	60.0 (7.5)	64.6 (6.7)	61.3 (7.4)	59.3 (7.5)	58.2 (7.4)	<0.001
BMI, mean (SD), kg/m^2	25.0 (3.7)	17.5 (0.8)	21.8 (1.4)	25.8 (1.1)	30.4 (2.2)	<0.001
Male, No. (%)	8491 (41.0)	271 (51.5)	3863 (47.8)	3137 (39.0)	1220 (30.2)	<0.001
Center, No. (%)						<0.001
Anqing	5211 (25.2)	350 (66.5)	3119 (38.6)	1406 (17.5)	336 (8.3)	
Lianyungang	15,483 (74.8)	176 (33.5)	4964 (61.4)	6637 (82.5)	3706 (91.7)	
SBP, mean (SD), mmHg						
baseline	166.9 (20.4)	164.3 (17.9)	166.0 (20.0)	167.1 (20.4)	168.4 (21.4)	<0.001
on-treatment	139.4 (10.9)	138.8 (10.8)	138.9 (11.0)	139.4 (10.8)	140.4 (11.0)	<0.001
DBP, mean (SD),mmHg						
baseline	94.1 (11.9)	88.0 (11.4)	91.8 (11.7)	95.0 (11.6)	97.7 (11.9)	<0.001
on-treatment	82.9 (7.5)	78.9 (7.7)	81.5 (7.4)	83.5 (7.2)	85.3 (7.2)	<0.001
Pulse, mean (SD),bpm	73.6 (10.1)	74.0 (11.0)	73.6 (10.2)	73.5 (10.1)	73.8 (9.9)	0.53
Smoking status (%)						<0.001
never	14,252 (68.9)	293 (55.7)	5015 (62.1)	5791 (72.0)	3153 (78.0)	
former	1567 (7.6)	35 (6.7)	604 (7.5)	649 (8.1)	279 (6.9)	
current	4867 (23.5)	198 (37.6)	2459 (30.4)	1601 (19.9)	609 (15.1)	
Alcohol drinking (%)						<0.001
never	14,265 (69.0)	343 (65.2)	5155 (63.8)	5665 (70.5)	3102 (76.8)	
former	1458 (7.0)	52 (9.9)	609 (7.5)	540 (6.7)	257 (6.4)	
current	4960 (24.0)	131 (24.9)	2313 (28.6)	1836 (22.8)	680 (16.8)	
Education (%)						<0.001
illiterate	13,221 (63.9)	365 (69.4)	5261 (65.1)	4999 (62.2)	2596 (64.3)	
primary	3446 (16.7)	103 (19.6)	1468 (18.2)	1296 (16.1)	579 (14.3)	
secondary or above	4015 (19.4)	58 (11.0)	1347 (16.7)	1745 (21.7)	865 (21.4)	
Stress (%)						0.035
mild	12,578 (60.8)	289 (54.90)	4846 (60.0)	4960 (61.7)	2479 (61.4)	
moderate	6921 (33.4)	204 (38.8)	2765 (34.2)	2627 (32.7)	1323 (32.8)	
severe	1189 (5.7)	33 (6.3)	464 (5.7)	454 (5.6)	237 (5.9)	
FPG, mean (SD), mmol/L	5.8 (1.7)	5.3 (1.6)	5.6 (1.6)	5.9 (1.8)	6.1 (1.7)	<0.001
TC, mean (SD), mmol/L	5.5 (1.2)	5.0 (1.2)	5.4 (1.2)	5.6 (1.2)	5.7 (1.2)	<0.001
TG, mean (SD), mmol/L	1.7 (1.2)	1.2 (0.5)	1.4 (0.8)	1.8 (1.0)	2.0 (1.8)	<0.001
HDL-C, mean (SD), mmol/L	1.3 (0.4)	1.6 (0.4)	1.5 (0.4)	1.3 (0.3)	1.2 (0.3)	<0.001
SCr, mean (SD), umol/L	66.0 (19.3)	67.6 (16.7)	67.3 (19.6)	65.6 (20.5)	64.0 (16.3)	<0.001
Hcy, mean (SD), umol/L	14.5(8.4)	14.3 (7.7)	14.5 (8.1)	14.5 (8.4)	14.3 (8.9)	0.534
Albumin, mean (SD), g/L	49.0 (5.9)	47.57 (6.6)	48.57 (6.0)	49.34 (5.7)	49.34 (5.6)	<0.001
Treatment (%)						0.832
Enalapril	10,352 (50.0)	271 (51.5)	4053 (50.1)	4025 (50.0)	2003 (49.6)	
Enalapril-Folic Acid	10,342 (50.0)	255 (48.5)	4030 (49.9)	4018 (50.0)	2039 (50.4)	

[1] For the determination of p-values, two-sample t-tests for continuous variables, chi-square tests for categorical variables. SBP, systolic blood pressure; DBP, diastolic blood pressure; FBG, fasting blood glucose; TC, total cholesterol; TG, triglycerides; SCr, serum creatinine; Hcy, homocysteine.

3.2. BMI and Mortality

The relationship between BMI and overall mortality for all patients with hypertension is shown in Table 2. During a median follow-up period of 4.5 years (88,466.64 person-years), 622 deaths occurred. Specifically, with increasing BMI, the all-cause mortality rate in underweight, normal weight, overweight and obese groups was 7.8%, 3.9%, 2.4% and 1.8%, respectively. According to the BMI category, the all-cause mortality rate per 1000 person-years was 17.63, 8.93, 5.76 and 4.24, respectively. In a crude Cox proportional-hazards regression model, the HRs were 1.97 (95% CI, 1.42–2.73) for underweight, 0.64 (95% CI, 0.54–0.77) for overweight and 0.47 (95% CI, 0.37–0.61) for obesity compared with normal weight. In model II, after adjusting for sex, age, center, baseline and on-treatment BP, smoking status, alcohol drinking, education, stress and serum biochemical measurements, the HRs were 1.56 (95% CI, 1.11–2.18) for underweight, 0.78 (95% CI, 0.64–0.95) for overweight and 0.64 (95% CI, 0.48–0.85) for obesity compared with normal weight.

Table 2. Hazard ratios for all-cause mortality according to BMI status [1].

BMI kg/m²	*N*	Event (%)	Curde Rate	All-Cause Mortality			
				Model 1	*p*-Value	Model 2	*p*-Value
Continuous	20,694	622 (3.0%)	7.03	0.90 (0.88, 0.92)	<0.001	0.94 (0.91, 0.96)	<0.001
<18.5	526	41 (7.8%)	17.63	1.97 (1.42, 2.73)	<0.001	1.56 (1.11, 2.18)	0.010
18.5–23.9	8083	312 (3.9%)	8.93	1		1	
24.0–27.9	8043	197 (2.4%)	5.76	0.64 (0.54, 0.77)	<0.001	0.78 (0.64, 0.95)	0.012
⩾28	4042	72 (1.8%)	4.24	0.47 (0.37, 0.61)	<0.001	0.64 (0.48, 0.85)	0.002

[1] Multivariable Cox proportional-hazards regression models were applied to calculate hazard ratios (HR) and 95% confidence intervals (CI) for the risk of all-cause mortality in each of the BMI groups. A BMI (kg/m²) of 18.5–23.9 was used as the reference to estimate all HRs. Crude rates are all-cause mortality per 1000 person-years. Model 1: crude; Model 2: adjustment for sex, age, center, baseline and on-treatment BP, smoking status, alcohol drinking, education, stress, fasting blood glucose, total cholesterol, triglycerides, serum creatinine, homocysteine, albumin.

Figure 1 shows the Kaplan-Meier curves of the cumulative hazards of all-cause mortality stratified by BMI categories. All-cause mortality between each of the four BMI groups was significantly different (log-rank test, $p < 0.001$). With increased BMI, the cumulative mortality risk gradually decreased, rendering the underweight group with the maximum mortality risk.

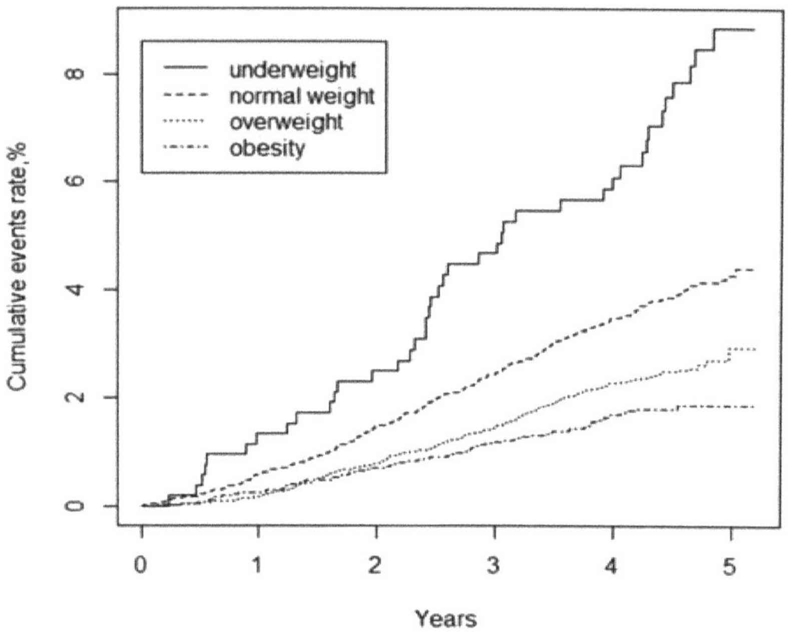

Figure 1. Kaplan-Meier curves of cumulative hazards of all-cause mortality stratified by BMI categories (underweight <18.5, normal weight 18.5–23.9, overweight 24.0–27.9, obesity ⩾28.0 kg/m²). log-rank test, $p < 0.001$.

Further stratified analyses were performed by important covariables including gender, center, smoking status, alcohol drinking status, education, stress and albumin levels (Table 3). There were no significant interactions in any of the subgroups ($p > 0.05$ for all comparisons). The beneficial effect appeared to be more pronounced in participants older than 60 years.

We subsequently repeated the analysis using narrower BMI categories (<18.5, 18.5–19.9, 20.0–21.9, 22.0–23.9, 24.0–25.9, 26.0–27.9, 28.0–29.9, 30–34.9, ⩾35 kg/m²) to delineate the relationship between BMI and mortality with greater precision. Compared to patients with normal BMI (between 22.0 and 23.9 kg/m²), patients with grade 1 obesity (30–34.9 kg/m²) had the lowest risk of all-cause mortality (Figure 2). However, all-cause mortality increased drastically for patients with severe obesity (⩾35 kg/m²).

Table 3. Multivariable hazard ratios for mortality [1].

Variables	N	Death, *n*	%	BMI Categories(kg/m^2)							Adjusted * *p* for Interaction
				<18.5		18.5–23.9	24.0–27.9		≥28		
				HR 95%CI	*p*-Value	HR 95%CI	HR 95%CI	*p*-Value	HR 95%CI	*p*-Value	
All Participants	20,694	622	3.0	1.56 (1.10, 2.14)	0.012	1	0.80 (0.66, 0.97)	0.026	0.66 (0.49, 0.87)	0.003	
Sex											0.692
Females	12,203	258	2.1	1.24 (0.66, 2.33)	0.505	1	0.78 (0.58, 1.05)	0.097	0.60 (0.41, 0.89)	0.010	
Males	8491	364	4.3	1.74 (1.16, 2.58)	0.007	1	0.82 (0.63, 1.07)	0.144	0.71 (0.46, 1.09)	0.119	
Center											0.719
Anqing	5211	218	4.2	1.58 (1.04, 2.38)	0.030	1	0.72 (0.49, 1.05)	0.090	0.88 (0.45, 1.72)	0.709	
Lianyungang	15,483	404	2.6	1.59 (0.88, 2.88)	0.125	1	0.84 (0.67, 1.06)	0.153	0.65 (0.47, 0.90)	0.009	
Age											0.588
<60	10,469	172	1.6	1.82 (0.78, 4.25)	0.167	1	0.82 (0.56, 1.19)	0.302	0.84 (0.52, 1.34)	0.463	
≥60	10,225	450	4.4	1.62 (1.13, 2.34)	0.009	1	0.75 (0.60, 0.95)	0.016	0.53 (0.36, 0.76)	<0.001	
Smoking Status											0.298
Never	14,254	327	2.3	1.40 (0.83, 2.37)	0.208	1	0.80 (0.61, 1.04)	0.090	0.62 (0.43, 0.89)	0.009	
Former	1570	75	4.8	3.76 (1.64, 8.67)	0.002	1	1.37 (0.75, 2.49)	0.305	1.28 (0.56, 2.90)	0.558	
Current	4869	219	4.5	1.33 (0.79, 2.25)	0.281	1	0.70 (0.50, 1.00)	0.052	0.60 (0.33, 1.09)	0.095	
Alcohol											
Never	14,265	355	2.5	1.54 (0.98, 2.43)	0.064	1	0.75 (0.58, 0.97)	0.026	0.63 (0.44, 0.89)	0.009	0.906
Former	1458	80	5.5	2.51 (1.17, 5.42)	0.019	1	0.85 (0.48, 1.48)	0.559	0.50 (0.20, 1.28)	0.148	
Current	4960	186	3.8	1.27 (0.65, 2.47)	0.482	1	0.93 (0.65, 1.34)	0.695	0.84 (0.46, 1.55)	0.581	
Education											0.599
Illiterate	13,221	411	3.1	1.43 (0.95, 2.15)	0.087	1	0.75 (0.59, 0.96)	0.021	0.67 (0.48, 0.94)	0.022	
Primary	3446	116	3.3	1.52 (0.70, 3.31)	0.290	1	0.98 (0.63, 1.53)	0.935	0.49 (0.22, 1.09)	0.080	
Secondary or above	4015	94	2.3	2.18 (0.88, 5.40)	0.093	1	0.78 (0.47, 1.29)	0.330	0.68 (0.33, 1.39)	0.290	
Stress											0.506
Mild	12,574	391	3.1	1.26 (0.79, 2.00)	0.333	1	0.73 (0.57, 0.94)	0.013	0.66 (0.47, 0.94)	0.019	
Moderate	6919	202	2.9	1.89 (1.13, 3.17)	0.016	1	0.91 (0.64, 1.29)	0.602	0.58 (0.33, 1.01)	0.054	
Severe	1188	28	2.4	2.97 (0.59, 14.93)	0.187	1	1.29 (0.49, 3.42)	0.604	0.90 (0.24, 3.32)	0.869	
Albumin, g/L											0.527
<49	11,813	412	3.5	1.48 (1.00, 2.18)	0.051	1	0.73 (0.57, 0.93)	0.012	0.68 (0.48, 0.97)	0.033	
≥49	8876	210	2.4	1.87 (0.98, 3.56)	0.058	1	0.87 (0.63, 1.20)	0.394	0.56 (0.34, 0.90)	0.016	

[1] Cox proportional-hazards regression models to test interaction terms between BMI and other factors, but none were found to be significant. * Adjustment for sex, age, center, baseline and on-treatment BP, smoking status, alcohol drinking, education, stress, fasting blood glucose, total cholesterol, triglycerides, serum creatinine, homocysteine, albumin; sex, center, age, smoking status, alcohol, education, stress and albumin were not adjusted for in each corresponding subgroup analyses.

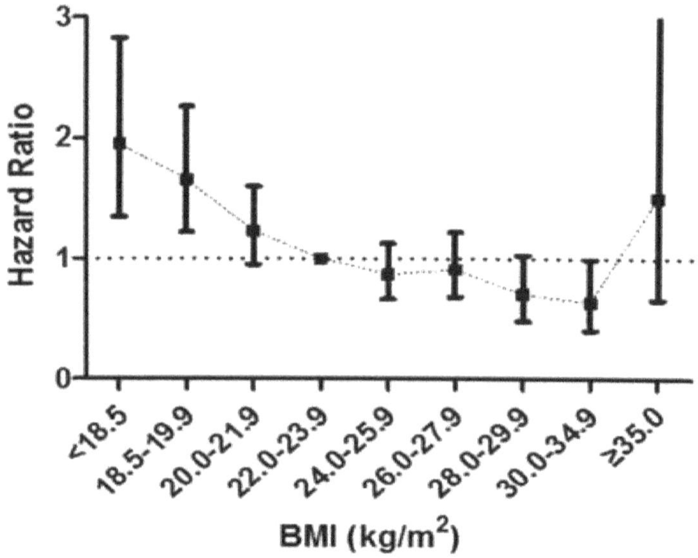

Figure 2. Hazard ratios for all-cause mortality according to narrower BMI categories. A BMI (in kg/m^2) of 22.0–23.9 was used as the reference to estimate all HRs. Adjustment for sex, age, center, baseline and on-treatment BP, smoking status, alcohol drinking, education, stress, fasting blood glucose, total cholesterol, triglycerides, serum creatinine, homocysteine, albumin.

4. Discussion

Our post-hoc analysis of this Chinese population with primary hypertension in the CSPPT showed the association between BMI and all-cause mortality followed a reversed J-shaped curve with increased risk at low and high BMI status. Even after adjusting for potential confounders, the results were similar. Compared to normal weight, the HRs were 1.56 (95% CI, 1.11–2.18) for underweight, 0.78 (95% CI, 0.64–0.95) for overweight and 0.64 (95% CI, 0.48, 0.85) for obesity. In this population, the optimal BMI was grade 1 obesity (30–34.9 kg/m^2). Stratified analyses were consistent in all important covariables. Moreover, overweight or obese patients older than 60 years showed the most benefit.

Many studies conducted on different populations showed a U-shaped or J-shaped association between BMI and all-cause mortality, which is consistent with our results when applied to the underweight participants only [4–8]. In these studies, the population age distribution and whether subgroup analyses were performed by age group might be two major reasons for the controversial results. Janssen *et al.* found that BMI was inversely associated with mortality risk in elderly Asians [16]. Compared to middle-aged adults, some previous studies found that the optimal BMI among the elderly shifted upwards [17,18]. This finding is similar to what has been observed in other Asian regions such as Taiwan [19], Hong Kong [20], India and Bangladesh [8], among others [4,5,7]. Many of the elderly participants from these studies were residents of live-in care facilities, and/or were diagnosed with a health ailment such as hypertension, or were from undeveloped communities compared with urban residents. However, the optimal range of BMI proposed among the elderly varies among studies. As the world's population ages and the number of hypertensive adults rises, our findings are important for health care professionals and policy-makers whose decisions affect elderly hypertensives.

Several potential explanations for the observed obesity paradox seen in our study exist. Firstly, reverse causality is a major problem in observational studies. For example, weight loss is classically experienced prior to death among the elderly who are ill. Secondly, socioeconomic status could confound the association between BMI and the risk of death, as people from less well-developed countries with a high BMI are more likely to have a higher socioeconomic status, allowing them better access to health care than those with a lower BMI [8]. However, the participants in our study are from rural communities, and a similar relation between BMI and socioeconomic status exists for them. Thirdly, in a meta-analysis of patients with existing coronary artery disease, those classified as overweight and obese had longer survival rates, potentially because of the benefit from the body's reservation of nutrition within the population of elderly suffering from illness [21]. Fourthly, intensive pharmacotherapy could play a large role in the reverse J-shaped relationship. It has been demonstrated that patients with intensive pharmacotherapy are more likely to reach targets for secondary prevention. In population studies conducted in the USA and Canada, obese patients are more likely to meet targets for BP, lipids, and glycemic control than normal-weight patients [22]. In addition, hypertensive participants are relatively less healthy compared to the general population, although in our study we excluded patients with stroke and MI. Mary *et al.* found that among elderly Chinese with poor health status, there was an inverse, dose-response relationship between BMI and mortality, and this relationship was more pronounced in the group with the most morbidity compared to subjects of normal weight [23]. Another interpretation is that BMI can be a marker of adiposity, fitness and muscle mass, so that BMI maintenance in older people serves as an overall marker of health. Song *et al.* accessed the sex-age-specific association between BMI and all-cause mortality in the general population, and showed that the optimal BMI increased according to age and the trend was consistent in both males and females [24]. Similarly, Woo *et al.* found that in older elderly (aged over 75 years), a higher BMI was a protection from mortality [17].

Our study also has several limitations. Firstly, our participants were all middle-aged or elderly hypertensives; therefore, the result of this study cannot be generalized to all populations. Secondly, with the strict exclusion of the history of cardiovascular disease, cardiovascular cause of death counted for only 14% of all-cause death, which is less than other studies conducted on Chinese hypertensive adults. The association between BMI and a specific cause of death cannot be analyzed. Thirdly, in the current study, relatively few elderly were $\geqslant$30 kg/m^2 (10% of total subjects) and $\geqslant$35 kg/m^2 (1%); thus, the impact of obesity cannot be adequately assessed. Moreover, although we have excluded subjects with a baseline diagnosis of coronary heart disease, stroke, cancer, or acquired organic diseases, some preexisting illness may modify the association between BMI and mortality risk. However, according to our investigation, after excluding those subjects with no history of disease at baseline and who survived the first two years of follow-up, the BMI and all-cause mortality association was consistent with all 4.5 years of this study.

5. Conclusions

In conclusion, this study revealed a reversed J-shaped association between BMI and all cause mortality in Chinese hypertensive adults. Relative to normal weight, underweight was associated with significantly higher mortality. Excessive weight was not associated with increased risk of mortality. A BMI classification of grade 1 obesity for Chinese hypertensive adults without stroke or MI showed the lowest mortality. Additional large-scale prospective studies with well-controlled confounding factors are needed to further address this important public health issue.

Acknowledgments: This research was supported by the Ministry of Science and Technology of the People's Republic of China (2012zx 09101105); the Major State Basic Research Development Program of China (973 program, No. 2012CB517703); and Projects of National Natural Science Foundation of China (grants 81437052).

Author Contributions: Y.H.: study supervision, access to all data in the study, integrity of data, and accuracy of the data analysis; W.Y., F.F.F., X.P.X., Z.Y.Z. and Y.H.: study concept and design and statistical analysis; X.P.X., B.Y.W., X.X., X.H.Q., H.X.X., G.F.T. and Y.H.: acquisition of data; W.Y., F.F.F., X.P.X., B.Y.W., Z.Y.Z. and Y.H.: analysis and interpretation of data; W.Y. and Y.H.: drafting of the manuscript; X.P.X., D.F.G. and D.Z. provided a critical review of the content of the manuscript, and revised the manuscript for important intellectual content; J.P.L., Y.Z., X.P.X., B.Y.W., H.X.X., G.F.T. and Y.H.: administrative, technical, or material support; and all authors: critical revision of the manuscript for important intellectual content.

Abbreviations

The following abbreviations are used in this manuscript:

BMI	body mass index
BP	blood pressure
CI	confidence interval
CSPPT	China Stroke Primary Prevention Trial
CV	major cardiovascular
DBP	diastolic blood pressure
FBG	fasting blood glucose
Hcy	homocysteine
HR	hazard ratio
MI	myocardial infarction
SBP	systolic blood pressure
SCr	serum creatinine
TC	total cholesterol
TG	triglycerides
WHO	The World Health Organization

References

1. Yang, Z.; Hall, A.G. The Financial Burden of Overweight and Obesity among Elderly Americans: The Dynamics of Weight, Longevity, and Health Care Cost. *Health Serv. Res.* **2008**, *43*, 849–868. [CrossRef] [PubMed]
2. World Health Organization. WHO Global Infobase, 2014. Available online: http://www.who.int/gho/ncd/risk_factors/overweight_text/en/ (accessed on 22 December 2015).
3. World Health Organization. *Physical Status: The Use and Interpretation of Anthropometry*; Report of a WHO Expert Committee; WHO Technical Report Series No. 854; World Health Organization: Geneva, Switzerland, 1995.
4. Flegal, K.M.; Graubard, B.I.; Williamson, D.F.; Gail, M.H. Excess deaths associated with underweight, overweight, and obesity. *JAMA* **2005**, *293*, 1861–1867. [CrossRef] [PubMed]
5. Flegal, K.M.; Kit, B.K.; Orpana, H.; Graubard, B.I. Association of all-cause mortality with overweight and obesity using standard body mass index categories: A systematic review and meta-analysis. *JAMA* **2013**, *309*, 71–82. [CrossRef] [PubMed]
6. Hu, F.B.; Willett, W.C.; Li, T.; Stampfer, M.J.; Colditz, G.A.; Manson, J.E. Adiposity as Compared with Physical Activity in Predicting Mortality among Women. *N. Engl. J. Med.* **2004**, *351*, 2694–2703. [CrossRef] [PubMed]
7. Winter, J.E.; MacInnis, R.J.; Wattanapenpaiboon, N.; Nowson, C.A. BMI and all-cause mortality in older adults: A meta-analysis. *Am. J. Clin. Nutr.* **2014**, *99*, 875–890. [CrossRef] [PubMed]
8. Zheng, W.; McLerran, D.F.; Rolland, B.; Zhang, X.; Inoue, M.; Matsuo, K.; He, J.; Gupta, P.C.; Ramadas, K.; Tsugane, S.; *et al.* Association between body-mass index and risk of death in more than 1 million Asians. *N. Engl. J. Med.* **2011**, *364*, 719–729. [CrossRef] [PubMed]
9. Haslam, D.W.; James, W.P. Obesity. *Lancet* **2005**, *366*, 1197–1209. [CrossRef]
10. WHO Expert Consultation. Appropriate body-mass index for Asian populations and its implications for policy and intervention strategies. *Lancet* **2004**, *363*, 157–163.
11. Chen, C.; Lu, F.C. The guidelines for prevention and control of overweight and obesity in Chinese adults. *Biomed. Environ. Sci.* **2004**, *17*, 1–36. [PubMed]
12. Liu, L.S. 2010 Chinese guidelines for the management of hypertension. *Zhonghua Xin Xue Guan Bing Za Zhi* **2011**, *39*, 579–615. [PubMed]
13. Huo, Y.; Li, J.; Qin, X.; Huang, Y.; Wang, X.; Gottesman, R.F.; Tang, G.; Wang, B.; Chen, D.; He, M.; *et al.* Efficacy of Folic Acid Therapy in Primary Prevention of Stroke Among Adults With Hypertension in China. *JAMA* **2015**, *313*, 1325. [CrossRef] [PubMed]
14. EmpowerStats. Available online: http://www.empowerstats.com (accessed on 25 March 2016).
15. R Software, Verson 3.2.1. Available online: http://www.R-project.org/ (accessed on 25 March 2016).
16. Janssen, I.; Mark, A.E. Elevated body mass index and mortality risk in the elderly. *Obes. Rev.* **2007**, *8*, 41–59. [CrossRef] [PubMed]

17. Woo, J.; Ho, S.C.; Sham, A. Longitudinal changes in body mass index and body composition over 3 years and relationship to health outcomes in Hong Kong Chinese age 70 and older. *J. Am. Geriatr. Soc.* **2001**, *49*, 737–746. [CrossRef] [PubMed]
18. Chung, W.; Ho, F.; Cheng, N.; Lee, M.; Yeh, C. BMI and all-cause mortality among middle-aged and older adults in Taiwan: A population-based cohort study. *Public Health. Nutr.* **2015**, *18*, 1839–1846. [CrossRef] [PubMed]
19. Lin, W.; Albu, J.; Liu, C.; Huang, H.; Pi-Sunyer, F.X.; Li, C.; Li, T.; Lin, C.; Huang, K. Larger Body Mass Index and Waist Circumference Are Associated with Lower Mortality in Chinese Long-Term Care Facility Residents. *J. Am. Geriatr. Soc.* **2010**, *58*, 2092–2098. [CrossRef] [PubMed]
20. Lee, J.S.W.; Auyeung, T.; Chau, P.P.H.; Hui, E.; Chan, F.; Chi, I.; Woo, J. Obesity Can Benefit Survival—A 9-Year Prospective Study in 1614 Chinese Nursing Home Residents. *J. Am. Med. Dir. Assoc.* **2014**, *15*, 342–348. [CrossRef] [PubMed]
21. Romero-Corral, A.; Montori, V.M.; Somers, V.K.; Korinek, J.; Thomas, R.J.; Allison, T.G.; Mookadam, F.; Lopez-Jimenez, F. Association of bodyweight with total mortality and with cardiovascular events in coronary artery disease: A systematic review of cohort studies. *Lancet* **2006**, *368*, 666–678. [CrossRef]
22. Chang, V.W.; Asch, D.A.; Werner, R.M. Quality of care among obese patients. *JAMA* **2010**, *303*, 1274–1281. [CrossRef] [PubMed]
23. Schooling, C.M.; Lam, T.H.; Li, Z.B.; Ho, S.Y.; Chan, W.M.; Ho, K.S.; Tham, M.K.; Cowling, B.J.; Leung, G.M. Obesity, physical activity, and mortality in a prospective Chinese elderly cohort. *Arch. Intern. Med.* **2006**, *166*, 1498–1504. [CrossRef] [PubMed]
24. Yi, S.; Ohrr, H.; Shin, S.; Yi, J. Sex-age-specific association of body mass index with all-cause mortality among 12.8 million Korean adults: A prospective cohort study. *Int. J. Epidemiol.* **2015**, *44*, 1696–1705. [CrossRef] [PubMed]

Disordered Eating Attitudes and Behavioral and Neuroelectric Indices of Cognitive Flexibility in Individuals with Overweight and Obesity

Caitlyn G. Edwards [1], Anne M. Walk [2], Sharon V. Thompson [1], Sean P. Mullen [2], Hannah D. Holscher [1,2,3] and Naiman A. Khan [1,2,4,*]

1 Division of Nutritional Sciences, University of Illinois, Urbana, IL 61801, USA; cgedwar2@illinois.edu (C.G.E.); svthomp2@illinois.edu (S.V.T.); hholsche@illinois.edu (H.D.H.)
2 Department of Kinesiology and Community Health, University of Illinois, Urbana, IL 61801, USA; amcclur3@illinois.edu (A.M.W.); spmullen@illinois.edu (S.P.M.)
3 Department of Food Science and Human Nutrition, University of Illinois, Urbana, IL 61801, USA
4 Neuroscience Program, University of Illinois, Urbana, IL 61801, USA
* Correspondence: nakhan2@illinois.edu

Abstract: Impairment in cognitive flexibility is a trait characteristic among individuals with diagnosed eating disorders. However, the extent to which these relationships exist in individuals with overweight or obesity remains unclear. Furthermore, there is a lack of knowledge characterizing the neural underpinnings of these relationships. The current study aimed to investigate disordered eating attitudes and cognitive flexibility among adults with overweight and obesity. The Eating Attitudes Test (EAT-26) and a task-switching paradigm were collected from 132 adults (50 males, Body Mass Index (BMI) = 32.0 ± 5.8 kg/m^2). Behavioral measures (accuracy and reaction time (RT)) and neuroelectric indices (amplitude and latency) of the P3 component were assessed. Hierarchical linear regressions, following adjustment of age, sex, intelligence quotient (IQ), weight status, and diet quality were developed using summative and subscale scores of the EAT-26. Higher EAT-26 summative scores, and the Dieting subscale, were related to longer RT. Only the Bulimia and Food Preoccupation subscale was related to longer P3 latency. The relationship between disordered eating attitudes and cognitive flexibility extends to individuals with overweight and obesity and is independent of age, sex, IQ, weight status, and diet quality. These findings are important, as differences in cognitive flexibility can lead to behavioral rigidity. Future work should aim to examine other neuroelectric components to identify where differences driving behavioral latencies may be occurring.

Keywords: feeding behavior; cognition; obesity; event-related potential; P3

1. Introduction

Despite many large-scale public health efforts targeted towards reducing excess energy intake and improving diet quality, many Americans fail to meet federally recommended dietary guidelines [1]. While there are many gaps in current knowledge concerning how to overcome the barriers to improving diet quality, there is limited research on the relationship between the mental or cognitive processes surrounding dietary regulation. Understanding these relationships is increasingly important, as our environment is inundated by aggressively advertised and hedonically rewarding high-fat/high-sugar foods, thus requiring constant control of the drive to consume foods beyond hunger and metabolic needs [2].

Exploration of cognitive flexibility, one of many interrelated, yet dissociable, components of cognitive control, may hold particular promise to understanding modulation of eating attitudes and behaviors. Cognitive control allows for the initiation, planning, regulation, and achievement of goal-oriented behavior [3]. Cognitive flexibility, as a component of cognitive control, can be thought of as the ability to appropriately adjust one's behavior according to a changing environment [4]. In our increasingly obesogenic environment, one where we are constantly barraged by images and marketing strategies aimed at overconsumption, cognitive flexibility becomes increasingly pertinent [5]. For some individuals, particularly those with obesity or disordered eating attitudes, adequately employing cognitive flexibility can be challenging in obesogenic settings that may require choosing less appealing food options in the name of health, in the face of more immediately rewarding options [6,7].

Although much work has been dedicated towards behavior change promotion, many individuals perpetually struggle to maintain healthful eating behaviors. Cognitive inflexibility potentially contributes to this lack of success. Previous work has indicated that impairment in cognitive flexibility is a trait characteristic among patients with diagnosed eating disorders [8–10]. This research is becoming increasingly relevant as 30 million adults in the United States report suffering from clinically significant disordered eating attitudes at some point in their lives [11]. Infrequently studied is the relationship between disordered eating attitudes and cognitive control among individuals who suffer from sub-clinical disordered eating thought patterns. Indeed, in a lifetime prevalence study of eating disorders, both males and females were more likely to suffer from a "subthreshold binge eating disorder" than either anorexia nervosa or bulimia nervosa [11]. While these subthreshold disordered eating attitudes have been briefly studied, the literature is sparse and particularly lacking in individuals with overweight and obesity [12]. It is possible, and probable, that individuals with these subthreshold disorders will similarly have difficulty adequately regulating their eating behaviors, potentially due to poor cognitive flexibility.

Cognitive flexibility is commonly assessed using behavioral measures (i.e., accuracy and reaction time (RT)) in task-switching paradigms, but previous literature relating these behavioral measures to disordered eating attitudes lacks proposed mechanisms of action. The use of the electroencephalography and the event-related potential (ERP) technique allows for examination of stimuli response with millisecond precision, allowing for examination of not only the behavioral responses but also the neural underpinnings of said responses. Specifically, the P300 (P3, P3b), a positive-going component occurring roughly 300–700 milliseconds (ms) post-stimulus onset, signifies the resources required for stimulus context updating and resource allocation [13]. In a task-switching paradigm, the P3 is largely thought to reflect how well one can activate currently relevant stimulus-response rules and deactivate previously relevant rules [14]. The P3 amplitude refers to the magnitude to which attentional resources are reconfigured to adapt to the change in stimulus-response rules, while the latency references the speed of this information processing [15]. Captured in these measures is an attentional (changes in stimuli that then require rule-set adaptation) as well as an intentional (changes in the rule-set then requiring selection of motor responses) switch [16]. Examining the P3 component in relation to disordered eating attitudes in a task-switching paradigm may provide novel insights into the potential neural mechanism by which disordered eating attitudes may contribute to poorer cognitive flexibility, or vise-versa.

An additionally important factor to consider when studying the relationship between eating attitudes and cognitive control is weight status. Individuals with overweight or obesity have been previously shown to exhibit poorer performance on cognitive control tasks [17,18]. Given the frequency of co-morbidity between disordered eating attitudes and obesity, poor dietary choices may be a consequence of cognitive flexibility decrements among individuals with overweight and obesity and disordered eating attitudes. This is additionally problematic given the emergence of recent evidence that individuals with a BMI ≥ 25 kg/m^2 may have greater than two-fold risk for disordered eating [19]. Disordered eating attitudes and behaviors have also been shown to be prevalent across both sexes [11]. However, there is a paucity of data linking disordered eating attitudes to specific aspects of cognitive control, particularly among adults with overweight and obesity. Accordingly, the aim of this study was to elucidate the relationship between eating attitudes and cognitive flexibility in a non-clinical group of men and women with overweight and obesity. We hypothesized that we would observe evidence of disordered eating attitudes in our non-clinical sample. We also hypothesized that higher disordered eating attitudes would be related to lower accuracy and longer RT in a task-switching paradigm. We further aimed to explain these increased RT's through the examination of the P3 component. We hypothesized that for this component, increased disordered eating attitudes would be related to lower amplitudes and longer latencies.

2. Materials and Methods

2.1. Participants and Procedures

Participant characteristics are described in Table 1. Data were collected from 132 adults (50 male), with BMIs ranging from 25.0 to 57.7 kg/m^2. As an ethnic breakdown of our sample, 1.5% of participants identified as American Indian or Alaskan, 10% identified as of Asian descent, 70% identified as white or Caucasian, 5% identified as Black or African American, and 4% identified as mixed or other. In terms of Social-economic status, 16% of our sample reported an annual household income between 0–$30,000, 56% reported between $30,000–$90,000, and 20% reported greater than $90,000. To qualify for the study, participants had to have a BMI $\geq$ 25.0 kg/m^2, be between 25–45 years of age, be free of diagnosed neurological disorders, and free of clinician-diagnosed depression and anxiety disorders. Participants were recruited using flyers posted in community settings, e-mails sent to University employees, as well as word-of-mouth recruitment. To ensure recruitment reached a wide variety of participants, recruitment focused on pursuing individuals outside of the University setting through bus advertisements, postcard mailing in rural neighborhoods, and school flyers in surrounding neighborhoods. Participants were compensated with gift cards upon completion of all study procedures. During the first laboratory visit, participants provided demographic data, completed the EAT-26, as well as height and weight measurements for BMI assessment. The Kaufman Brief Intelligence Test was administered to assess IQ [20]. Participants also completed the National Cancer Institute's Diet History Questionnaire II to assess overall diet quality [21]. During the second laboratory visit, cognitive testing was conducted following a 10-hour fast in the morning hours to reduce the potentially confounding effects of acute meal consumption on cognitive performance [22]. All participants provided verbal and written consent in accordance with the University of Illinois' Institutional Review Board and the Declaration of Helsinki.

Table 1. Demographic characteristics, weight status, and EAT-26 variables [1].

Variable	Group	Female	Male
N	132	82	50
Age, years	33.88 ± 6.00	34.28 ± 5.98	33.22 ± 6.06
IQ	108.48 ± 12.22	107.18 ± 11.67	110.60 ± 12.91
BMI, kg/m [2]	32.03 ± 5.81 *	33.18 ± 5.39	30.14 ± 6.05
HEI-2015 [3]	54.33 ± 13.71	53.49 ± 13.56	55.72 ± 13.96
EAT-26 Summative Score	6.73 ± 5.82 *	7.72 ± 7.26	5.12 ± 4.55
Dieting Subscale	4.69 ± 4.38	5.22 ± 4.94	3.82 ± 3.10
Bulimia and Food Preoccupation Subscale	1.45 ± 2.75	1.56 ± 3.20	1.56 ± 3.20
Oral Control Subscale	1.26 ± 1.65	1.37 ± 1.76	1.08 ± 1.44

[1] Values are means ± standard deviation unless otherwise stated; [2] Determined by the Center for Disease Control Body Mass Index (BMI) classifications; [3] Calculated using National Cancer Institute Healthy Index (HEI) 2015 Assessment; * Independent *t*-tests revealed significant differences between sex ($p < 0.05$).

2.2. Intelligence Quotient

KBIT-2 is a test of general intellectual abilities that has been nationally normed for ages 4–90 years [23]. The test is comprised of three subtests: Verbal Knowledge, Riddles, and Matrices. A composite score of the three subtests is then used as a measure of general intellectual abilities.

2.3. *Habitual Diet Quality*

The Healthy Eating Index-2015 (HEI-2015) was calculated using the Dietary History Questionnaire II with portion sizes to assess diet quality. Data were analyzed using National Cancer Institute's Diet*Calc (Diet*Calc Analysis Program, Version 1.5.0., National Cancer Institute, Epidemiology and Genomics Research Program, Bethesda, MD, USA) software and HEI-2015 scores were generated using HEI-2015 macros in Statistical Analysis System (SAS version 9.4; SAS Institute, Inc., Cary, NC, USA.). HEI scores range from 0–100, based on compliance to 2015–2020 Dietary Guidelines for Americans recommendations. The Healthy Eating Index contains 13 components, including nine adequacy (minimum standard) and four moderation (maximum allowed) components. The component scores were summed to calculate the total HEI score, which was used for analysis. HEI-2015 was calculated to account for the possibility that disordered eating attitudes may influence overall diet quality, which in turn may affect cognitive control processes [24,25].

2.4. *Anthropometric Measures*

Height and weight measurements were completed to calculate BMI (weight (kg)/height (m^2)). Height and weight were assessed using a stadiometer (model 240; SECA, Hamburg, Germany) and a digital scale (WB-300 Plus; Tanita, Tokyo, Japan). Participant height and weight were assessed while wearing light clothing and no shoes.

2.5. *Eating Attitudes Test-26*

Disordered eating attitudes were assessed using the self-report 26 question EAT-26 [26]. The EAT-26 has been validated for use in both populations with and without diagnosed eating disorders [27]. The composite EAT-26 score is a continuous variable summative of three subscales: A Dieting subscale, a Bulimia and Food Preoccupation subscale, and an Oral Control subscale. The three subscales tap into different aspects of disordered eating attitudes. The Dieting subscale assesses behaviors related to over concern with weight and calorie content of foods, the Bulimia and Food Preoccupation subscale assesses preoccupations with food and bulimic tendencies, and the Oral Control subscale assesses aspects of self-control [27]. A score on the summative score, as well as the subscales scores, indicates a larger degree of disordered eating attitudes.

2.6. *Switch Task*

Cognitive Flexibility was assessed using a Switch task [14,16]. The Switch task is comprised of three blocks, two homogenous and one heterogeneous. To emulate a real-world scenario where individuals may be forced to switch between rule-sets, the purpose of the homogeneous block is to learn an association, or rule, on certain stimuli (Figure 1). The first homogeneous block is entitled "Less than/greater than" and participants viewed a series of numbers between 1 and 10 inside of a solid box. Participants responded with a right button press if the number was less than 5, and a left button press if the number was greater than 5, thus associating a solid box with the less than/greater than rule-set. The second homogenous block is entitled "Odd/even" and participants viewed a series of numbers between 1 and 10 inside of a dashed box. Participants responded with a right button press if the number was even, and a left button press if the number was odd, thus associating a dashed box with the odd/even rule-set. A test block of 90 trials with jittered inter-stimulus interval (ISI) of either 1600, 1800, or 2000 ms was administered for both homogeneous blocks. In the heterogeneous condition, participants are shown numbers in both solid and dashed boxes. After a practice block of 50 trials, 200 trials of randomized less than/greater than and odd/even stimuli (i.e., randomized homogeneous blocks) were presented and participants were required to switch back and forth between the previously learned mental rule-sets. A Switch trial in the heterogeneous block is defined as a trial in which the previous stimuli belonged to a different mental set than the one presented, or a number was presented inside of a dashed box and followed by a number in a solid box. A NonSwitch trial is defined as a trial in which the previous stimuli belonged to the same mental set as the stimuli presented, or a number was presented inside of a dashed box and followed by another number inside a dashed box. Measures of accuracy and RT for homogeneous and heterogeneous blocks, and for both Switch and NonSwitch trials of the heterogeneous block, were assessed. Global Switch Cost for accuracy was calculated as overall accuracy of the homogenous trials—overall accuracy of the heterogeneous trials, and for RT as overall RT of the heterogeneous trials—overall RT of the homogenous trials.

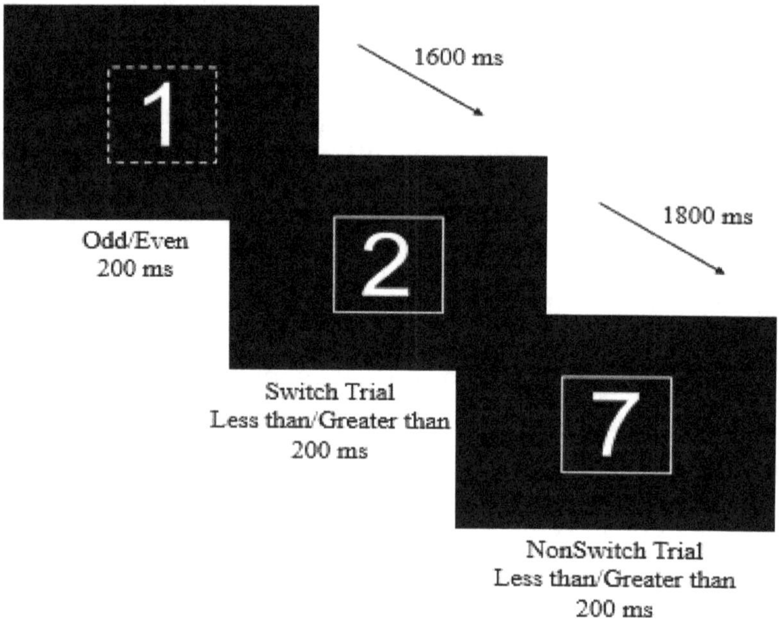

Figure 1. Task stimuli and parameters for the Switch task. Participants completed three task blocks, two homogeneous (within rule-set and dashed/solid boxes) and one heterogeneous (between rule-set and dashed/solid boxes).

2.7. ERP Assessment

Electroencephalographic (EEG) activity was recorded via a Neuro-scan Quik-cap (Compumedics, Neuroscan, Charlotte, NC, USA) with 64 scalp electrodes arranged in the international 10-10 system. Electrooculographic (EOG) activity was recorded with a set of four electrodes placed at the outer canthus of each eye and above and below the left orbit. A midline sensor placed between Cz and CPz served as a reference and AFz served as the ground. Using a Neuroscan SynampsRT amplifier (Compumedics, Neuroscan, Charlotte, NC, USA), the continuous EEG signal was digitized at a sampling rate of 500 Hz, amplified 500 times to an online low-pass 70-Hz filter with a direct current and a 60-Hz notch filter. Impedance values for all electrodes were maintained $\leq$10 kohms.

Offline, continuous data were re-referenced to averaged mastoids and merged with behavioral data. An independent components analysis (ICA) was used to systematically reject eye-blink artifacts from the data. Data were submitted to a 0.1-Hz high-pass filter before being submitted to the ICA. ICA and vertical EOG channel correlations greater than 0.35 were considered eye-blinks and were thus rejected. The ICA-corrected EEG data were segmented for each trial beginning −200 ms prior to stimulus onset and continuing 1200 ms post onset. The −200 ms to stimulus onset was used for baseline correction. Data were filtered using a 30-Hz zero phase shift low-pass filter.

Based on evidence observed from post-hoc topographic images, a 6-sensor region of interest (ROI) comprised of C1, CZ, C2, CPZ, CP1, and CP2 electrodes was used for P3 assessment. Topographic grand average plots were constructed using a stylized topographic map plugin for EEGLAB/ERPLAB [28]. Only correct trials from individuals who reported >50 usable trials in both homogenous and heterogeneous trial types were used for analyses. The P3 component was defined as the localized peak and corresponding latency occurring between 300–600 ms post-stimulus onset. Amplitude was measured as a change score from the pre-stimulus baseline and peak latency was defined as the time point of the maximum amplitude.

2.8. Statistical Analysis

Statistical analyses were performed with SPSS Statistics version 24 (IBM, Armonk, New York). Internal consistency for the EAT-26 instrument was assessed using Cronbach's Alpha. Pearson product-moment correlations were conducted to examine bivariate relationships between demographic factors (age, IQ, and sex (females coded as 0 and males coded as 1)), HEI-2015, BMI, EAT-26, and cognitive control variables. Due to non-normality as assessed via Shapiro-Wilk $p < 0.05$, log transformations of all EAT-26 variables were used for all analyses. Hierarchical linear regression analyses were used to determine the contribution of the summative EAT-26 score and each subscale to the cognitive control outcomes. Factors correlated with any one of the cognitive control outcomes were included in step 1 of the regression model. Overall model fit was assessed using ANOVA significance ($p < 0.05$) and tests for multicollinearity were conducted for each subscale. Based on published research demonstrating large effect sizes among clinical samples [9,29], we conducted an a priori power calculation. Specifically, we applied a moderate effect size ($r = 0.30$), two-sided α of 0.05, and 80% power resulting in a minimum sample size target of 81 participants to conduct the multiple regression analyses. For ERP waveform illustrative purposes in Figure 2, participants with "low" (<11) and "high" (>11) EAT-26 responses. An independent *t*-test was conducted among these groups with a significance threshold of $p < 0.05$, and they were plotted for comparison purposes in Figure 2.

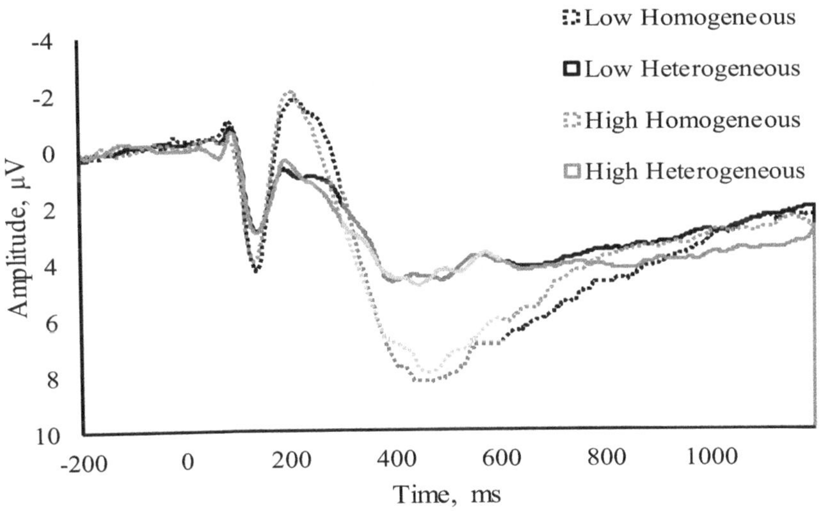

(a)

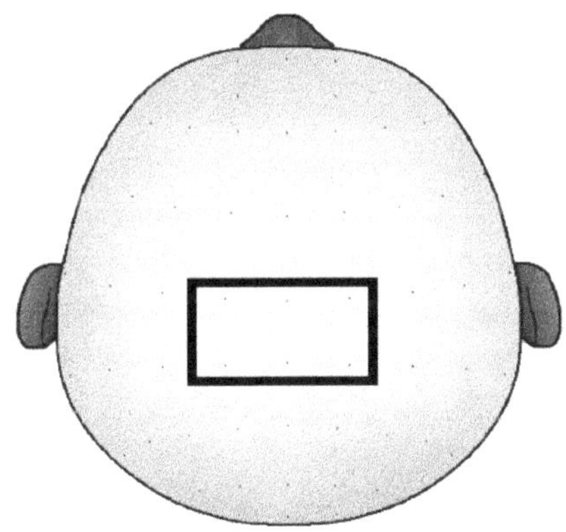

(b)

Figure 2. (**a**) Waveform depictions of "low" (n = 105) and "high" (n = 29) EAT-26 scores of the homogenous and heterogeneous Switch task trials, and (**b**) a topographic representation of the 6 electrode sites (C1, CZ, C2, CPZ, CP1, and CP2) used in the P3 region of interest (ROI).

3. Results

3.1. EAT-26

Mean scores from all participants for summative scores and subscales are reported in Table 1. Only 13% of study participants reported a summative EAT-26 score of 0, therefore, 87% of our sample reported some degree of disordered eating attitudes. Three percent of individuals reported scores of 20 or above (the score at which clinician referral is recommended) and 20% of individuals scored above an 11 (the score at which a doctor referral has been proposed for individuals belonging to non-clinical populations) [23,24]. While the EAT-26 score cannot be used to diagnose an eating disorder without also being coupled with an evaluation by a physician, these results indicate that our sample may be largely comprised of individuals who display subthreshold disordered eating attitudes, or disordered eating attitudes at levels that do not qualify for clinical diagnosis. Cronbach's alpha conducted on the Dieting, Bulimia and Food Preoccupation, and Oral Control subscales yielded scores of 0.79, 0.73, and 0.50, respectively.

3.2. Bivariate Correlations

Negative relationships were observed between age and the Bulimia and Food Preoccupation subscale ($r = -0.26$, $p = 0.003$) and between IQ and the Dieting subscale ($r = -0.18$, $p = 0.04$). EAT-26 variables were unrelated to BMI, sex, and HEI-2015 scores ($p > 0.05$).

Regarding the behavioral Switch task outcomes, sex was related to RT of the NonSwitch ($r = 0.30$, $p = 0.001$) and Switch trials ($r = 0.20$, $p = 0.02$), indicating that males took longer to respond on these trials. IQ was related to accuracy of both the NonSwitch ($r = 0.38$, $p < 0.001$) and Switch trials ($r = 0.30$, $p = 0.001$). No relationships were observed between BMI, age, or HEI-2015 scores and behavioral Switch task outcomes of accuracy nor RT. The correlations between EAT-26 variables and Switch task variables are described in Table 2.

Table 2. Bivariate Correlations between EAT-26 variables and Switch task behavioral variables.

	Summative EAT-26	Dieting Subscale	Bulimia and Food Preoccupation Subscale	Oral Control Subscale
		Homogeneous		
Overall Accuracy	−0.09	−0.08	−0.10	0.06
Overall RT	0.25 **	0.26 **	−0.10	0.16
		Heterogeneous		
NonSwitch Accuracy	−0.17	−0.22 *	0.04	0.03
NonSwitch RT	0.16	0.19 *	−0.12	0.03
Switch Accuracy	−0.19 *	−0.22 **	0.00	−0.02
Switch RT	0.15	0.20 *	−0.04	0.10
		Switch Cost		
Global Accuracy	0.16	0.21 *	−0.07	0.01
Local Accuracy	0.04	0.03	0.05	0.07
Global RT	−0.01	0.03	−0.02	−0.05
Local RT	0.05	0.10	0.07	0.13

RT—Reaction Time; ** Correlation is significant at the 0.01 level (2-tailed). * Correlation is significant at the 0.05 level (2-tailed).

Regarding the ERP Switch task outcomes and EAT-26 variables, the EAT-26 summative score was not correlated with any of the ERP variables (all p's > 0.05). The Dieting subscale was positively associated with the Global Switch Cost calculation for accuracy ($r = 0.17$, $p = 0.05$). An inverse trend was also observed between the Dieting subscale and peak P3 amplitude in the homogeneous trials ($r = -0.17$, $p = 0.06$). The Bulimia and Food Preoccupation subscale was negatively correlated with peak P3 latency in the homogenous trials ($r = -0.23$, $p < 0.01$) and trending in its relationships with the NonSwitch ($r = -0.17$, $p = 0.06$) and Switch ($r = -0.15$, $p = 0.09$) trials. The Oral Control subscale was not correlated with any of the ERP variables. In terms of demographic variables, IQ was associated with peak P3 latency in the homogenous trials ($r = -0.18$, $p = 0.04$) and HEI-2015 scores were positively associated with peak P3 amplitude of the Switch trials ($r = 0.18$, $p = 0.04$). Sex, BMI, and age were not correlated with any of the ERP variables. Complete correlations between ERP outcomes and EAT-26 variables are reported in Table 3.

Table 3. Bivariate Correlations between EAT-26 variables and Switch task ERP variables.

	Summative EAT-26	Dieting Subscale	Bulimia and Food Preoccupation Subscale	Oral Control Subscale
		Homogeneous		
Amplitude	−0.09	−0.17 †	0.05	0.01
Latency	0.01	0.03	−0.23 **	0.11
		Heterogeneous		
NonSwitch Amplitude	0.08	0.03	0.09	0.04
NonSwitch Latency	0.01	−0.01	−0.17 †	−0.02
Switch Amplitude	0.10	0.06	0.06	0.05
Switch Latency	0.40	0.01	−0.15	0.06
		Switch Cost		
Global Amplitude	0.13	0.17 *	0.12	−0.01
Local Amplitude	0.00	0.02	−0.09	−0.07
Global Latency	−0.10	−0.08	0.00	−0.16
Local Latency	0.07	0.10	0.04	0.11

** Correlation is significant at the 0.01 level (2-tailed). * Correlation is significant at the 0.05 level (2-tailed).
† Correlation is trending at $p < 0.07$ (2-tailed).

3.3. *Regression Analyses*

Age, sex, BMI, IQ, and HEI-2015 scores were entered into step 1 for each model, as they were shown to be associated with cognitive control outcomes at the bivariate level. Sex was pertinent to the aim of our study, and BMI, age and IQ have been previously associated with cognitive control tasks [3]. For each dependent variable, a standardized step 1 was used, followed by 4 different step 2 regression analyses. The summative EAT-26 and each subscale were therefore entered as separate step 2 variables. Tests for multicollinearity indicated that a low level of multicollinearity was present between the Summative EAT-26 and subscales (variance inflation factor (VIF) Dieting subscale = 1.37, Bulimia and Food Preoccupation subscale = 1.13, Oral Control subscale = 1.31).

Full behavioral regression values are reported in Table 4. For the behavioral Switch task variables, no step 2 variable was associated with accuracy in the homogeneous trials (all $p > 0.05$), indicating that disordered eating attitudes are not associated with accuracy in these trial types. The model for RT in the homogenous trials was significantly improved with the addition of EAT-26 summative score ($\Delta R^2 = 0.06$, $\beta = 0.25$) as well as with the Dieting subscale ($\Delta R^2 = 0.06$, $\beta = 0.26$). The addition of the Dieting subscale was associated with an improved model for overall heterogeneous accuracy ($\Delta R^2 = 0.3$, $\beta = -0.17$) as well as Switch accuracy ($\Delta R^2 = 0.3$, $\beta = -0.17$) and trending for the NonSwitch accuracy ($\Delta R^2 = 0.02$, $\beta = -0.15$). These results indicate that individuals with higher Dietary subscale scores took longer to respond on both homogeneous and heterogeneous trial types and performed worse on measures of heterogeneous accuracy. Similarly, the model for RT of the NonSwitch trials was significantly improved with the addition of EAT-26 summative scores ($\Delta R^2 = 0.04$, $\beta = 0.20$) and with the addition of the Dieting subscale ($\Delta R^2 = 0.04$, $\beta = 0.19$). RT of the Switch trials was significantly improved following the inclusion of the summative EAT-26 ($\Delta R^2 = 0.03$, $\beta = 0.18$) and the Dieting subscale ($\Delta R^2 = 0.04$, $\beta = 0.20$). These results indicate that individuals with higher summative EAT-26 scores took longer to respond on these trial types, and that the Dieting subscale was even further associated with an increased RT, as indicated by the significant ΔR^2. The Dieting subscale was trending with Global Accuracy Cost ($\Delta R^2 = 0.02$, $\beta = 0.16$), though no relationships were observed for Global RT Cost, nor Local Switch Costs.

Table 4. Hierarchical Regression between pertinent variables and Switch task cognitive outcomes.

	Homogeneous RT			NonSwitch RT			Switch RT		
Step and Variable	β	ΔR^2	**Model** p	β	ΔR^2	**Model** p	β	ΔR^2	**Model** p
Step 1									
Sex	0.07			0.30 **			0.20 *		
BMI	−0.03			−0.05			−0.11		
IQ	−0.10	0.02	0.68	−0.12	0.14	$p < 0.01$	−0.10	0.08	0.05
Age	0.09			0.18 *			0.12		
HEI-2015	0.05			0.02			−0.01		
Step 2									
Summative EAT-26	0.25 **	0.06 **	0.08	0.20 *	0.04 *	$p < 0.001$	0.18*	0.03 *	0.02
Dieting Subscale	0.26 **	0.06 **	0.07	0.20 *	0.04 *	$p < 0.001$	0.20 *	0.04 *	0.01
Bulimia and Food Preoccupation Subscale	−0.08	0.01	0.69	−0.10	0.01	$p < 0.001$	−0.01	0.00	0.09
Oral Control Subscale	0.15	0.02	0.41	0.03	0.00	$p < 0.001$	0.09	0.01	0.06

RT—Reaction Time. ** Correlation is significant at the 0.01 level (2-tailed). * Correlation is significant at the 0.05 level (2-tailed).

The model for latency of the homogeneous P3 trials was significantly improved by the addition of the Bulimia and Food Preoccupation subscale ($\Delta R^2 = 0.04$, $\beta = -0.20$). Intriguingly, apart from this, no models were predictive of Switch task ERP variables in either the homogenous or heterogeneous task conditions, nor in terms of Global or Local Switch Costs (all $p > 0.05$). Therefore, while relationships were observed between disordered eating attitudes and behavioral accuracy and RT, relationships were largely not seen regarding the P3, indicating that these behavioral decrements may not be driven by differences in P3 amplitude or latency. Waveform depictions are presented in Figure 2.

4. Discussion

We aimed to elucidate relationships between disordered eating attitudes and cognitive flexibility in a non-clinical sample of adults with overweight and obesity. As hypothesized, behavioral latencies in a cognitive flexibility task were correlated with higher disordered eating attitudes, specifically the EAT-26 Dieting subscale. Furthermore, the contribution of disordered eating attitudes was generalized such that it was evident for both the homogenous and heterogeneous task conditions. Importantly, this relationship occurred even after controlling for potential confounding factors such as sex, age, BMI, diet quality, and intellectual abilities. However, the only statistically significant relationship observed between measures of disordered eating attitudes and ERP P3 variables was with the Bulimia and Food Preoccupation subscale. These results suggest that the neural mechanisms by which disordered eating attitudes influence cognitive flexibility may be evident without decrements captured by the P3 ERP component, and that future work should examine possible alternative neurophysiological mechanisms of this relationship.

Our findings are consistent with previous literature indicating that individuals with eating disorders and with overweight or obesity exhibit differential patterns during cognitive flexibility task performance [30,31]. Both homogenous and heterogeneous trial types of the Switch task were related with disordered eating attitudes, as indicated by longer RTs and lower accuracies among individuals with higher Dieting subscale scores. These results also extend previous work relating eating attitudes to cognitive flexibility by demonstrating that cognitive impairment related to disordered eating risk is not limited to clinical populations but is also present among otherwise healthy individuals with overweight and obesity [30]. Interestingly, the relationship between RT and disordered eating attitudes was observed across both the EAT-26 summative score as well as the Dieting subscale for all trial types, suggesting both a generalized and specific negative influence of disordered eating attitudes on processing speed.

While the EAT-26 is a widely used eating disorder screening tool, there is substantially less work evaluating the independent subscales. Evidence in support of the specificity between the Dieting subscale and cognitive flexibility reinforces the theory of functional differences across disordered eating symptoms. The Dieting subscale is thought to reflect "negative body image and avoidance of fattening foods" [32]. Orbitello et al. reported that, in a sample of non-clinical individuals with overweight and obesity, a high Dieting subscale score was a risk factor for eating disorders not otherwise specified (previously EDNOS, now other specified feeding or eating disorder (OSFED)) [27]. Our results reveal that participants with higher Dieting subscale scores took longer to respond in both homogenous and heterogeneous task conditions. Our results indicate that, not only do a large number of participants identify with the Dieting subscale, but also that they exhibit cognitive rigidity patterns similarly evident in clinical studies of patients with eating disorder diagnoses. These results point to a need for more studies examining cognitive barriers to behavior change among community populations.

Intriguingly, in contrast to our hypothesis, the only relationships between EAT-26 variables and P3 outcomes that maintained significance after controlling for pertinent demographic and body composition variables were between the Bulimia and Food Preoccupation subscale and latency in the homogenous task trials. Yet, no relationships were observed between the Bulimia and Food Preoccupation subscale and behavioral variables. This is interesting, as bivariate relationships were observed between the Dieting subscale and the peak amplitude during homogeneous trials, yet this relationship did not persist in regression modeling. To the authors this implies that there may be some relationship between these variables, albeit not very strong. The homogeneous trials are also thought of as the "easier" task trials, in that you are staying within one rule-set, and thus it is intriguing that results were observed here.

The P3 component is largely thought to reflect contextual updating of task-set configurations, or how well one can activate currently relevant stimulus-response rules and deactivate previously relevant rules (in this case the difference prompted by the solid or dashed boxes) [14]. As outlined below, various explanations may explain these relationships. In the present task, motor responses were held constant across conditions, meaning that our task was better able to capture an attentional switch rather than an intentional switch. The lack of associations indicates that decrements in behavioral performance are perhaps not reliant on stimulus evaluation or contextual updating and may instead draw mechanistic foundations from measures of an *intentional* switch, including task-specific motor response remapping, or inhibition of response alternatives. Support for this explanation can also be drawn from the correlations between RT and P3 latency variables. While RT is an index of both duration of stimulus evaluation process as well as response selection, the P3 latency is only reflective of stimulus evaluation [16]. Our results revealed correlations between RT and P3 latency in the homogenous conditions ($r = -0.31$, $p < 0.01$), but no relationships between RT and P3 latency in the Switch and NonSwitch conditions ($r = 0.12$, $p = 0.18$; $r = 0.07$, $p = 0.43$). While interpretations of this result may vary, one can view these relationships as another indication that an individual's eating attitudes do not have bearing on the stimulus evaluation component of the P3, indicating a need for investigation of disordered eating attitudes using tasks designed to evaluate intentional switches involved in behavior. Another explanation for a lack of a relationship between disordered eating attitudes and P3 outcomes may be that, in this task, while we observed global switch effects we did not observe local switch effects (Figure 1). Further tasks using the ERP technique in conjunction with task-switching paradigms are thus warranted.

While this study draws its strength from the novel use of the ERP technique in conjunction with eating attitude assessment in a large non-clinical sample of individuals with overweight and obesity, our study was not without limitations. Primarily, our study was cross-sectional, and thus any conclusions drawn are correlational, rather than causational. Thus, cognitive flexibility could have been driven by the disordered eating attitudes, or disordered eating attitudes could be maintained due to cognitive rigidity. Further longitudinal work is thus needed to elucidate these relationships. Nevertheless, we were able to shed light on a relatively concordant relationship between eating attitudes and behavioral measures of cognitive flexibility in a non-clinical group of men and women with overweight or obesity.

5. Conclusions

We observed statistically significant relationships between disordered eating attitudes and behavioral RT, yet not neuroelectric indices, on a cognitive flexibility task in a sample of men and women with overweight and obesity. Importantly, these relationships were independent of age, sex, BMI, IQ, and overall dietary quality. More experimental work is necessary to explore the relationship between eating attitudes and cognitive flexibility to determine the cognitive underpinnings of eating behavior regulation and inform future therapeutic approaches to improving adherence to healthful diet habits in the general population with overweight and obesity.

Author Contributions: C.G.E. and N.A.K. wrote the manuscript. C.G.E. and S.V.T. collected the data. A.M.W., S.P.M., and H.D.H. reviewed and commented on subsequent drafts of the manuscript.

Acknowledgments: We would like to thank the undergraduate research team of the Body Composition and Nutritional Neuroscience laboratory.

References

1. Krebs-Smith, S.M.; Guenther, P.M.; Subar, A.F.; Kirkpatrick, S.I.; Dodd, K.W. Americans do not meet Federal Dietary Recommendations. *J. Nutr.* **2010**, *140*, 1832–1838. [CrossRef]
2. Hofmann, J.; Ardelt-Gattinger, E.; Paulmichl, K.; Weghuber, D.; Blechert, J. Dietary restraint and impulsivity modulate neural responses to food in adolescents with obesity and healthy adolescents. *Obesity* **2015**, *23*, 2183–2189. [CrossRef] [PubMed]
3. Diamond, A. Executive Functions. *Annu. Rev. Clin. Psychol.* **2013**, *64*, 135–168. [CrossRef] [PubMed]
4. Dajani, D.R.; Uddin, L.Q. Demystifying cognitive flexibility: Implications for clinical and developmental neuroscience. *Anal Chem.* **2015**, *25*, 368–379. [CrossRef] [PubMed]
5. Ziauddeen, H.; Alonso-Alonso, M.; Hill, J.O.; Kelley, M.; Khan, N.A. Obesity and the neurocognitive basis of food reward and the control of intake. *Adv. Nutr.* **2015**, *6*. [CrossRef] [PubMed]
6. Mobbs, O.; Van der Linden, M.; d'Acremont, M.; Perroud, A. Cognitive deficits and biases for food and body in bulimia: Investigation using an affective shifting task. *Eat. Behav.* **2008**, *9*, 455–461. [CrossRef] [PubMed]
7. Hendrikse, J.J.; Cachia, R.L.; Kothe, E.J.; Mcphie, S.; Skouteris, H.; Hayden, M.J. Attentional biases for food cues in overweight and individuals with obesity: A systematic review of the literature. *Obes. Rev.* **2015**, *16*, 424–432. [CrossRef]
8. Roberts, M.E.; Tchanturia, K.; Stahl, D.; Southgate, L.; Treasure, J. A systematic review and meta-analysis of set-shifting ability in eating disorders. *Psychol. Med.* **2007**, *37*, 1075–1084. [CrossRef] [PubMed]
9. Rosval, L.; Steiger, H.; Bruce, K.; Israël, M.; Richardson, J.; Aubut, M. Impulsivity in women with eating disorders: Problem of response inhibition, planning, or attention? *Int. J. Eat. Disord.* **2006**, *39*, 590–593. [CrossRef] [PubMed]
10. Perpiñá, C.; Segura, M.; Sánchez-Reales, S. Cognitive flexibility and decision-making in eating disorders and obesity. *Eat. Weight Disord. Stud. Anorexia Bulim. Obes.* **2016**, *22*, 435–444. [CrossRef]
11. Hudson, J.I.; Hiripi, E.; Pope, H.G.; Kessler, R.C. The Prevalence and Correlates of Eating Disorders in the National Comorbidity Survey Replication. *Biol. Psychiatry* **2007**, *61*, 348–358. [CrossRef] [PubMed]
12. Wolz, I.; Fagundo, A.B.; Treasure, J.; Fernandez-Aranda, F. The processing of food stimuli in abnormal eating: A systematic review of electrophysiology. *Eur. Eat. Disord. Rev.* **2015**, *23*, 251–261. [CrossRef] [PubMed]
13. Polich, J.; Kok, A. Cognitive and biological determinants of P300: An integrative review. *Biol. Psychol.* **1995**, *41*, 103–146. [CrossRef]
14. Kray, J.; Li, K.Z.H.; Lindenberger, U. Age-related changes in task-switching components: The role of task uncertainty. *Brain Cogn.* **2002**, *49*, 363–381. [CrossRef] [PubMed]
15. Hillman, C.H.; Kramer, A.F.; Belopolsky, A.V.; Smith, D.P. A cross-sectional examination of age and physical activity on performance and event-related brain potentials in a task switching paradigm. *Int. J. Psychophysiol.* **2006**, *59*, 30–39. [CrossRef] [PubMed]
16. Kieffaber, P.D.; Hetrick, W.P. Event-related potential correlates of task switching and switch costs. *Psychophysiology* **2005**, *42*, 56–71. [CrossRef] [PubMed]
17. Sellaro, R.; Colzato, L.S. High body mass index is associated with impaired cognitive control. *Appetite* **2017**, *113*, 301–309. [CrossRef] [PubMed]
18. Yang, Y.; Shields, G.S.; Guo, C.; Liu, Y. Executive function performance in obesity and overweight individuals: A meta-analysis and review. *Neurosci. Biobehav. Rev.* **2018**, *84*, 225–244. [CrossRef] [PubMed]
19. Waaddegaard, M.; Davidsen, M.; Kjøller, M. Obesity and prevalence of risk behaviour for eating disorders among young Danish women. *Scand. J. Public Health* **2009**, *37*, 736–743. [CrossRef] [PubMed]
20. Kaufman, A.S.; Kaufman, N.L. *K-BIT: Kaufman Brief Intelligence Test*; American Guidance Service: Circle Pines, MN, USA, 1990.
21. *Diet History Questionnaire, Version 2.00*; National Cancer Institute: Bethesda, MD, USA, 2010.
22. Hoyland, A.; Lawton, C.L.; Dye, L. Acute effects of macronutrient manipulations on cognitive test performance in healthy young adults: A systematic research review. *Neurosci. Biobehav. Rev.* **2008**, *32*, 72–85. [CrossRef] [PubMed]
23. Naugle, R.I.; Chelune, G.J.; Tucker, G.D. Validity of the kaufman brief intelligence test. *Psychol. Assess.* **1993**, *5*, 182–186. [CrossRef]

24. Walk, A.M.; Edwards, C.G.; Baumgartner, N.W.; Chojnacki, M.R.; Covello, A.R.; Reeser, G.E.; Hammond, B.R.; Renzi-Hammond, L.M.; Khan, N.A. The role of retinal carotenoids and age on neuroelectric indices of attentional control among early to middle-aged adults. *Front. Aging Neurosci.* **2017**, *9*, 1–13. [CrossRef] [PubMed]
25. Khan, N.A.; Raine, L.B.; Drollette, E.S.; Scudder, M.R.; Hillman, C.H. The relation of saturated fats and dietary cholesterol to childhood cognitive flexibility. *Appetite* **2015**, *93*, 51–56. [CrossRef] [PubMed]
26. Garner, D.M.; Olmsted, M.P.; Bohr, Y.; Garfinkel, P.E. The Eating Attitudes Test: Psychometric features and clinical correlates. *Psychol. Med.* **1982**, *12*, 871–878. [CrossRef] [PubMed]
27. Orbitello, B.; Ciano, R.; Corsaro, M.; Rocco, P.L.; Taboga, C.; Tonutti, L.; Armellini, M.; Balestrieri, M. The EAT-26 as screening instrument for clinical nutrition unit attenders. *Int. J. Obes.* **2006**, *30*, 977–981. [CrossRef]
28. Pontifex, M.B. Stylized Topographic Map Plugin for EEGLAB/ERPLAB. Available online: http://education.msu.edu/kin/hbcl/software.html (accessed on 22 September 2018).
29. Tchanturia, K.; Davies, H.; Roberts, M.; Harrison, A.; Nakazato, M.; Schmidt, U.; Treasure, J.; Morris, R. Poor Cognitive Flexibility in Eating Disorders: Examining the Evidence using the Wisconsin Card Sorting Task. *PLoS ONE* **2012**, *7*, 1–5. [CrossRef]
30. Zastrow, A.; Kaiser, S.; Stippich, C.; Walther, S.; Herzog, W.; Tchanturia, K.; Belger, A.; Weisbrod, M.; Treasure, J.; Friederich, H.-C. Neural correlates of impaired cognitive-behavioral flexibility in anorexia nervosa. *Am. J. Psychiatry* **2009**, *166*, 608–616. [CrossRef] [PubMed]
31. Wu, M.; Brockmeyer, T.; Hartmann, M.; Skunde, M.; Herzog, W.; Friederich, H.-C. Set-shifting ability across the spectrum of eating disorders and in overweight and obesity: A systematic review and meta-analysis. *Psychol. Med.* **2014**, *44*, 3365–3385. [CrossRef]
32. Masuda, A.; Latzman, R.D. Psychological flexibility and self-concealment as predictors of disordered eating symptoms. *J. Context. Behav. Sci.* **2012**, *1*, 49–54. [CrossRef]

15

Investigating Philosophies Underpinning Dietetic Private Practice

Claudia Harper [1,*] and Judith Maher [2]

1 The Boden Institute of Obesity, Nutrition, Exercise and Eating Disorders, Sydney Medical School, The University of Sydney, Level 2, Charles Perkins Centre, John Hopkins Drive, Camperdown, NSW 2006, Australia

2 Faculty of Science, Health, Education and Engineering, University of the Sunshine Coast, 90 Sippy Downs Dr, Sippy Downs, QLD 4556, Australia; jmaher@usc.edu.au

* Correspondence: claudia.harper@sydney.edu.au

Academic Editors: Amanda Sainsbury and Felipe Luz

Abstract: There is limited theory or knowledge regarding dietitians' practice philosophies and how these philosophies are generated and incorporated into their professional practices. For the purposes of this study, a conceptual framework will explain and define the 'philosophies' as three different types of knowledge; episteme, techne, and phronesis. This study aimed to develop an explanatory theory of how dietitians in private practice source, utilise, and integrate practice philosophies. A grounded theory qualitative methodology was used to inform the sampling strategy, data collection, and analytical processes. Semi-structured interviews with dietitians in private practice were undertaken and data were collected and analysed concurrently. The results show that dietitians form collaborative relationships with their clients, in order to nurture change over time. They use intrinsic and intertwined forms of episteme, techne, and phronesis, which allow them to respond both practically and sensitively to their clients' needs. The learning and integration of these forms of knowledge are situated in their own practice experience. Dietitians adapt through experience, feedback, and reflection. This study highlights that private practice offers a unique context in which dietitians deal with complex issues, by utilising and adapting their philosophies.

Keywords: grounded theory; health care professionals; diet therapy; knowledge utilization; philosophy; relationships; patient-provider; theory development

---

1. Introduction

The profession of dietetics, consistent with medicine, nursing, and other allied health care providers, is firmly based in 'Evidence-Based Practice' (EBP). Sackett et al., the forefather of EBP, stated that EBP is the "conscientious, explicit and judicious use of current best evidence in making decisions about the care of individual patients" [1] (p. 71). The rationale behind EBP, which originated in the medical field, was to increase patient safety and to ensure that the best known intervention was being employed [1]. Health practitioners and their auditors feel confident that, when using EBP guidelines, the applied therapy is based on sound theory and evidence. In Australia, the accrediting professional body/organisation for Dietitians, the Dietitians Association of Australia (DAA), explicitly requires that EBP is used [2,3].

The DAA and the International Confederation of Dietetic Associations (ICDA) states that dietitians need to utilize EBP in conjunction with both the "dietitians' expertise and judgment, and the clients' or communities' unique values and circumstances to guide decision-making in dietetics" [2,4]. This is particularly true for dietitians in private practice; an area of practice which has been poorly researched, despite the rapidly growing numbers in this sector in recent years [5]. In addition, although encouraging a practice that integrates clinical judgment and patient values with EBP, accreditation requirements for dietetic university programs heavily emphasize a biomedical reductionist model of practice [6]. Despite these codes of practice, there is no description of the level of expertise needed to effectively carry out this practice and there is little knowledge of whether or how dietitians should do this in practice [2,4].

Nutrition and food behavior is a complex area with many competing influences, posing challenges to the formulation and application of applicable EBP. Such influences include, but are not limited to: 'taste and food preferences, weight concerns, physiology, time and convenience, environment, abundance of foods, economics, media/marketing, perceived product safety, culture, and attitudes/beliefs' [7].

While there are no questions about whether or not EBP works under the conditions that the research was pursued, there is a realization that these conditions are rarely reproduced in individual circumstances [8]. Additionally, evidence based on a single intervention is not congruent in a clinical setting, where a range of treatment approaches are often required [8]. Other health modalities have also noted that EBP constrains practice to quantifiable aspects and that there are areas within the patient-practitioner relationship that have been overlooked.

Perspectives and studies on exerting change in nutrition behavior have been primarily generated in the public health sector and, as such, possible problems and solutions have also largely been discussed in this context. On a public health scale, EBP has failed to exert meaningful change in the health behavior of targeted populations [9]. Buchanan suggests this could be due to social science attempting to apply a natural science perspective to the complexity of human behavior [9]. In effect, natural or biomedical science cannot adequately study, explain, or address phenomena in which the subjects have volition to choose their own actions [9]. Others call for more social research to explore the areas that are poorly understood when it comes to applying successful interventions within the social and environmental contexts of nutrition and health behavior [10,11].

Schubert et al. and Buchanan suggest that the analytical approach to nutrition science fails to recognize diet and nutritional disease as a complex set of processes outside of predictable scientific models [9,10]. Further, research is greatly removed from the human level, where dietitians interact with their clients and their dietary practices within the consultation process [10]. Studies that have explored nutrition and dietetic consultation practices generally focus on dietitians working in the hospital or community health arenas, and on singular aspects of practice. Some of these aspects include verbal and non-verbal communication skills [12], trust in communication between dietitians and clients [13], patients' experiences of dietetic consultations [14], dietitians use of EBP [15–17], and dietitians' opinions of client-centered nutrition counselling. Most studies investigate what dietary interventions are needed to effect nutritional change; however, less attention is paid to counselling approaches in dietetic consultation [14]. To date, no studies have explored the knowledge types in relation to nutrition and dietetic practices.

Proponents within medicine and nursing have noted gaps in research where EBP has failed to address important areas of practice that exist on the human level, in consultation with the patient [18–21]. They have proposed a practice framework which incorporates three philosophies that arguably underpin the skillsets and behaviors of practitioners whom are able to practice in a holistic way, working to address the particular needs of the patient [18–24]. These philosophies encompass reflective practice and clinical judgement, as well as skills that are not easily identifiable in a quantitative way [18,22,24,25]. These philosophies; episteme, techne, and phronesis, are identified as types of knowledge and originate from Aristotle's Nicomachean Ethics [26].

Practitioners who possess the knowledge types episteme and techne are said to be competent practitioners. However, those practitioners who possess phronesis, in addition to episteme and techne, utilize knowledge and skillsets that show expert characteristics [25,27–29]. It has been shown within nursing, that practitioners exhibiting the use of these three concepts, are better able to respond contextually and appropriately to their patients [30,31]. Others have noted that practice and research which incorporates phronesis with episteme and techne, may help bridge the gap between theory and practice, and encompass knowledge and skills that are not effectively conceived within a biomedical science paradigm [18,21,23,29].

Episteme, translated to epistemology, refers to 'the branch of philosophy which investigates the origin, nature, method and limits of human knowledge' [32]. In essence, episteme encompasses what is seen as true scientific knowledge based on evidence, which is the basis of dietetic practice. The term epistemology has come to be understood as scientific knowledge which is universal, invariable, and context independent. The most highly respected form of scientific knowledge in healthcare comes from randomly controlled clinical trials, in which theories are tested and found to be true or untrue.

Techne denotes production, namely art, workmanship, or skill (the 'know how'). It describes the endeavor of using technical rationality to produce a certain outcome [28]. Technical rationality describes a practice of systematically performing a set of discrete tasks, in order to produce a generic product [28]. This ensures that the practice is efficient, standardized, and 'practitioner proof' [28]. In this way, it can be replicated and controlled, and lends itself to practice criteria that are easily assessed and accounted for [28]. This aligns with clinical reasoning in medicine, in that, decisions made objectively whilst remaining neutral and which are based on the strongest evidence, should produce results free from conflict; with respect to multiple values and interests [28]. By utilizing both episteme and techne in practice, evidential knowledge is combined with a good technique. However, relying on technique alone may be inappropriate within complex contemporary situations [29]. Expert judgement in contextual situations requires practical judgement, and phronesis helps fill the gaps that good technique alone cannot address [21,29].

Phronesis is most often translated as 'practical wisdom' or prudence, and denotes the ability or character trait of being able to use one's collective knowledge in a different way, in order to produce the most optimal outcome of a specific situation [32]. A phronetic practitioner is able to draw on their knowledge, recognize what is needed in that situation, and deal with it effectively [28]. This ability requires a high level of perception and flexibility, in combination with an understanding of which epistemic and technical knowledge to apply for the best outcome [28]. Benner et al. state that phronesis is necessary to evaluate and integrate evidence and techne [18]. Phronetic action is not easily formulated as it requires creative insight and the ability to actuate knowledge with appropriateness to the situation [18,28]. Phronesis is concerned with the highest good in a situation and requires moral deliberation [33]. Phronesis is dependent on experiential learning, is changeable, and develops in practical endeavors [18,33]. It is also described as being ethical and reflective in practice, and develops through interactions with others [29,34].

Based on the above, our aim was to investigate which forms of knowledge dietitians use, and how these are developed and incorporated within the practices of dietitians in private practice. We are using Gustavsson's description of knowledge to guide us: "Knowledge is not merely theoretical, it is also practical, it is about what we know, what we do and how we act" [35].

In this text, we alternate between the use of the terms, patient and client, as well as, participant and dietitian.

2. Method

Constructivist grounded theory, developed by Charmaz, was used to explore what types of knowledge dietitians use in private practice in Australia [36]. How these knowledge philosophies are acquired, developed, and integrated into practice, was also investigated. Consistent with Blumer and Charmaz, sensitizing concepts were used to shape the research topic and guide the questions [36,37]. We used Aristotle's philosophical concepts of knowledge to provide us with a starting point for our investigation. These three types of knowledge, stemming from Aristotle's intellectual virtues, are: episteme, techne, and phronesis [38]. Our awareness of these knowledge philosophies assisted our discernment between diverse types of knowledge, despite their acquisition and use being simultaneous and interconnected.

It is important to note, however, that these concepts were not used to force the data into preconceived perspectives. According to Charmaz, researchers using constructivist grounded theory construct theories through interactions, perspectives, and practices [36]. Charmaz explicitly states that theories formulated by researchers using constructive methodology, are an interpretive description of the phenomena under study [36]. This study was approved by the University of the Sunshine Coast Human Ethics Committee.

2.1. Recruitment and Sampling

Accredited Practicing Dietitians (APD) in private practice, registered with the Dietitians Association of Australia (DAA), were identified via the DAA website. The DAA is the regulatory body for dietitians in Australia. It is a requirement that practicing dietitians register with the DAA, in order to gain APD status. Dietitians may then be listed on their website and searched for by the public. It is assured that all dietitians listed as an APD on the DAA website hold the credentials to practice as a dietitian.

Invitation emails were sent to 89 dietitians listed as APDs on the DAA website, inviting them to take part in the study. The first round of dietitians were chosen randomly and, as analysis progressed, the recruitment of dietitians became more specified, with the aim of testing emerging concepts within broader sample characteristics. To add robustness to our categories, once we had noted similar concepts within less experienced dietitians, more experienced dietitians were targeted, in order to expand our sample. For example, when a theme of dietitians experiencing a 'fast learning curve' and then a levelling out of this learning, emerged in dietitians with less than five years of experience, dietitians with more than 20 years experience were asked whether they remembered a similar process. As a result, an additional theme of 'lifelong learning' emerged in those dietitians with more experience.

Eleven dietitians, registered as APDs at the time of this study, agreed to participate in the study. This represents a 12% response rate. The length of time that had been spent working as a dietitian in private practice spanned between seven months and 30 years. All but one dietitian was self-employed. Two dietitians included in the sample were male. The dietitians in this study were a mixture of generalist and specialist dietitians, and two dietitians held double degrees, with the additional degree being held in another allied health modality. One dietitian held a Diabetes Educator status.

2.2. Data Collection and Analysis

Data were collected via semi structured interviews with dietitians, who responded affirmatively to invitation emails. A pilot interview was conducted prior to the commencement of data collection. The pilot interview indicated that the interview format was appropriate for gathering rich data associated with our subject matter. One-on-one, in depth, semi structured interviews were conducted in person (eight interviews), or on the telephone (three interviews). Telephone interviews were conducted to gain access to dietitians who were not close enough to interview in person. This also helped broaden the sample. The interviews were recorded with a recording device and a recording service was used to record the phone interviews. All interviews were transcribed by the researcher verbatim. This process allowed the researcher to become more familiar with the data.

In the interview, participants were asked to describe an interesting or recent case which they had worked on. The purpose of this was to explore a case that the participants could recollect in more detail. Subsequent questions allowed an exploration of the participant's thoughts, decisions, and reasoning, before, during, and after the case. At times, the interview process became reflective, due to the participant needing to reflect on why they chose to do things in a certain way, or how they arrived at the decisions that they had made. As data collection and analysis proceeded, and emerging concepts became apparent, additional questions were asked, in order to develop the categories more fully. For example, when data analysis indicated that being a self-employed business owner significantly contributed to the subject matter, this area was explored in more detail in subsequent interviews.

Observations and perceptions made during the interview were recorded as field notes at a convenient time and were used to provide further context on the emerging categories. During transcription and throughout analysis, further thoughts surrounding the data were recorded as memos and used to add depth to the analytical process [36].

Consistent with grounded theory, data analysis occurred concurrently with data collection [36]. In the initial open coding phase, preliminary codes were ascribed to words, lines, or incidents within the data. The data were preliminarily open-coded in Microsoft WordPerfect10 (Microsoft, Washington, DC, USA). We then used NVivo10 qualitative software (QSR International Pty Ltd, Melbourne, Australia) to store and group the data. Codes were crosschecked across the data set, to ensure the accuracy of the emerging concepts. Codes that appeared frequently or seemed significant across the data, were focused into categories.

Theoretical coding, according to Charmaz, conceptualizes possible relationships between the categories that were developed during the previous analytical stage [36]. For instance, the category 'applying evidence contextually and collaboratively' subsumed a number of codes that described strategies and information which dietitians used to determine appropriate therapies in practice. One other category, 'non prescriptive', encompassed various approaches to nutrition therapy favored by the dietitians. These categories were then encompassed within the conceptual category, 'collaborative therapy', as a way in which dietitians make decisions on nutrition therapy. Other major categories, 'nurturing change' and 'evolution and adaptation', also subsumed various processes and strategies.

Because our area of interest was the types of knowledge that dietitians use, the contextual information detected during this study, along with observational memos, were used to create a model of the knowledge philosophies that underpin the key strategies and skills which dietitians used in this study. This model of private practice also described the contexts and processes within which dietitians acquired, developed, and integrated these knowledge philosophies into practice skills.

3. Results

In the presentation of our results, we will first describe the overview of our theoretical model of private practice, summarized in Figure 1. This model of private practice was generated from the data, as themes which were common across the data set became apparent, and were elevated and organized into concepts and overarching categories.

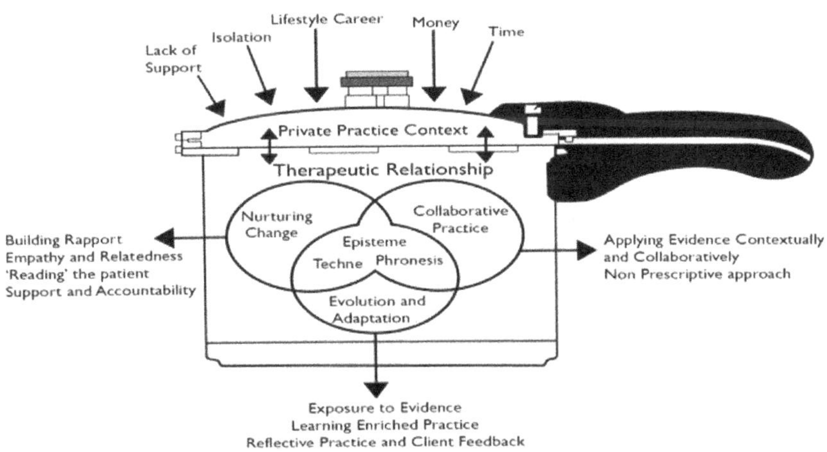

Figure 1. Philosophies Underpinning Dietetic Private Practice.

We will then, in turn, explain each component of the model, beginning with describing the unique context of private practice. We will describe the therapeutic relationships and the individual key strategies and processes that dietitians utilize to foster these in private practice. Finally, we will elucidate the knowledge philosophies underpinning these processes and show how these philosophies are integrated within processes that allow dietitians to adapt and evolve their practices.

3.1. Overview

As depicted in Figure 1, private practice is a complex and pressured environment within which dietitians adapt and evolve their practices. The unique context of private practice (described below) compels dietitians to modify their practices and foster mutually beneficial therapeutic relationships with their patients.

Synergistically, the therapeutic relationships themselves provide a context in which dietitians hone the skills and strategies needed within their practices. The key strategies used by dietitians with their patients: 'nurturing change' and 'collaborative practice', are continuously being refined using the third strategy of 'evolution and adaptation'. Underpinning and intertwined within these strategies, the three intellectual virtues: episteme, techne, and phronesis, were evident. These knowledge types remain at the center of this model. This is due to their presence being fundamental to the way in which dietitians adapt and evolve their strategies, in relation to the therapeutic relationships that are cultivated in the context of private practice. We will consider these concepts separately, explaining each of them in turn. Firstly, we will set the scene in the context of private practice.

3.2. Private Practice Context

Private practice dietetics appears to be a unique context within which dietitians acquire skills and use knowledge specific to that setting. It presents as a complex and pressured environment, within which dietitians adapt and evolve their practices. Private practitioners experience concerns over money and time, a lack of support, isolation, and enmeshment of their work and personal life. The private practitioners in this study acknowledged the challenging aspects of working in a private practice, which involved many hours of unpaid work, running a business, and doing the necessary paperwork that goes along with being both a dietitian, and being a business owner. Unpaid time was spent on business endeavors, preparing and updating education material, reading, keeping up to date, and professional development. Positive aspects of working in private practice included the freedom to choose which areas of interest they would focus their practice on and being one's own boss. These positive aspects were more prevalent among more established dietitians. The dietitians in this study indicated that running a business was more suitable for their perceived personalities.

Dietitians in this study spoke of the necessity of entering private practice due to the lack of work for dietitians. The more established dietitians expressed concerns that new graduates are entering private practice with no support or experience, and who are accepting an income well below what they should, thus creating a negative impression of the dietetic profession as a whole. Dietitians expressed that there was a lack of education on the complex aspects of private practice. These aspects included the wide array of conditions encountered, business acumen, people skills needed for dealing with frequently emotional patients, and the psychological aspects of feeling emotionally drained or experiencing death in long term patients with whom close therapeutic relationships have been established.

A sense of isolation from peers was experienced by the dietitians that worked alone. Some spoke of being comfortable with this isolation and had no desire to change. Others had sought out opportunities to connect with other dietitians, to varying degrees. Competition with other local dietitians, in some cases, was expressed as paradoxical to making connections.

The participants expressed the desire to deliver the best service that they could, and were continuously adapting their practice and knowledge base in an effort to better serve their client base. On account of this, dietitians spoke of the all-encompassing nature of being a dietitian in private practice. When they weren't actively working in their practice, they were learning, reading, and thinking about nutrition and business. In effect, this created a career which could be described as a 'lifestyle career', as it was often difficult to 'turn off', even when outside of the practice. The high exposure which nutrition, food, and cooking has within society through various outlets, also added to this feeling. Those that also lived in the community which they worked in described the balancing act of seeing clients both professionally and in a more casual setting, and being conscious of the relationship which they had with their clients. Overall, private practice provided a rich context in which dietitians worked and in which they learned the skills which are needed to be successful.

3.3. *Therapeutic Relationship*

The therapeutic relationship is the foundation of the practitioner-patient alliance. Research suggests that this relationship has two parts: building a relationship and facilitating positive action [39]. A successful therapeutic relationship requires the practitioner to build a good rapport, show empathy, and gain the trust of their client [39]. Braude states that within the intersubjective space between the practitioner and patient, elements exist that are beyond the cognitions of the practitioner and patient [20]. Despite being beyond cognition, these nonverbal, tacit clues that exist within the context of the therapeutic relationship, provide valuable information to the practitioner, which they draw upon to appropriately respond to their patient [20].

Dietitians in private practice recognized the importance of developing a therapeutic relationship as the foundation of their practice. They have developed strategies that directly relate to fostering a mutually satisfying therapeutic relationship with their clients. The motivations for dietitians in private practice to foster these relationships are multi-faceted. The participants in this study described the importance of the therapeutic relationship for facilitating change and positive outcomes for their clients. Furthermore, they noted that positive outcomes were more likely in clients who received ongoing support through follow-up consultations over time. Follow-up consultations and the resultant positive outcomes were mediated by the therapeutic relationships that dietitians fostered from the outset of contact. Additionally, dietitians in this study were aware that building these relationships were crucial to their professional reputation with both doctors and patients, and that, in turn, they had a direct effect on their income. In this way, the therapeutic relationship was vital to both the client's wellbeing and the practitioner's livelihood.

3.4. *Collaborative Therapy*

Collaborative therapy refers to the key strategy that dietitians in this study used to formulate their education focus and nutrition interventions with their clients. Using a non-prescriptive approach, and applying evidence both contextually and collaboratively, are ways in which the dietitians in this study worked collaboratively with their clients. These processes were the most commonly described approaches across the data set and they are elucidated below.

3.4.1. Evidence Applied Contextually and Collaboratively

Dietitians in this study described working with their patients to design therapies that were informed by EBP, but that were, more importantly, collaboratively formulated with the patient. The clients' social contexts were often barriers to implementing strict EBPs and necessitated a flexible approach. One dietitian showed awareness of the clinical guidelines for a low salt diet, but access to suitable foods and the clients' lifestyle prohibited recommending a diet which was strictly based on clinical guidelines:

> 'It wasn't a clinical low salt diet, it's quite difficult to access that sort of food here unless you're going to cook absolutely everything from scratch which wasn't quite realistic for her. We also discussed how to, you know, eat out, get take away in a sensible manner. She had become quite reliant on take away for small periods of time there, she had her children, came back home and was doing lots of events of the evening, so she needed to do that sort of thing so it was about, so if you need to do take away how can we do that well?' (Dietitian 7)

The primary goal of the dietitians was to ascertain the client's abilities, requirements, and wishes, and to collaborate with their client in order to tailor a suitable intervention protocol. Facilitating client autonomy within this collaborative process, where possible and practical, was seen by dietitians as a necessary part of gaining trust, enhancing a rapport, and increasing compliance with their clients. They described the approach of telling a client what they had to do as having the potential of alienating the client and getting them off side. One dietitian described a client who arrived with a diet plan that she wanted to follow, and which had previously allowed her to successfully lose weight. The dietitian chose to facilitate this to show support for the client and encourage follow-up visits. Over time, taking into consideration her previous failures, the dietitian hoped to work with the client to make her diet more easily sustainable over the long term:

> '(She) had specifically come to me because she said she wanted some accountability and just a little bit of support along the way so, in many ways I was guided by what she wanted to do. . . given her previous failures, that we would have to look at something that I think would be a bit more sustainable for her. But in the first appointment I decided to let her run with what she wanted to start with because I wanted to show, demonstrate to her that I was, you know, being supportive of what she wanted to do.' (Dietitian 8)

Evidence applied contextually and collaboratively as episteme and techne. Episteme as a knowledge type underpinning practice is evident in the use of evidence-based guidelines for nutrition interventions and counselling techniques. Techne, as a knowledge type, is present when dietitians have the technical acumen to use this knowledge and apply it appropriately to suit their clients' needs. In this way, episteme and techne underpin the DAA competency standards which state that, for dietitians to be competent, they must be able to use client care in collaboration with clients.

3.4.2. Non Prescriptive

The dietitians in this study most often used a non-prescriptive diet approach during intervention. Increasing awareness whilst eating and educating to increase nourishment within an often imperfect diet, was seen as more desirable than promoting prescriptive diets. Some others spoke of supplying a diet plan to their clients, when they felt that the client preferred that approach. One participant described how being non-prescriptive worked well for her clients:

> 'It's not prescriptive; it's them figuring it out for themselves. That's how I work anyway and it works really well.' (Dietitian 3)

Non-prescriptive as episteme and techne. Using a non-prescriptive diet for clients would be underpinned by episteme and techne, in the use of evidence which signifies that changes are needed in the diet and using the techniques to apply changes in a non-prescriptive way.

3.5. Nurturing Change

Nurturing change refers to the key strategy that the dietitians in this study used to foster an environment in which their clients felt heard and supported. The processes that constitute 'nurturing change' are, 'building rapport', 'empathy and relatedness', 'reading the patient', and 'support and accountability'. These relational and interpersonal skills were the most commonly described processes across the data set. They are individually considered below.

3.5.1. Building Rapport and Relationships

The dietitians in this study were conscious of establishing a good relationship with their clients. They were aware that, prior to any education or intervention being delivered or being successful, they need to establish a relationship in which the client feels comfortable and feels as though they are engaged in the consultation process. The techniques that they use to build a rapport and relationships vary, according to the dietitian and the client.

The dietitians reported changing their approach, depending on the type of client that they had. They use a range of techniques to show the client that they are interested, respectful, and willing to listen. In doing so, they were more confident that the client would be more engaged with them and more likely to return to see them. Repeat visits were seen as much more conducive to successful outcomes for the client, as well as being advantageous for the business. One dietitian spoke of the importance of engaging the client and making them comfortable, in order to be able to help them:

> 'I know if I can't engage that patient that I'm not going to be able to help them so it's of primary importance to make sure you are on that level with the patient and they're happy with you, you know, if they're not happy with you, or comfortable with me I'm not going to be able to help them so I need to kind of establish that right from the beginning.' (Dietitian 6)

Another dietitian described being aware that more than one consultation is usually needed to help a client achieve positive outcomes, and that facilitating follow-up visits hinged on establishing a rapport and connection, right from the first consult:

> 'Generally I try and establish a really good rapport and connection with the person because I know that if I can establish that rapport then I know that I can keep them coming back and I know that I can help them, whereas if we can't establish that connection, so that's what I sort of try to establish in that first consult.' (Dietitian 9)

Building rapport and relationships as episteme and techne. Although not stated explicitly in the competency standards, building a rapport with clients is a fundamental element of counselling models and is implied in dietetic counselling practice. In this way, episteme and techne are evident as knowledge types underpinning the techniques used to a build rapport and relationships when counselling clients.

3.5.2. Empathy and Relatedness

All participants described the amount of emotionality that they encounter in consultations with their clients. Some dietitians felt this emotionality was due to the more personal and unregimented atmosphere of the private practice consultation process. This atmosphere was contrasted with consults in hospital wards by dietitians who had experience in both areas. Depression is often encountered and crying was encountered on a very regular basis by all dietitians in this study. Dietitians in this study felt that being respectful and empathetic during these encounters was crucial. Often, dietitians described crying as flattering and showing trust, and also as cathartic, moving the consultation in a more beneficial direction. All dietitians reported that when the emotionality became counterproductive to moving forward, they would encourage clients to seek professional help. The dietitians in this study recognized the importance of understanding the client from their perspective and being able to relate to their circumstances. The older dietitians also described scenarios in which having personal experience helped them relate to their client's situation. The younger dietitians revealed how they had grown more comfortable with clients' emotions over time. Anger was also encountered, although to a much lesser extent, and was usually dealt with by listening to the clients' concerns and reassuring them that they are there to help. A dietitian describes becoming comfortable with dealing with crying patients over time:

> 'I go through many boxes of tissues in a week, but it's a tough situation and I remember when I first had my client cry on me, I didn't know what to do, I didn't know what to say but I think through experience you get to know it's part of the whole process—it's part of that process of change because it's a realization.' (Dietitian 2)

An older dietitian described being able to relate to different life stages of her clients, after having the same experiences:

'I think that it allows you to relate to people at that stage, so when I had young children I could relate to how tired and busy young mums are, when I had teenage daughters I could relate to, you know, so the mother drags the teenage daughter in sits her in the chair and says 'she eats terribly, fix her diet' you know, so you can relate to fact that the child is sitting there going, 'yeah mum I don't want to be here' so yeah.' (Dietitian 4)

Empathy and relatedness as phronesis. Being empathic is a necessary element of being a skillful counsellor [40]. Svenaus (2003) draws a direct comparison between empathy and phronesis, and suggests that empathy is a fundamental component of being a phronetic practitioner who seeks the good for his patient in each situation [41]. In this way, phronesis underpins the practice of being empathetic in the context of this situation.

3.5.3. 'Reading' the Patient

The dietitians in this study frequently alluded to 'picking up' signals from their clients which helped them decide how to proceed within the consultation. They used a variety of ways to describe this process. These included, 'gut feel', 'intuition', 'reading the person', 'instinct', 'clever questioning', and 'tone'. These non-verbal cues or the tone of the conversation, despite being hard for the dietitians to describe, played a significant role in how the dietitians chose to proceed and respond throughout the consultation. During the interviews, the dietitians could recall how the patient was feeling and described asking direct questions, if they weren't sure.

Most dietitians described this as a natural ability that they had, but which they honed over time:

'Yeah, I guess I think I naturally can read people pretty well that sort of one area I can adapt the way I speak with people, so yeah that instinct as well—it kind of gets better as you go.' (Dietitian 2)

Most dietitians described using this perceptive ability to help them make clinical decisions:

'I think you've really just got to tailor everything to the individual and that's all on gut feel. I don't know that's the way I operate anyway—it's—it is a bit gut feel.' (Dietitian 1)

Reading the patient and phronesis. Braude suggests that perception connects cognition and consciousness, and that it is important for clinical reasoning [20]. He suggests that these perceptions are present within the therapeutic relationship and contends that, when perception and intuition are combined with the explicit, phronesis is a fitting concept to apply to clinical decisions [20]. Phronesis, then, underpins the practice of using tacit clues which are implicit within the consultation process, to assist in being responsive to the patients' needs.

3.5.4. Support and Accountability

Dietitians who saw clients regularly over a period of time, reported that their roles moved more towards providing support and accountability, rather than nutritional advice or changes. These consultations became less structured than the first consultations. This dynamic was the most successful in helping their clients change nutritional and lifestyle habits. Slow, long term incremental changes were seen as being more successful in the long run, and repeat visits gave these dietitians the freedom to more successfully support clients and make necessary changes:

'For review consultations, subsequent consultations, probably a lot more of my energy would be focused on motivational interviewing, health coaching and supportive counselling, that sort of thing. So it's gradual changes occurring but I think they're coming about from her having that accountability of coming in and seeing me every week and that's her decision.' (Dietitian 10)

3.6. *Evolution and Adaptation*

Acquisition, development, and integration encompass how dietitians are exposed to knowledge, how they seek it out, and how they learn and integrate information and strategies in their practice.

3.6.1. Exposure

In line with the concept of dietetics in private practice being a lifestyle career, dietitians are constantly exposed to nutritional information from the media, social media, supermarkets, newspapers, and magazines, as well as their own clients. They report that, in addition to these sources, they also seek out information on Google Scholar and access online resources provided through dietetic professional organizations, in particular, Practice Based Evidence in Nutrition (PEN). The DAA website provides registered dietitians with online forum style 'interest groups', in which dietitians can discuss various topics relating to nutrition and dietetics. Most of the participants in this study found that these forums were an interesting and valuable source of information, and also participated in these groups. Mentors were also described as being useful and valuable sources of information, with some dietitians continuing to choose mentoring options long after the DAA stipulation of one year. In cases where opportunities to speak to other dietitians were taken or sought out, these contacts were described as very helpful. Professional development is a necessity for all accredited dietitians, and dietitians in private practice most often sought learning opportunities in areas that taught motivational interviewing or other courses that concentrated on the psychological aspects of dietetic counselling, rather than the nutritional aspects. One dietitian described how social media and the interest groups provided a constant stream of information:

> 'I like loads of different nutrition and dietetic sorts of pages, and it's probably the quickest and easiest way along with email to [get information]. I've always got social media or my emails up there where the interest group stuff is coming through all the time so, yeah so they probably are the two quickest and easiest ways that I'm sort of updating things all the time.' (Dietitian 5)

All dietitians used PEN and google scholar as sources of evidence:

> '(The) first port of call would probably be PEN, so the data base associated with the DAA and then I'd probably just go google scholar somewhere like that and start looking up papers.' (Dietitian 11)

Exposure as episteme and techne. Episteme and techne, as knowledge types, underpin having a knowledge base of evidential information and the technique to search for and discern relevant sources of evidence and information, and integrate them into practice.

3.6.2. Learning Enriched in Practice

The development of sound nutrition and practice philosophies occurred most quickly and thoroughly within the context of the consultation process, with secondary input coming from exposure to other information sources. New graduates entering private practice reported a steep learning curve which levelled out in a matter of months with increased exposure to the consultation process, although all dietitians reported continuous learning and improvement over their career span. Dietitians described that building these skills occurred over time with experience, but that they were also building on pre-existing skills and knowledge that they felt they naturally possessed. All dietitians reported constantly adapting their practice and approach, in relation to the perceived needs of their clients. Over time, this process becomes embedded in practice and becomes intrinsic within the dietitian, permitting them become continuously responsive to the changing environment of private practice. One participant described how, through experience, existing skills improve:

> 'I think just through experience, I think you know as an initial dietitian you know you can do everything that an experienced dietitian can do just about but you can't, you can't

convert that into that kind of people skill connection. You can have people skills but through experience you get to know what people respond to, and I think that's where it's definitely built from. I'd like to think that my people skills are really good and have always been really good but you still can't put that into a consultation situation until you've been able to do it many times I think.' (Dietitian 7)

Learning enriched in practice as phronesis. Phronesis requires experiential learning across time, as is evident in our participants, where knowledge is honed, corrected, or rejected [18]. Phronesis is a knowledge type that is essentially changeable and particular to situations. Therefore, it requires experiential learning, during which it can be improved, corrected, and responsive to real events [18].

3.6.3. Reflective Practice and Client Feedback

Practice philosophies are integrated through the process of reflective practice and client feedback. Reflective practice was carried out via mentoring, and through thinking about their performance and what they needed to change. One dietitian set a specific time each week to reflect on where her gaps in knowledge were and how she could improve them. All the dietitians spoke in a reflective manner during the interviews and they were self-aware in knowing their strengths and weaknesses. They described their character traits and their personality types, and how these fitted with private practice and consultations with clients. The participants also reflected on circumstances with patients, both inside and outside of consultations. They thought about and described how they felt about them, how they thought the patient felt, and at times, how they might do things differently, if a similar circumstance happened in future.

Client feedback was provided in the forms of both physical biomarkers and the observation that clients who are happy with the service they are receiving will return for follow-up visits, and that these repeat clients had better success rates. Physical biomarkers were seen as a secondary source of success to any psychological aspects that had changed positively in the client over time and which helped to ensure the continued compliance of any implemented healthy lifestyle changes. One participant described how reflecting on practice culminated in changing strategies with patients:

> 'But I feel it just sort of comes around like, when you really reflect on your consultations and you go—ok well you know once you see 30 people you get an idea about what are some common things that come up with clients...and you sort of reflect on that and come up with some strategies that you know are going to help them.' (Dietitian 3)

One dietitian reflected on how she would react differently, if a similar situation happened in the future:

> 'So I guess that first consult, when I reflect back on it was really, you know, probably faced with somebody else in that situation I wouldn't have done anything, I would've said you know "this is what it is" maybe explained it—off to hospital you go.' (Dietitian 2)

Reflective practice as phronesis. The participants were able to reflect and respond within the consultation in response to cues, as well as reflect on previous circumstances involving patients. They used these reflective skills to help them respond appropriately, increase self-awareness, and improve future performance. In this way, phronesis, which is aligned with reflective practice, underpinned these actions. Phronesis is said to underscore reflection as a means to guide wise action, assist with navigating the various contexts of practice, and ultimately gain practical wisdom [29].

4. Discussion

The theoretical model of the philosophies of dietitians in private practice, integrates the experiences, practices, and perspectives of 11 dietitians working in private practices in Australia. It describes the key strategies and processes that dietitians use in the context of private practice and the therapeutic relationships which were found to be important mediators. It also highlights the underlying knowledge types that dietitians utilize when performing and learning these key strategies. Most studies exploring episteme, techne, and in particular, phronesis, as philosophies underpinning health care, concentrate on medicine and nursing [21,30,31,42,43]; they do not account for the context of private practice or the complexities faced by dietitians when helping patients choose and/or change lifelong eating habits.

The processes that the dietitians used in this study shared similarities with health care and counselling models that are a small part of dietetic student curricula [38,40]. This study supports the accepted notion that the counselling relationship is a fundamental aspect of a successful counselling relationship [41]. We extend and enhance this concept by exploring the processes specific to dietetics, as well as by identifying a philosophical/knowledge construct that may be useful in framing the explicated processes and strategies.

The key strategy, 'collaborative therapy', shares similarities with what is generally known as 'patient or client centered care' [14,44,45]. Nutrition and dietetics suffer from a lack of definition surrounding client-centered care, as it pertains to nutrition counselling [14,44]. The contextual and collaborative approach for applying interventions in this study was, at times, in conflict with applying a straight forward, evidence-based guideline. Despite a lack of time and skill being the most cited barriers to using EBP, the dietitians in this study described the client's contextual situation as the main driver, when deciding on intervention strategies ahead of EBP [15,46,47]. This disparity could be due to the longer consultation that private practice affords and the possibility of follow-up appointments affording a slower approach to education and therapy. Barriers cited when applying this contextual approach elsewhere, specifically professional norm and organizational culture, are not present in this study, which highlights the professional freedom that dietitians have in private practice, when delivering patient-centered care [44,48]. This contextual approach to intervention was strongly favored by clients of dietitians in a qualitative examination of client preferences [14]. This study confirms that dietitians in private practice are not only aware of the mitigating factors that affect the food choice and practices of their clients, but also strive to collaboratively develop interventions with these in mind. Hancock et al. (2012) found that most patients favored a non-prescriptive approach, although a small subset preferred a specific diet plan [14]. The dietitians in our study appeared aware of which approach their clients preferred and this is reflected in the strategies which they use in response to these perceived preferences.

Building a rapport was shown to be an important aspect of practice in our study. This finding is consistent with research that shows that building a rapport is important for establishing a counselling relationship [41,42]. The practice of building a rapport helps to build trust in clients, allowing for more positive outcomes and relationships [42]. Hancock et al. (2012) found that dietetic clients cited rapport building as being important in their dealings with dietitians [14]. Further to these findings, our study revealed that the context of private practice provided the motivation to establish a rapport with clients, and a rich learning environment in which to foster the skills to do so.

The practices of dietitians in this study support the findings by Cant and Aroni, who found that dietitians strive to show empathy in their consultations by listening, in order to understand the patient's situation [12]. This is further supported by Goodchild et al., who noted that empathic moments are common throughout dietetic consultations and that these moments are rarely missed by dietitians [49]. Patients reported a higher satisfaction in consultations where responses to emotional opportunities by dietitians were coded as more empathic [49]. Rogers (1940) contends that demonstrating empathy towards the client is an integral part of the counselling process [45]. The dietitians in this study also used their own experiences to relate to the patient empathically. It is suggested that using one's own experience to relate to the patient may optimize the empathic response and, in turn, improve the patient's satisfaction [14]. It is argued that empathy as a character trait is needed, to enable an understanding of the needs and wishes of patients [41]. To use empathy as a phronetic, the practitioner would need to seek to understand and desire ethical solutions that align with the patients' goals for the most beneficial outcome in that situation [41]. This requires the practitioner to be highly cognizant of the patients' version of what their own best health and wellbeing is. Further study on this concept within dietetics would be beneficial to ascertain levels of empathetic responses within consultations that take into account the patients' viewpoint of their own best health outcome.

Our study showed that nonverbal communication featured heavily in the way that dietitians responded to their patients. Further, the participants described using perception or intuition when dealing with their clients, and that perceptiveness was intrinsic to them. Nonverbal communication is largely involved with conveying feelings and attitudes, and is often beyond our conscious awareness [12]. Nonverbal communication may account for 65% of meaning in interpersonal communications [50]. The present study confirms the Cant and Aroni finding, that dietitians are aware of nonverbal communication and place an importance on this being nonthreatening [12]. Intuition and perception in dietitians has not been previously researched; however, research on nurses has recognized its presence in nursing practice. Intuition and perception in clinical practice is a form of understanding or knowing something about the situation or patient, without logical thought processes or being explicitly told by the patient [51,52]. Rew and Barrow, in the reviewing literature, found that intuition was vital for complex decision making [53]. A review by King and Appleton found evidence that nurses used intuition (i.e., gut feelings) to initiate action [54]. Rigid adherence to protocol tended to devalue intuition and perception in clinical reasoning [54]. Feasibly, due to having less procedural and departmental constraints, the dietitians in our study were able to recognize and verbalize that intuition and/or perception played an important role when interacting with their clients.

Dietitians in this study saw successful outcomes by providing long term support and accountability to their clients. Hancock et al. found that, in a community and hospital setting, patients reported that support felt limited, due to the length or frequency of the appointment, or the continuity of the dietitian [14]. In a private practice situation, this scenario is avoided and, as such, the dietitians in this study reported successful outcomes for patients that they had seen, or were seeing, long term, both in biomedical markers and habit changes. This indicates that private practice is well placed to provide successful outcomes to those clients who can access long term private practice dietetic support.

The sources of evidence that participants used in this study are in contrast to Thomas et al., who found that pediatric dietitians had access to Medline, Cochrane, and CINAHL, and that 39% used Medline as their main source of information [17]. Dietitians in this study report using online searches (google scholar), and online resources provided by DAA and DAA interest groups, as their main sources of information when sourcing evidence. This is most likely due to the lack of access that private practice dietitians have to other sources of literature that require payment. There are no studies documenting other types of information that are sourced, such as social media, and this study uncovers the phenomenon of dietitians in private practice being inundated by nutrition and food information.

The newer dietitians in this study reported that, upon entering the practice, their communication and counselling skills increased quickly with continuous consultation experience. This supports Cant et al., who found only a small variation in communication practices of recently qualified and more senior dietitians [12]. Situational or experiential learning is at the core of learning for professionals, and health professional training courses require a period of placement types within their profession before graduation [55,56]. This study supports the concept that skill acquisition for professionals is embedded in practice, and highlights the importance of ongoing exposure to clinical settings by professionals as a means to improve and maintain their skills.

As part of the accreditation process, new graduates must enter a mentoring partnership for one year [57]. Part of that process is reflective by design, as the mentoring partnership requires the graduate to explore his/her practice with the mentor [58]. There is little research on the mentoring partnerships in Australia; however, research has shown that the mentoring partnership can facilitate lifelong learning through supporting the habit of reflective practice [58]. Palermo et al. found that mentor attributes of facilitating trusting relationships and providing effective feedback, were important components of mentoring [59]. This study supports this finding, with dietitians in this study reporting positive relationships and experiences with their mentor, and this positive experience compelled some dietitians to seek ongoing mentoring after the mandatory period was over, throughout their career.

Reflective practice is an essential skill for being an APD and dietitians are expected to autonomously continue this practice throughout their career [6]. Reflective practice allows practitioners to learn from experience. Ajjawi et al. found that self-evaluation and reflection in allied health professionals were important for monitoring and correcting clinical reasoning and communication [60]. Proponents of including phronesis as a necessary element, along with episteme and techne, for a model of good practice, and the traits of an expert practitioner, contend that to be phronetic is to be reflective [18,21,29]. Schon and Benner posit that the ability to reflect in and on practice, and change actions within constant contextual shifts within practice, distinguishes an expert from a technically proficient practitioner [25,61]. Kinsella contends that merely reflecting on practice, such as journaling and blogging, is aligned towards techne, and that to aspire to expertise resultant change and critical judgments must be able to be processed and arrived at within the context of the moment [22]. It was evident in this study that dietitians use high level reflective practice both in and out of the consultation experience to improve their interpersonal skills, clinical judgement, and their business models. This study supports the implications that dietitians continue to reflect on practice throughout their career and use those skills to improve services to their clients. This indicates that private practitioners subscribe to the DAA's stipulations and agree with the value of reflective practice.

5. Episteme, Techne, and Phronesis

This model of private practice revealed that dietitians use intertwining and embedded forms of episteme, techne, and phronesis in their practice and throughout the consultation practice. It was clear in this study that the dietitians used episteme, techne, and phronesis when using key strategies and processes, and that these philosophies also underpinned how the participants improved and integrated these strategies into practice. The key strategies that the dietitians employed, although discussed separately, are used in a simultaneous manner in response to the environment. Similarly, it is not possible to separate episteme, techne, and phronesis as underpinning forms of knowledge skills in practice, although at times, one form of knowledge may be predominant over another, depending on the situation. In line with other studies, elements of practice that are not easily described or assessed were evident when dietitians adapted their approach to clients within consultations, in response to both extrinsic and intrinsic cues. This study supported the use of the concept of phronesis through the dietitian's practices of perception, empathy, and reflective practice.

Phronesis was useful in exploring the therapeutic relationship that is a complex interpersonal experience where dietitians use tacit, theoretical, and evidential knowledge, to appropriately respond to clients. In this space, dietitians simultaneously reflect, respond, and learn. These responses become intrinsically embedded over time. It is also clear that the therapeutic relationship was a crucial platform for using, learning, and integrating these strategies, and that the context of private practice is an important mediator of nurturing the therapeutic relationship. Episteme, techne, and phronesis as a framework for professional practice, provided a useful lens to view dietetic practice, particularly the contexts and elements of practice that are not easily described, but that are crucial to being an expert practitioner.

6. Strengths and Limitations of the Study

The study's findings reveal the key strategies and underpinning philosophies that dietitians use during private practice. To our knowledge, this is the first investigation of dietitians' philosophies in private practice and shows a unique perspective of private practice in Australia. A strength of this study is that it reveals the dynamics and intricacies within the consultation process, including facets within the therapeutic relationship and strategies used that are frequently invisible. An important strength of this study is that it provides in-depth knowledge of private practice issues and reveals how dietitians nurture and protect the therapeutic relationship. The therapeutic relationship was shown to be an important learning environment and mediator of successful outcomes for patients, as well as crucial for a successful private practice business. Notably, the context of private practice was revealed as a stimulus for developing key strategies to nurture the therapeutic relationship. Further study in these areas would greatly benefit the area of dietetic private practice in Australia. The aspects of practice that contributed to successful outcomes for patients, such as empathy, perception, and reflective practice, are scarce in nutrition and dietetic studies. This study contributed important information on key strategies that are understudied, and that are poorly understood in the context of dietetic private practice.

This study used a lens of episteme, techne, and phronesis, to understand the different types of knowledge that dietitians use when performing key strategies and processes. In addition to using evidence and techniques that meet competency standards, other aspects of practice, such as, perception, intuition, empathy, and reflection in and on practice were evident, and as such, phronesis is a useful lens with which to view these aspects. In this regard, phronesis could add valuable dimensions to dietetic practice when gauging the differences between competent and expert dietitians. The framework of episteme, techne, and phronesis as knowledge types, provided a useful lens to explain a patient-centered holistic practice style and to examine how these key strategies are learnt and integrated into practice. This grounded theory study produced a model of private practice that shows concepts and relationships that could be explored quantitatively.

These strengths are countered by the fact that the practice and nutrition strategies were only investigated from the dietitian's perspective. How patients experienced their care and approach was not a focus of this study, and there is a need for studies that consider the patients' perspective of their care. Another limitation is that, although terms such as 'client centred approach', 'mindfulness', and 'intuition' have been used by the dietitians in this study, no further enquiry was made as to how similar in meaning these were to each other, when used by another dietitian. Due to the interview question, this model depicts what usually happens, from the dietitians view of a 'case study'; that is, a long-term client. No data of how one-off 'Medicare' (public healthcare) patients were treated was included. Although the dietitians reported that these patients were treated similarly, the same outcomes were not seen with these short-term patients, due to the short length of care. The sample size ($n = 11$) was small; however, the sample represented a broad cross section of the profession and the concepts remained static across the sample, adding to the strength of the results. In this way, generality is plausible, but not possible with this sample size. Possibly due to the burden of the interview process on the participants, recruitment for this study was difficult, and the sample may be skewed towards dietitians who were interested in the subject matter and the trajectory of dietetics in Australia in general.

7. Conclusions

Dietetic private practice in Australia is a complex environment in which dietitians must employ high level professional, technical, and interpersonal skills. Private practice dietitians form collaborative relationships with their clients to nurture change over time and are able to provide continuity of care without departmental constraints. Thus, private practice is well placed to provide successful outcomes to those clients who can access long term private practice.

The context of private practice was revealed to be an important element of how and why dietitians develop and integrate knowledge over time. Further study aimed at uncovering more detailed information of how dietitians experience different aspects of private practice would be advantageous, to further develop our understanding of the challenges that dietitians face in private practice. The nuances that seem unique to private practice seem to facilitate a practitioner's ability to respond in a client-centered manner, over a short period of time. Dietitians used intertwined forms of episteme, techne, and phronesis, to collaboratively nurture change in clients.

Episteme, techne, and phronesis offer a broader model of practice that has considerable applicability for nutrition and dietetics. Framing practice research within these concepts could be useful for addressing the complex aspects that are specific to the nutrition and dietetic profession.

Acknowledgments: The author disclosed receipt of the following financial support for the research, authorship, and publication of this article: Honours Funding, University of the Sunshine Coast.

Author Contributions: Judith Maher conceived and designed the research; Claudia Harper performed the research; Claudia Harper and Judith Maher analyzed the data; Claudia Harper wrote the paper; Judith Maher edited the paper. This paper was undertaken as an Honours Project by Claudia Harper. Judith Maher acted as the supervisor. The Figure was produced by: Heather Ngata, QUT Art Student.

References

1. Sackett, D.L.; Rosenberg, W.M.C.; Muir Gray, J.A.; Haynes, R.B.; Richardson, W.S. Evidence based medicine: What it is and what it isn't. *BMJ* **1996**, *312*, 71–72. [CrossRef] [PubMed]
2. DAA. Available online: http://daa.asn.au/wp-content/uploads/2013/09/Dietitian-Scope-of-Practice-2015.pdf (accessed on 31 August 2014).
3. Hise, M.E.; Kattelmann, K.; Parkhurst, M. Evidence-Based Clinical Practice: Dispelling the Myths. *NCP* **2005**, *20*, 294–302. [CrossRef] [PubMed]
4. International Confederation of Dietetic Associations. ICDA Code of Ethics and Code of Good Practice. Available online: http://www.internationaldietetics.org/Downloads/ICDA-Code-of-Ethics-and-Code-of-Good-Practice.aspx (accessed on 28 August 2014).
5. Ball, L.; Larsson, R.; Gerathy, R.; Hood, P.; Lowe, C. Working profile of Australian private practice Accredited Practising Dietitians. *Nutr. Diet.* **2013**, *70*, 196–205. [CrossRef]
6. DAA. The National Competency Standards for Dietitians in Australia. Available online: http://daa.asn.au/wp-content/uploads/2015/12/NCS-Dietitians-Australia-1.0.pdf (accessed on 23 August 2014).
7. Freeland-Graves, J.H.; Nitzke, S. Position of the Academy of Nutrition and Dietetics: Total Diet Approach to Healthy Eating. *J. Acad. Nutr. Diet.* **2013**, *113*, 307–317. [CrossRef] [PubMed]
8. Grimmer, K.; Bialocerkowski, A.; Kumar, S.; Milanese, S. Implementing evidence in clinical practice: The 'therapies' dilemma. *Physiotherapy* **2004**, *90*, 189–194. [CrossRef]
9. Buchanan, D. Two Models for Defining the Relationship between Theory and Practice in Nutrition Education: Is the Scientific Method Meeting Our Needs? *J. Nutr. Educ. Behav.* **2004**, *36*, 146–154. [CrossRef]
10. Schubert, L.; Gallegos, D.; Foley, W.; Harrison, C. Re-imagining the 'social' in the nutrition sciences. *Public Health Nutr.* **2012**, *15*, 352–359. [CrossRef] [PubMed]
11. Swift, J.A.; Tischler, V. Qualitative research in nutrition and dietetics: Getting started. *J. Hum. Nutr. Diet.* **2010**, *23*, 559–566. [CrossRef] [PubMed]
12. Cant, R.; Aroni, R. Exploring dietitians' verbal and nonverbal communication skills for effective dietitian-patient communication. *J. Hum. Nutr. Diet.* **2008**, *21*, 502–511. [CrossRef] [PubMed]
13. Cant, R. Constructions of competence within dietetics: Trust, professionalism and communications with individual clients. *Nutr. Diet.* **2009**, *66*, 113–118. [CrossRef]
14. Hancock, R.E.E.; Bonner, G.; Hollingdale, R.; Madden, A.M. 'If you listen to me properly, I feel good': A qualitative examination of patient experiences of dietetic consultations. *J. Hum. Nutr. Diet.* **2012**, *25*, 275–284. [CrossRef] [PubMed]
15. Byham-Gray, L.D.; Gilbride, J.A.; Dixon, L.B.; Stage, F.K. Evidence-Based Practice: What Are Dietitians' Perceptions, Attitudes, and Knowledge? *J. Am. Diet. Assoc.* **2005**, *105*, 1574–1581. [CrossRef] [PubMed]
16. Taylor, M.A. Evidence-based practice: Are dietitians willing and able? *J. Hum. Nutr. Diet.* **1998**, *11*, 461–472. [CrossRef]
17. Thomas, D.E.; Kukuruzovic, R.; Martino, B.; Chauhan, S.S.; Elliott, E.J. Knowledge and use of evidence-based nutrition: A survey of paediatric dietitians. *J. Hum. Nutr. Diet.* **2003**, *16*, 315–322. [CrossRef] [PubMed]

18. Benner, P.; Hughes, R.; Sutphen, M. Clinical Reasoning, Decisionmaking and Action: Thinking Critically and Clinically. In *Patient Safety and Quality: An Evidence-Based Handbook for Nurses*; Hughes, R., Ed.; Agency for Healthcare Research and Quality: Rockville, MD, USA, 2008; Volume 1, pp. 1–109.
19. Beresford, M.J. Medical reductionism: Lessons from the great philosophers. *QJM Int. J. Med.* **2010**, *103*, 721–724. [CrossRef] [PubMed]
20. Braude, H.D. Conciliating cognition and consciousness: The perceptual foundations of clinical reasoning. *J. Eval. Clin. Pract.* **2012**, *18*, 945–950. [CrossRef] [PubMed]
21. Flaming, D. Using phronesis instead of 'research-based practice' as the guiding light for nursing practice. *Nurs. Philos.* **2001**, *2*, 251–258. [CrossRef]
22. Kinsella, E.A. Professional knowledge and the epistemology of reflective practice. *Nurs. Philos.* **2009**, *11*, 3–14. [CrossRef] [PubMed]
23. Miles, A. On a medicine of the whole person: Away from scientistic reductionism and towards the embrace of the complex in clinical practice. *J. Eval. Clin. Pract.* **2009**, *15*, 941–949. [CrossRef] [PubMed]
24. Thorgaard, K.; Jensen, U.J. Evidence and the end of medicine. *Med. Health Care Philos.* **2011**, *14*, 273–280. [CrossRef] [PubMed]
25. Benner, P. *From Novice to Expert: Excellence and Power in Clinical Nursing Practice*; Prentice Hall: Upper Saddle Rive, NJ, USA, 2001.
26. Aristotle. Metaphysics. In *The Complete Works of Aristotle*; Ross, W.D., Tr., Ed.; Princeton University Press: Princeton, NJ, USA, 1984; Volume 2.
27. Dreyfus, H.; Dreyfus, S. *Mind over Machine: The Power of Human Intuition and Expertise in the Era of the Computer*; Free Press: New York, NY, USA, 1986.
28. Dunne, J. Professional judgement and the predicaments of practice. *Eur. J. Mark.* **1999**, *33*, 707–720. [CrossRef]
29. Kinsella, E.A. Practitioner Reflection and Judgement as Phronesis: A Continuum of Reflection and Considerations for Phronetic Judgement. In *Phronesis as Professional Knowledge: Practical Wisdom in the Profession*; Kinsella, E.A., Pitman, A., Eds.; Sense Publishers: Rotterdam, The Netherlands, 2012.
30. James, I.; Andershed, B.; Gustavsson, B.; Ternestedt, B.-M. Knowledge Constructions in Nursing Practice: Understanding and Integrating Different Forms of Knowledge. *QHR* **2010**, *20*, 1500–1518. [CrossRef] [PubMed]
31. Nieminen, A.L.; Mannevaara, B.; Fagerstrom, L. Advanced practice nurses' scope of practice: A qualitative study of advanced clinical competencies. *Scand. J. Caring Sci.* **2011**, *25*, 661–670. [CrossRef] [PubMed]
32. Hirst, R.J. *Philosophy: An outline for the Intending Student*; Routledge & Kegan Paul Ltd.: London, UK, 1968.
33. Gadamer, H.G. Practical philosophy as a model of human sciences. *Res. Phenomol.* **1979**, *9*, 74–85. [CrossRef]
34. Gustavsson, B. What do we mean by lifelong learning and knowledge? *Int. J. Educ. Res.* **2002**, *21*, 13–23. [CrossRef]
35. Gustavsson, B. Revisiting the philosophical roots of practical knowledge. In *Developing Practice Knowledge for Health Professionals*; Higgs, J., Richardson, W.S., Abrandt Dahlgren, M., Eds.; Butterworth Heinemann: Edinburgh, UK, 2004; pp. 35–51.
36. Charmaz, K. *Constructing Grounded Theory: A Practical Guide Through Qualitative Analysis*; Sage Publications: London, UK, 2006.
37. Blumer, H. *Symbolic Interactionism*; Prentice-Hall: Englewood Cliffs, NJ, USA, 1969.
38. Bauer, K.; Sokolik, C. *Basic Nutrition Counselling Skill Development*; Wadsworth/Thomson Learning: Belmont CA, USA, 2002.
39. Aristotle. *The Ethics of Aristotle [Electronic Resource]: (the Nichomachean Ethics, Chase's Translation, Newly Revised)*; W. Scott: London, UK, 1890.
40. Gable, J. *Counselling Skills for Dietitians*; Blackwell Publishing: Oxford, UK, 2007.
41. Svenaeus, F. Hermeneutics of medicine in the wake of Gadamer: The issue of phronesis. *Theor. Med. Bioeth.* **2003**, *24*, 407–431. [CrossRef] [PubMed]
42. Daniel Davis, F. Phronesis, clinical reasoning, and Pellegrino's philosophy of medicine. *Theor. Med.* **1997**, *18*, 173–195. [CrossRef]
43. Tyreman, S. Promoting critical thinking in health care: Phronesis and criticality. *Med. Health Care Philos.* **2000**, *3*, 117–124. [CrossRef] [PubMed]
44. MacLellan, D.L.; Berenbaum, S. Dietitians' Opinions and Experiences of Client-Centred Nutrition Counselling. *Can. J. Diet. Pract. Res.* **2006**, *67*, 119–124. [CrossRef] [PubMed]

45. Rogers, C.R. The processes of therapy. *J. Consult. Psychol.* **1940**, *4*, 161–164. [CrossRef]
46. Metcalfe, C.; Lewin, R.; Wisher, S.; Perry, S.; Bannigan, K.; Moffett, J.K. Barriers to Implementing the Evidence Base in Four NHS Therapies: Dietitians, occupational therapists, physiotherapists, speech and language therapists. *Physiotherapy* **2001**, *87*, 433–441. [CrossRef]
47. Upton, D.; Upton, P. Knowledge and Use of Evidence-based Practice by Allied Health and Health Science Professionals in the United Kingdom. *J. Allied Health* **2006**, *35*, 127–133. [PubMed]
48. Deschênes, S.-M.; Gagnon, M.-P.; Légaré, F.; Lapointe, A.; Turcotte, S.; Desroches, S. Psychosocial Factors of Dietitians' Intentions to Adopt Shared Decision Making Behaviours: A Cross-Sectional Survey. *PLoS ONE* **2013**, *8*, e64523. [CrossRef] [PubMed]
49. Goodchild, C.E.; Skinner, T.E.; Parkin, T. The value of empathy in dietetic consultations. A pilot study to investigate its effect on satisfaction, autonomy and agreement. *J. Hum. Nutr. Diet.* **2005**, *18*, 181–185. [CrossRef] [PubMed]
50. Putnis, P.; Petelin, R. *Professional Communication: Principles and Applications*; Prentice Hall: Sydney, Australia, 1996.
51. Mitchell, G.J. Intuitive Knowing: Exposing a Myth in Theory Development. *Nurs. Sci. Q.* **1994**, *7*, 2–3. [CrossRef] [PubMed]
52. Young, C.E. Intuition and nursing process. *Holist. Nurs. Pract.* **1987**, *1*, 52–62. [CrossRef] [PubMed]
53. Rew, L.; Barrow, E.M. Intuition: A neglected hallmark of nursing knowledge. *Adv. Nurs. Sci.* **1987**, *10*, 49–62. [CrossRef]
54. King, L.; Appleton, J.V. Intuition: A critical review of the research and rhetoric. *JAN* **1997**, *26*, 194–202. [CrossRef]
55. Benner, P. Using the Dreyfus model of skill acquisition to describe and interpret skill acquisition and clinical judgment in nursing practice and education. *Bull. Sci. Technol. Soc.* **2004**, *24*, 188–199. [CrossRef]
56. O'Reilly, S.L.; Milner, J. Transitions in reflective practice: Exploring student development and preferred methods of engagement. *Nutr. Diet.* **2015**, *72*, 150–155. [CrossRef]
57. DAA. Guide to the APD Program, Continuing Professional Development and Mentoring. Available online: http://daa.asn.au/wp-content/uploads/2014/09/Guide-to-APD-September-2014.pdf (accessed on 16 July 2014).
58. Hawker, J.; McMillan, A.; Palermo, C. Enduring mentoring partnership: A reflective case study and recommendations for evaluating mentoring in dietetics. *Nutr. Diet.* **2013**, *70*, 339–344. [CrossRef]
59. Palermo, C.; Hughes, R.; McCall, L. An evaluation of a public health nutrition workforce development intervention for the nutrition and dietetic workforce. *J. Hum. Nutr. Diet.* **2010**, *23*, 244–253. [CrossRef] [PubMed]
60. Ajjawi, R.; Higgs, J. Learning to Reason: A Journey of Professional Socialisation. *Adv. Health Sci. Educ.* **2008**, *13*, 133–150. [CrossRef] [PubMed]
61. Schön, D.A. *The Reflective Practitioner: How Professionals Think in Action*; Basic Books: New York, NY, USA, 1983.

Feedback-Based Treatments for Eating Disorders and Related Symptoms

Claudio Imperatori [1,*], Miranda Mancini [1], Giacomo Della Marca [2], Enrico Maria Valenti [1,3] and Benedetto Farina [1]

1 Department of Human Sciences, European University of Rome, Via degli Aldobrandeschi 190, 00163 Roma, Italy; mancini.miranda@gmail.com (M.M.); enricomaria.valenti@gmail.com (E.M.V.); benfarina@gmail.com (B.F.)
2 Sleep Disorders Unit, Institute of Neurology, Catholic University, 00153 Rome, Italy; giacomodellamarca@gmail.com
3 Department of Dynamic and Clinical Psychology, Sapienza University of Rome, 00185 Rome, Italy
* Correspondence: imperatori.c@libero.it

Abstract: The effectiveness of biofeedback and neurofeedback has been investigated in a range of psychiatric disorders. However, to date, there are few studies on the clinical usefulness of feedback-based techniques for eating disorders (EDs) and EDs-related symptoms (e.g., food craving). A systematic search of PubMed, Scopus and PsychINFO identified 162 articles. Among these, thirteen studies exploring the therapeutic use of biofeedback and neurofeedback in EDs or EDs-related symptoms were included. Biofeedback and neurofeedback were implemented respectively in five and eight of all reviewed articles. No studies incorporated different feedback modalities or both biofeedback and neurofeedback. The considered studies provide preliminary data of the usefulness of feedback-based techniques in the treatment of several dysfunctional eating behaviors (e.g., food craving, rumination). Although no significant effect has been reported for other important EDs-related symptoms (i.e., body image disturbance), feedback-based techniques are also associated with significant modifications of both sympathetic reaction to food-related stimuli and brain activity in several regions of the reward system (e.g., insula). Taken together the results of the present review suggest that feedback-based treatments may be useful in the treatment of several dysfunctional eating behaviors operating both on top-down and bottom-up individual coping strategies. Methodological and clinical issues are also discussed.

Keywords: biofeedback; EEG-Neurofeedback; fMRI-Neurofeedback; eating disorders; psychophysiology; eating disorders-related symptoms

---

1. Introduction

Eating disorders (EDs) are severe and disabling conditions caused by multiple factors (e.g., genetic and psychosocial) [1], which are associated with significant functional impairments [2], high mortality risk [3] and treatment difficulties [4]. The last edition of the Diagnostic and Statistical Manual of Mental Disorders (DSM-5) [5] includes a substantially revised section on EDs [6,7], now named "Feeding and Eating Disorders". This section includes the following diagnoses: pica, rumination disorder (RD), avoidant/restrictive food intake disorder (ARFID), anorexia nervosa (AN), bulimia nervosa (BN), binge eating disorder (BED), and other specified feeding or eating disorder (OSFED).

EDs and related symptoms are common in both children and adolescents [8,9]. In adults, the lifetime prevalence is about 0.6% for AN, 1% for BN, and 3% for BED [2,3]. Furthermore, it has been recently reported that, following the transition to DSM-5, the prevalence of OSFED has decreased, and that AN, BN and BED have increased in non-clinical samples [10]. Similarly, EDs-related symptoms, such as food craving (i.e., an intense desire to consume a specific food that is difficult to resist); Refs. [11–13] or loss of control over eating, are widely reported amongst the general population. For example, in a non-clinical sample it has been reported [14] that 28% of women and 13% of men reported food craving at least once a week during the past 6 months. This symptom is also commonly experienced in AN [15,16], BN [16–19], and BED [20,21]. Moreover, it has been reported that food craving severity is positively associated with both body mass index (BMI) [13,22–25], drop-out from weight loss programs [25–27], and a meta-analysis [28] on 3292 individuals showed that it significantly contributes to dysfunctional eating behaviours and weight gain.

Similarly, loss of control over eating is a relatively frequent experience among both adolescents from the general population (i.e., about 17%) [29], adults with obesity (i.e., BMI $\geq$ 30 kg/m^2) and patients with EDs [30]. Additionally, it was positively associated with other psychopathological symptoms (e.g., non-suicidal self-injury, body dissatisfaction, higher depressive symptoms) [31].

Multidisciplinary approaches, combining medical, dietetic and psychological interventions are generally recommended in the treatment of EDs [32]. However, it is known that current treatments for EDs are often related to treatment difficulties [4] and poor long-term efficacy [1,33,34]. For example, it has been reported that several treatments, such as nutritional rehabilitation and psychological approaches (e.g., cognitive-behavioral therapy, family-based therapy), are associated with high relapse rates in adolescents with AN [33]. Similarly, binge eating remission rates at the end of treatments are only found in 30–40% of patients with BN [1]. Therefore, the necessity of additional treatment modalities for these mental disorders has been proposed [35].

Feedback-based treatments (i.e., biofeedback and neurofeedback) have been suggested as additional treatment modalities for EDs [36]. Feedback is considered a crucial component of mental health interventions, increasing motivation, facilitating the learning process and modifying dysfunctional thoughts and behaviors [37]. Over the last thirty years there has been an increasing number of disorders, including EDs, for which biofeedback and neurofeedback have been investigated with more or less empirically supported results [38,39].

Biofeedback and neurofeedback are operant-conditioning based trainings that allow individuals to learn how to regulate neurophysiological activity in response to real-time feedback, in order to improve health and performance [38]. Biofeedback refers to an intervention that helps individuals to control or change their physiologic functioning (e.g., heart rate, electrodermal activity, respiratory rate, muscle tension and peripheral temperature) [40]. Neurofeedback refers to a form of biofeedback involving different modalities, such as electroencephalography (EEG) or real-time functional magnetic resonance imaging (rt-fMRI), that trains individuals to control or modify their brain activity [41]. Compared to other neuro-stimulation techniques (i.e., transcranial direct current stimulation), which may be associated with several mild and transient adverse effects [42], feedback-based treatments are not related with side effects [43] and seems to be easy and affordable techniques for general practices and clinicians [44,45].

During a typical feedback-based session, neurophysiological activity (e.g., brain and or electrodermal activity) is "fed back" to the individual using a brain-computer interface, providing continuously updated information about their success in regulating their neurophysiological parameters [36]. The successful self-regulation of the individuals' physiology represents an immediate and effective positive reinforcement, creating a positive loop between the machine's feedback and the patient's successful self-regulation [40]. Therefore the three necessary components for a feedback-based session are: (i) a therapist explaining the equipment and its use, (ii) a patient and (iii) a monitoring machine that provides accurate neurophysiological information [38]. Although training sessions and modalities may be different according to the individual needs and/or the diagnosis [40], general protocol guidelines are provided [38].

2. Study Rationale

The clinical efficacy of biofeedback and neurofeedback has been investigated in a range of psychiatric disorders [38,39]. However, to date, there are few studies on the clinical usefulness of feedback-based techniques for EDs or EDs-related symptoms. Therefore, the present systematic review (PRISMA checklist is reported in Table S1) was carried out to explore the current therapeutic use of biofeedback and neurofeedback in EDs and EDs-related symptoms (i.e., food craving, binge eating, loss of control over eating). Specifically, in this study we investigated: (i) the type of feedback-based protocol applied, and (ii) the usefulness of feedback-based techniques assessed through clinical scales and/or neurophysiological measures.

3. Methods

3.1. Inclusion/Exclusion Criteria

We used the P.I.C.O.S. (Population, Interventions, Comparators, Outcomes, and Study Design) criteria to identify relevant studies. This review focused on feedback-based interventions for EDs and related symptoms. Therefore, original articles reporting data from studies investigating the potential therapeutic effects of different biofeedback (i.e., heart rate, electrodermal activity, respiratory rate, muscle tension and peripheral temperature) and neurofeedback modalities (i.e., EEG, fMRI) in this field were initially considered. Studies involving children and adolescents were also taken into consideration. Book chapters, conference papers, reviews, dissertations, and case reports were not included. Articles in which either feedback-based treatments for EDs or EDs-related symptoms were not the focal point were also excluded. Moreover, feedback-based studies investigating EDs-related symptoms (i.e., food craving, binge eating, overeating) in non-clinical or subthreshold sample were initially considered. Both randomized and non-randomized controlled studies, as well as pre-/post-intervention comparison reports were considered.

According to guidelines for the evaluation of the clinical efficacy of psychophysiological interventions [46], as well as with previous systematic reviews focused of feedback-based treatments in psychiatric disorders [39,47], articles that provided the following information were included in the study: (i) feedback modality type, (ii) sample (i.e., including age, sex, medication status, BMI, recruitment), (iii) study design (including type, number and duration of protocol sessions, as well as description of study conditions), (iv) collection and analysis of neurophysiological (e.g., EEG power spectrum, electrodermal activity etc.), behavioral (e.g., number of binge episodes) and/or psychological outcomes measure (i.e., clinical scales). Furthermore, according to Schoenberg and David [39], studies that did not report 2 or more components of points (ii) and (iii), and/or articles that did not specify points (i), (iv) and (v) were excluded.

3.2. Search Strategy

Potentially relevant studies were initially identified by searching publications from the year 1970 to 5 August 2018 through the following databases: PubMed, Scopus and PsychInfo. Only English articles were taken into account. The following search terms were entered into the databases: "biofeedback" OR "neurofeedback" AND "anorexia nervosa", "bulimia nervosa", "binge eating disorder", "pica", "rumination disorder", "avoidant/restrictive food intake disorder", "food intake disorder", "food craving", "binge eating", "overeating", "eating psychopathology". Articles resulting from the search strategy were examined for relevance by screening titles and abstracts. Then, articles that appeared to meet inclusion criteria were further evaluated by two independent researchers (C.I. and M.M.) in order to assess all inclusion/exclusion criteria. In case of disagreement, a senior researcher (B.F.) resolved any discrepancies and decided whether or not the study was going to be included. A detailed flow diagram of selection of studies is reported in Figure 1.

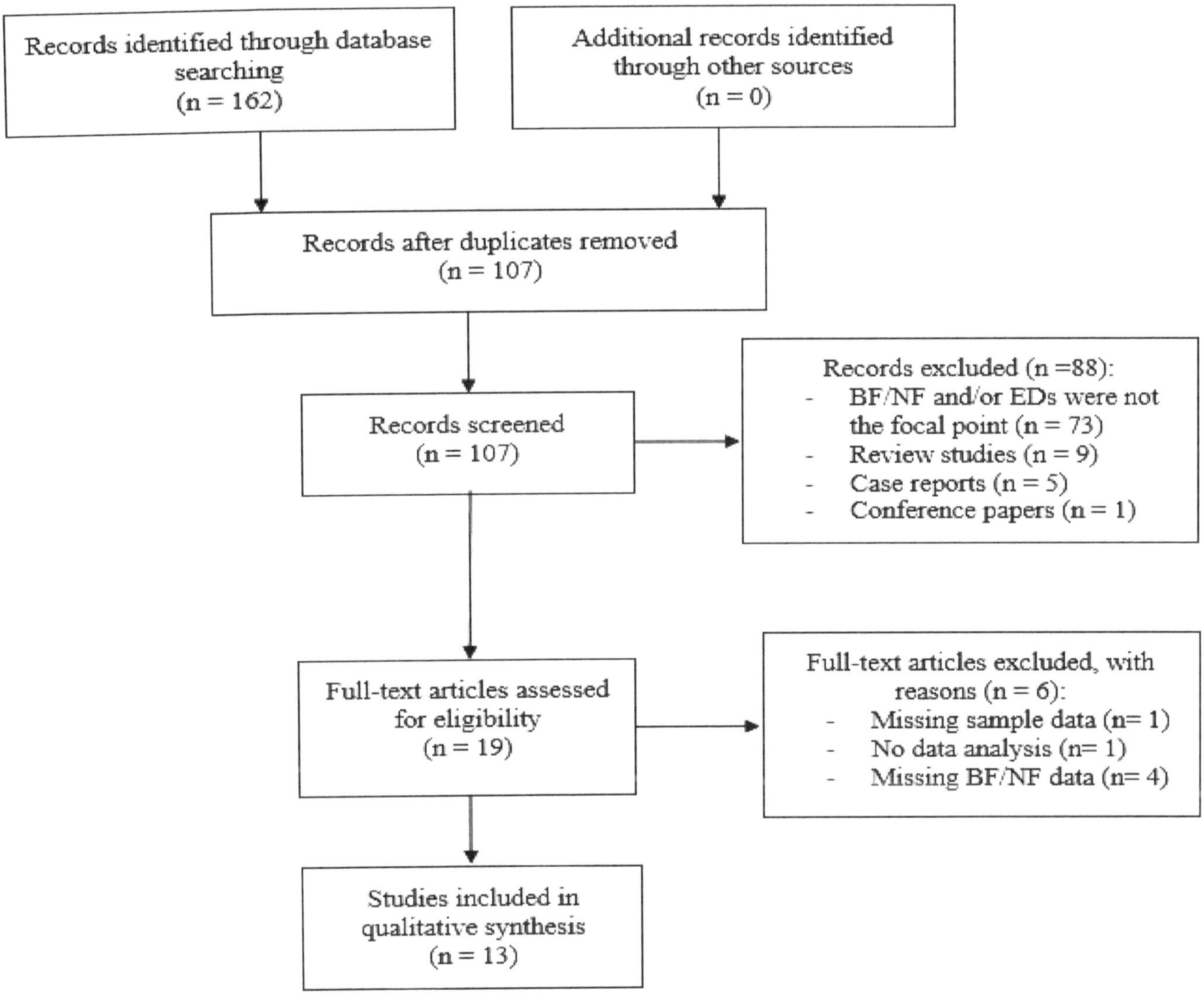

Figure 1. Flow diagram of selection of studies. Abbreviation: BF = Biofeedback; NF = Neurofeedback; EDs = Eating Disorders.

4. Results

The initial search resulted in 162 articles. Duplicate articles were eliminated, leaving 107 screened studies. Of these articles, 19 met initial inclusion criteria and were assessed for eligibility. Six articles were subsequently excluded with reasons (e.g., missing information pertaining to methods/outcome measures, no description of biofeedback modality, no statistical analysis etc.).

Thirteen articles fulfilled the quality assessment and are considered in this review (Table 1).

Table 1. Characteristics of the included studies (n = 13).

Authors	Participants	Design		Outcome Measures	Main Results
	(a) Sample (b) N (sex) (c) Age (mean ± sd. or range) (d) BMI (mean ± sd. or range) (e) Psychotropic medication (yes/no)	(a) Group (type of intervention) (b) Randomized (yes/no) (c) Blind (single/double)	(d) N of sessions (e) Duration (f) Follow-up (yes/no)	(a) Psychological/Behavioral (b) Physiological	(a) Psychological: ↑ = sign. increase; ↓ = sign. decrease; x = no change (b) Physiological: ↑ = sign. increase; ↓ = sign. decrease; x = no change (c) Stability at follow-up (yes/no)
Biofeedback Studies					
Pop-Jordanova 2000	(a) preadolescents with obesity; preadolescents with AN (b) 76 (F); 27 (F) (c) 12.75 ± 1.75; 14.25 ± 2.99 (d) bodyweight over 95th percentile; bodyweight below the 3rd percentile (e) n/a	(a) one group: ED-BF and supportive psychotherapy (b) no (c) n/a	(d) 5 (e) n/a (f) no	(a) n/a (b) EDA	(a) n/a (b)↓ of EDA in children with obesity and AN (c) n/a
Meule et al., 2012	(a) non-clinical sample (b) 56 (47 F, 9 M) (c) 24.12 ± 3.79 (d) 22.65 ± 3.19 (e) n/a	(a) 3 groups: (i) BFG (n = 14 high cravers): HRV-BF (ii) CG_1 (n = 14 high cravers): no intervention (iii) CG_2 (n = 28 low cravers): no intervention (b) pseudo-randomization * (c) single	(d) 12 (e) 20 min. (f) no	(a) FC [1]; eating disorder symptoms [2]; FA [3]; self-regulatory success in dieting; emotion regulation; locus of control (b) HR; HRV	(a) ↓ FC only in BFG; ↓ in eating and weight concerns only in BFG; x in other eating disorder symptoms, emotion regulation, FA, locus of control and self-regulatory success in dieting (b) ↓ in HRV in CG_1 (c) n/a
Teufel et al., 2013	(a) obese individuals (b) 30 (F) (c) 48.67 ± 11.93 (d) 35.5 ± 5.3 ** (e) no	(a) 3 groups: (i) BFG_1 (n = 10): ED-BF focused on food stimuli (ii) BFG_2 (n = 10): ED-BF focused on unspecific food stimuli (iii) CG (n = 10): no intervention (b) yes (c) single	(d) 8 (e) 21 min. (f) 3 months	(a) self-efficacy, stress, ability to relax, eating disorder symptoms[4]; BMI (b) EDA to food stimuli	(a) ↑ of food-related self-efficacy and perceived stress in BFGs; ↑ ability to relax in BFGs; x in BMI and, eating disorder symptoms (b) ↓ in EDA to food stimuli in BFGs (c) yes (a + b); ↓ loss of control during eating in BFG_2
Barba et al., 2015	(a) patients with RD (b) 28 (17 F, 11 M) (c) age range (14–76) (d) 22 ± 2 (e) yes (n = 4)	(a) 2 groups: (i) BFG (n = 15): EMG-BF (ii) CG (n = 4): no intervention (b) n/a (c) single	(d) 3 plus instructions for daily exercise (e) n/a (f) 1, 3, 6 months	(a) regurgitation episodes and associated abdominal symptoms. (b) EMG of abdominothoracic muscles	(a) ↓ in regurgitation episodes and associated abdominal symptoms immediately after treatment and after 6 month follow up (b) ↓ of intercostal and anterior wall muscle activity (c) yes (a + b)
Halland et al., 2016	(a) patients with RD (b) 16 (9 F, 7 M) (c) 37 ± 13 (d) 26.5 ± 5 (e) yes	(a) one group: DB-BF (b) no (c) n/a	(d) n/a (e) n/a (f) no	(a) rumination episodes (b) postprandial intragastric and esophagogastric junction pressure	(a) ↓ rumination episodes (b) ↑ of esophagogastric junction pressure; ↓postprandial intragastric pressure (c) n/a

Table 1. *Cont.*

Authors	Participants	Design		Outcome Measures	Main Results
		Neurofeedback Studies			
Schmidt & Martin 2015	(a) subthreshold sample of restrained eaters (b) 27 (F) (c) 34.54 ± 10.40 ** (d) 27.35 ± 5.24 ** (e) no	(a) 2 groups: (i) NFG (n = 14): EEG beta training NF (↓ 23–28 Hz activity at Cz) (ii) CG (n = 13): no intervention (b) yes (c) single	(d) 10 (e) 45 min. (f) 3 months	(a) overeating episodes and related distress; FC [1]; perceived dieting success; perceived stress; well-being (b) n/a	(a) ↓ overeating episodes and related distress in NFG; ↑ of perceived dieting success in NFG; x in FC, perceived stress, and well-being (b) n/a (c) yes (overeating episodes and related distress); ↓ of FC in NFG
Lackner et al., 2016	(a) adolescents with AN (b) 22 (F) (c) age range (12–18) (d) 15.41 ± 1.66 ** (e) yes (n = 1)	(a) 2 groups: (i) NFG (n = 10): EEG alpha training NF (↑ 8–12 Hz activity at Pz) and usual maintenance treatment CG (n = 12): usual maintenance treatment (b) yes (c) single	(d) 10 (e) 20 min (f) no	(a) psychological wellbeing, eating disorder symptoms [4,5,6], emotional competence, psychopathology (b) resting EEG power	(a) ↑ of disinhibition, ↑ of hunger;↓ restriction and dieting in NFG; ↓ of interpersonal sensitivity and ↑ emotional competence in NFG; x in BMI and psychopathology (b) ↑ EEG theta power (eyes closed) in NFG; x in EEG alpha power (c) n/a
Schmidt & Martin 2016	(a) subthreshold sample of binge eaters (b) 57 (F) (c) 44.77 ± 15.15 (d) 28.77 ± 5.47 (e) no	(a) 3 groups: (i) NFG (n = 18): EEG beta training NF (↓ 23–28 Hz activity at Cz) (ii) CG_1 (n = 18): mental imagery (iii) CG_2 (n = 21): no intervention (b) yes (c) single	(d) 10 (e) 45 min (f) 3 months	(a) subjective binge eating episodes and related, perceived stress, FC [7], self-efficacy (b) n/a	(a) ↓ binge eating episodes in NFG; ↓ of distress resulting from binge in NFG and CG_1; ↓ of FC in NFG and CG_1; ↓ of perceived stress and ↑ of dietary self-efficacy in NFG (b) n/a (c) yes (↓ binge eating episodes and related distress)
Ihssen et al., 2017	(a) non-clinical sample (b) 10 (F) (c) 21.4 ± 2.3 (d) 23.53 ± 2.66 (e) no	(a) one group: rt-fMRI-NF during exposure to appetitive food pictures (b) no (c) n/a	(d) 1 (e) 280 s (f) no	(a) subjective hunger, state FC [8], general FC [9], feelings of satiety (b) functional activation in brain areas	(a) ↓ of subjective hunger; ↑ of state FC; x in feelings of satiety; x in general FC (b) ↓ activation in reward brain areas (e.g., amygdala, insula, PFC) (c) n/a
Imperatori et al., 2017	(a) non-clinical sample (b) 50 (36 F, 14 M) (c) 22.90 ± 2.68 (d) 21.93 ± 3.41 (e) no	(a) 2 groups: (i) NFG (n = 25): EEG alpha/theta training NF (↓ 8–12.5 Hz and ↑ 4.5–7.5 Hz activity at Pz) (ii) CG (n = 25): no intervention (b) yes (c) single	(d) 10 (e) 27 min (f) 4 months	(a) FC [1], eating disorder symptoms [2], psychopathology (b) resting EEG power	(a) ↓ in FC in NFG; x in eating disorder symptoms and psychopathology (b) ↑ of alpha power in reward brain areas (e.g., insula, parahippocampal gyrus) (c) yes (a; b was not assessed)

Table 1. *Cont.*

Authors	Participants	Design		Outcome Measures	Main Results
Fattahi et al., 2017	(a) overweight (b) 30 (F) (c) age range (20–50) (d) n/a (e) n/a	(a) 2 groups: (i) NFG (n = 15): EEG alpha/theta training NF (↓ 8–12.5 Hz and ↑ 4.5–7.5 Hz activity at Pz) (ii) CG (n = 15): no intervention (b) yes (c) single	(d) 10 (e) 30–45 min (f) no	(a) FC [1] and mental health (b) n/a	(a) ↓ in FC and ↑ mental health in NFG (b) n/a (c) n/a
Spetter et al., 2017	(a) overweight/obese individuals (b) 8 (M) (c) 31.8 ± 4.4 (d) 29.4 ± 1.4 (e) no	(a) one group: rt-fMRI-NF during exposure to appetitive food pictures (b) n/a (c) n/a	(d) 4 (e) 9 min (f) no	(a) hunger and mood related ratings, food choice task, calorie intake (b) brain functional connectivity	(a) x in food choice task and in calorie intake assessment; x in hunger, fullness, satiety and appetite; ↓ in fear and agitation (b) ↑ functional connectivity between dlPFC and vmPFC (c) n/a
Leong et al., 2018	(a) obese individuals with FA symptoms (b) 21 (F) (c) 43.01± 13.97 ** (d) 33.5 ± 7.44 ** (e) no	(a) 2 groups: (i) NFG (n = 11): infraslow EEG-NF (modulation of slow wave activity at the PCC) (ii) CG (n = 10): placebo (b) yes (c) double	(d) 6 (e) 10 min (session #1) 20 min (other sessions) (f) 4 weeks	(a) state FC [10] (b) resting EEG power	(a) ↓ of state FC (b) ↑ in infraslow activity in the PCC (c) n/a

Abbreviations: n = number; BMI = body mass index; AN = anorexia nervosa; F = females; ED-BF = electrodermal biofeedback; n/a = not applicable; EDA = electrodermal activity; M = males: BFG = biofeedback group; HRV-BF = heart rate variability biofeedback; CG = control group; FC = food craving; FA = food addiction; HR = heart rate; HRV = heart rate variability; RD = rumination disorder; EMG-BF = electromyography biofeedback; EMG = electromyography; DB-BF = diaphragmatic breathing biofeedback; NFG = neurofeedback group; EEG = electroencephalography; rt-fMRI-NF = real-time functional magnetic resonance imaging neurofeedback; PFC = prefrontal cortex; dlPFC = dorsolateral prefrontal cortex; vmPFC = ventromedial prefrontal cortex; PCC = posterior cingulate cortex. Notes: * = 3 participants that could not participate in the study because of time constraints were then assigned to the control group; ** = pooled standard deviation; [1] = assessed with the Food Craving Questionnaire-Trait [48]; [2] = assessed with the Eating Disorder Examination Questionnaire [49]; [3] = assessed with Yale Food Addiction Scale [50]; [4] = assessed with Three Factor Eating Questionnaire [51];[5] = assessed with Eating Disorder Cognition Questionnaire [52]; [6] = assessed with Body Image Avoidance Questionnaire [53]; [7] = assessed with the Food Craving Questionnaire-Trait-reduced [24]; [8] = assessed with a single item ("How strong is your desire to eat?") rated on a five-point scale; [9] = assessed with the modified Trait and State Food Craving Questionnaire [54]; [10] = assessed with the Food Craving Questionnaire-State [48].

Biofeedback and neurofeedback were implemented respectively in five and eight of all reviewed articles. No studies incorporated different feedback modalities (e.g., electrodermal and electromyography biofeedback) or both biofeedback and neurofeedback. None of the studies investigated in this review reported relevant side effects for both biofeedback and neurofeedback training.

Mean number of sessions per study was 7.42 (range 1–12). Among reviewed article, three studies were focused on non-clinical samples [55–57], two on subthreshold samples [58,59], two on adolescents with AN [60,61], two on patients with RD [62,63] and 5 on overweight/obese individuals [61,64–67].

Eight studies were randomized [56–60,64,65,67], but only one was a double-blind trial [65]. Four studies did not have a control condition [55,61,63,66]. No treatment/waiting list was the most frequently (n = 7) control condition used [56–59,62,64,67], and only one study implemented a placebo condition (i.e., simulation protocol) [65] or an alternative treatment [59] (i.e., mental imagery).

Due to the high heterogeneity of samples, outcome measures and feedback modality, a meta-analysis was not performed.

4.1. *Biofeedback Studies*

Biofeedback was investigated in five of all reviewed articles. Of these, two studies implemented electrodermal biofeedback (ED-BF) [61,67], one heart rate variability biofeedback (HRV-BF) [57], one electromyography biofeedback (EMG-BF) [62], and one diaphragmatic breathing biofeedback (DB-BF) [63].

Barba et al. [62] and Halland et al., [63], investigated the usefulness of EMG-BF and DB-BF in patients with RD respectively. Both studies reported significant changes in clinical (e.g., decrease in regurgitation and rumination episodes) and physiological (e.g., decrease of intragastric pressure) outcomes.

Two studies examined the potential therapeutic effects of ED-BF in obese patients with overeating. Pop Jordanova [61], in a pre-post study design, showed that 5 sessions of ED-BF were associated with a decrease of electrodermal activity in a sample of girls with obesity (n = 76) and AN (n = 27). In a sample of obese women (n = 30), Teufel et al. [67], through a randomized controlled study, reported that compared to a waiting list, both ED-BF focused on food stimuli and ED-BF focused on unspecific stimuli were associated with an increased ability to tolerate food-related stress (e.g., decrease of electrodermal activity and increase self-efficacy in dealing with food). Although these results remained stable after 6-months follow-up, no significant changes were observed in BMI and in ED-related symptoms (e.g., tendency to lose control of food intake).

Finally, in a study on non-clinical sample of cravers (n = 56), Meule et al., [57], reported that, compared to a waiting-list, 12 sessions of HRV-BF were associated with a decrease of food craving as well as with a decrease of eating and weight concerns. No significant changes were observed in physiological measures (e.g., HRV) and in other EDs-related symptoms (e.g., shape concern, binge frequency).

4.2. *Neurofeedback Studies*

Neurofeedback was investigated in eight of all reviewed articles. Of these, six studies implemented EEG [56,58–60,64,65] and two rt-fMRI [55,66].

Two randomized controlled studies investigated the usefulness of EEG beta training neurofeedback (i.e., decrease beta activity at Cz electrode) in female subthreshold samples of restrained eaters ($n = 27$) [58] and binge eaters ($n = 57$) [59]. Both studies reported that, compared to a waiting-list, 10 sessions of neurofeedback were associated with a decrease in overeating episodes and related distress. These results remained stable after 3-months follow-up.

Two randomized controlled studies investigated the effectiveness of EEG alpha/theta training neurofeedback (i.e., raise posterior theta over alpha amplitude with eyes closed without falling asleep) in reducing food craving, in a non-clinical sample ($n = 50$) [56] and in a sample of overweight women ($n = 30$) respectively [64]. It has been observed that, compared to a waiting-list, 10 sessions of neurofeedback were associated with a decrease of food craving severity [56,64] as well as with an improvement of mental health [64]. A significant increase of resting EEG alpha power in several brain areas involved in food craving (e.g., insula) and food cue reactivity (e.g., parahippocampal gyrus) was also documented [56]. Although changes in food craving persisted after 4-months follow-up, no significant modifications were reported in other EDs-related symptoms (e.g., weight and shape concerns) and in the general level of psychopathology [56].

Lackner et al. [60] examined the potential therapeutic effects of EEG alpha training neurofeedback (i.e., raise posterior alpha activity) in female adolescents with AN ($n = 22$). It has been observed that, compared to the standard treatment, 10 sessions of neurofeedback were associated with an improvement in several ED-related symptoms (e.g., decrease of restriction and dieting behavior) and with an increase of emotional competence. Although modifications of resting EEG power were also documented (i.e., increase of theta power), no significant modifications were reported in psychopathological symptoms (with the exception of interpersonal sensitivity), in BMI and in body image related symptoms.

Two studies investigated the usefulness of rt-fMRI neurofeedback during the exposure to appetitive food pictures, respectively in a non-clinical sample of women ($n = 10$) [55] and in overweight/obese men ($n = 8$) [66]. Both studies showed that rt-fMRI neurofeedback could modify brain activity [55] and brain connectivity [66] in crucial areas involved in the reward system (e.g., amygdala and prefrontal cortex). Although no significant improvement was reported in food craving or in calorie intake assessment, a decrease of subjective hunger [55] and negative mood [66] related to food stimuli was reported.

Finally, in the only double-blind, placebo-controlled neurofeedback study, Leong et al. [65], investigated the effectiveness of infraslow EEG neurofeedback (i.e., the modulation of slow wave activity (0–0.1 Hz)) in obese women with food addiction symptoms. Compared to placebo condition, it has been reported that 6 sessions of neurofeedback were associated with an increase of infraslow activity in the posterior cingulate cortex as well as with a decrease of state food craving.

4.3. Risk of Bias

Risk of bias in the reviewed articles was performed according to Cochrane standards of practice [68]. Two reviewers (CI and GDM) independently assessed the risk for bias. In case of disagreement, a senior researcher (BF) resolved any discrepancies. Risk for bias was mainly related to the lack of both blinding and control conditions. Assessment of bias in the included studies are reported in Figures 2 and 3.

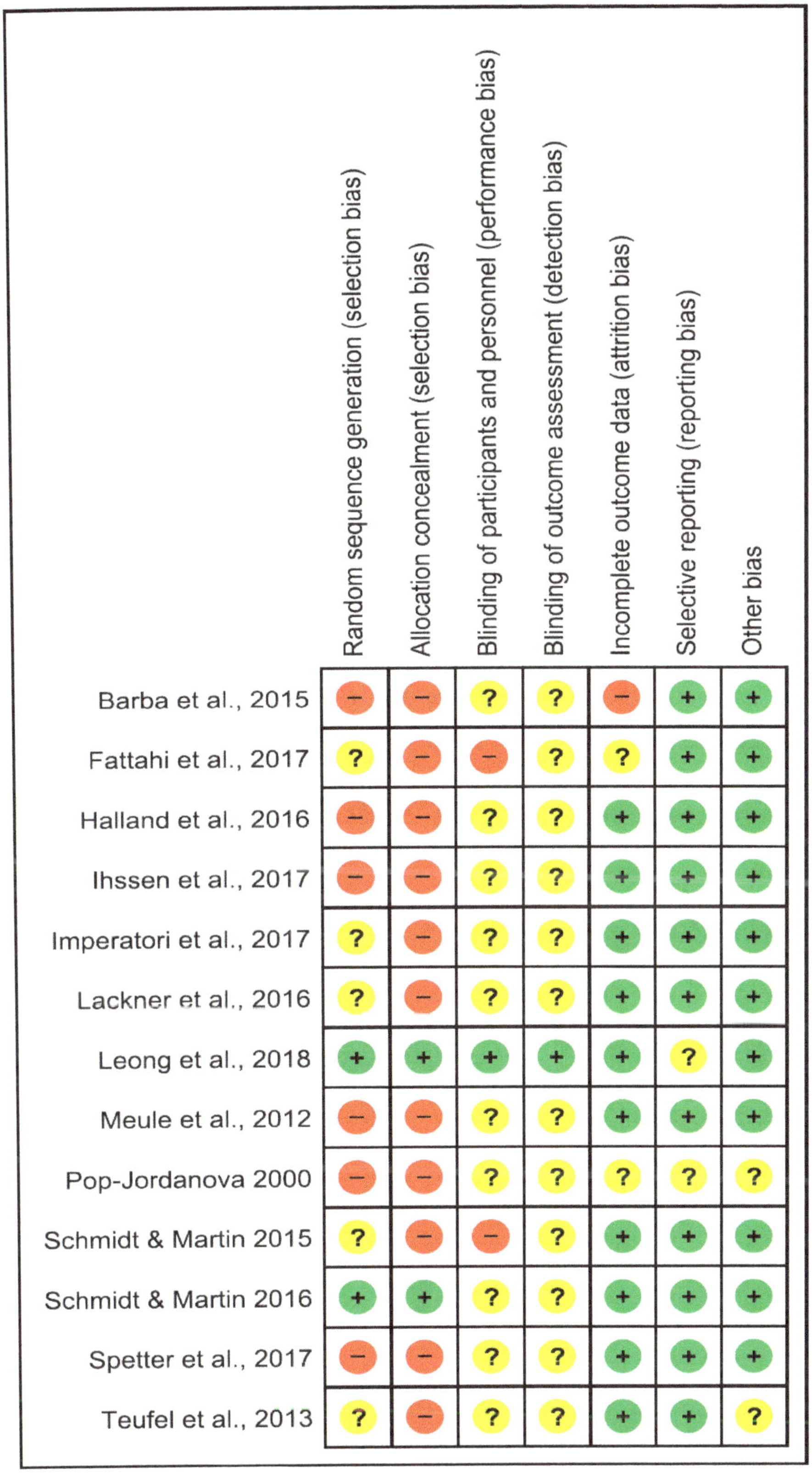

Figure 2. Risk of bias summary: review authors' judgements about each risk of bias item for each included study. Green, yellow and red circles represent low, unclear and high risk of bias respectively.

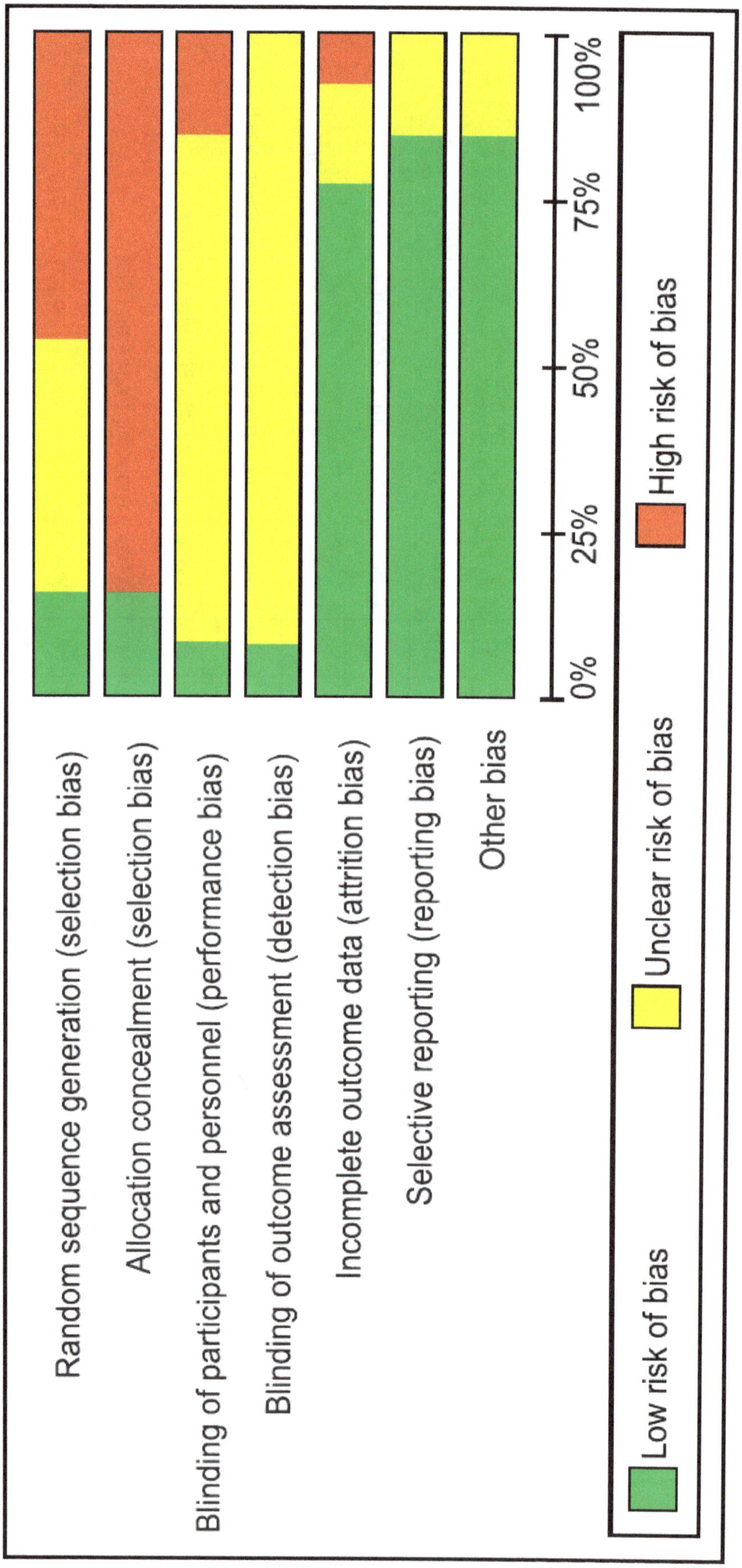

Figure 3. Risk of bias graph: review authors' judgements about each risk of bias item presented as percentages across all included studies.

5. Discussion

The main aim of the present systematic review was to report how feedback-based treatment (i.e., biofeedback and neurofeedback) have been used in the treatment of EDs and EDs-related symptoms. To the best of our knowledge, this is the first systematic review that investigates both biofeedback and neurofeedback applications in this field.

The review identified 13 articles, five focused on biofeedback and eight focused on neurofeedback, providing preliminary data of the usefulness of feedback-based techniques in the treatment of several dysfunctional eating behaviors (Table 2). Specifically, it has been reported that both neurofeedback and biofeedback training may decrease food craving severity [56–58,64,65], overeating episodes [58,59], regurgitation [62] and rumination [63] episodes, restricting behavior [60], eating and weight concerns [57]. Furthermore, this review showed that feedback-based techniques are associated with significant modifications of both sympathetic reaction to food-related stimuli [61–63,67] and brain activity in several regions of the reward system (e.g., prefrontal cortex, amygdala, insula) [55,56,60,65,66].

Table 2. Usefulness of feedback-based techniques for the treatment of dysfunctional eating behaviors.

Clinical Eating-Related Problem	Feed-Based Technique	Number of Sessions
Food craving	HRV-BF; Beta-NF; Alpha/Theta-NF; Infraslow-NF	6 to 10
Binge eating episodes	Beta-NF	10
Regurgitation episodes	EMG-BF	3
Rumination episodes	DB-BF	n/a
Restricting behavior	Alpha-NF	10
Eating and weight concerns	HRV-BF; Alpha-NF	12–10

HRV-BF = heart rate variability biofeedback; NF = Neurofeedback; EMG-BF = electromyography biofeedback; DB-BF = diaphragmatic breathing biofeedback; n/a = not applicable.

These results seem to suggest that both biofeedback and neurofeedback increased the ability to better tolerate stress and the ability to cope with situations involving food. Indeed, the most common goal of feedback-based treatments implemented for EDs and EDs-related symptoms is the reduction of stressful arousal and the increase of top-down control abilities. For example, the aim of EEG alpha training [60] is to enhance individual alpha frequency, which is usually associated with alert relaxation [69], in the parietal area (i.e., Pz electrode). Similarly, the goal of EEG beta training [58,59] is to down-regulate beta activity, which is positively associated with ruminative states of stressful arousal [70]. Consistently, the aim of alpha/theta training is to raise posterior (i.e., Pz electrode) theta over alpha amplitude in order to produce a state of deep relaxation, enhancing top-down mental functions [71], such as mentalization [72]. Finally, an rt-fMRI neurofeedback has been implemented to increase functional connectivity between brain areas (i.e., dorsolateral prefrontal cortex and ventromedial prefrontal cortex) that regulate the top-down control of appetite for high-calorie foods [66].

Interestingly, it has also been suggested that the target of neurofeedback is to increase bottom-up strategies in order to decrease the salience attached to food [65], or down-regulate brain regions activation (i.e., amygdala) during exposure to food cues [55]. Therefore, taken together these data suggest that feedback-based treatments implemented for EDs and EDs-related symptoms can operate both on top-down and bottom-up strategies in order to foster the neural mechanisms underlying successful coping during stressful food-related situations.

On the other hand, this review showed no significant effect of feedback-based techniques in improving other important EDs-related symptoms, such as body image disturbance, a crucial core of AN and BN [5], which seems to affect also BED [73]. No significant modifications associated with both biofeedback and neurofeedback were also reported for BMI in both patients with AN and overweigh/obesity. These results confirm the need of multidisciplinary approaches, combining medical, dietetic and different kind of psychological interventions in the treatment of EDs and

ED-related symptoms [32]. For example, combining EEG alpha training neurofeedback [60] with cognitive-behavioral exposure-based body image therapy [74] may be useful in the treatment of EDs.

It is also interesting to note that, compared to feedback-based interventions in other psychiatric disorders [39], no studies considered in the present review incorporated different biofeedback modalities or both biofeedback and neurofeedback. Therefore, it is possible that combining HRV-biofeedback [57] and EEG alpha/theta neurofeedback [56,64] may be more effective in reducing food craving severity in both clinical and non-clinical samples. Similarly, the combination of two neurofeedback training methods, such as EEG alpha/theta training and EEG beta training, or the combination of feedback-based techniques with other cognitive-behavioral techniques (e.g., cognitive restructuring, exposure therapy and response prevention) may be more effective in improving a wider range of ED-related symptoms (i.e., binge eating episodes, food craving).

Although the present review provided preliminary results of the usefulness of feedback-based techniques in the treatment of EDs and EDs-related symptoms, several methodological issue should be considered.

First, up to date, there are few randomized, double-blind, placebo-controlled studies investigating the effectiveness of both biofeedback and neurofeedback in large clinical samples. Indeed, among reviewed randomized trials (n = 8) the most frequent control condition implemented was the no treatment/waiting list, and only one study was double-blind. Consequently, most of the studies included in the present review had a high risk of bias, which was mostly related to the lack of both blinding and control conditions (e.g., mock feedback). This is in line with a recent systematic review investigating the potential therapeutic effects of neurofeedback training in psychiatric disorders associated with criminal offending [47]. Therefore, future studies should compare biofeedback and neurofeedback with sham procedures in order to rule out the placebo effect. Secondly, compared to feedback-based interventions in other psychiatric disorders [39], the mean number of sessions was relatively lower (i.e., 7.42). Although it has been reported that patients may benefit by undergoing 8 to 12 sessions [40], the possibility that a greater number of sessions (i.e., from 20 to 30) may maximize both biofeedback and neurofeedback results should be assessed. Furthermore, the stability of psychological/behavioral and neurophysiological (e.g., EEG power) outcomes should also be investigated taking into account long-term follow-up (i.e., at least one year). Finally, although the present review did not provide relevant differences associated with both age and gender, future studies should also investigate the relationship between feedback-based interventions outcomes (e.g., adherence to treatment, symptoms improvement) and several socio-demographic data (e.g. adolescent vs adults with EDs, and/or men vs women with EDs).

Study Limitations and Conclusions

There are several limitations of the present review that should be considered. Firstly, the search strategy was limited to articles published in English. Secondly, due to the high heterogeneity of samples, outcome measures and feedback modalities, a meta-analysis in order to quantify the effectiveness of both biofeedback and neurofeedback was not performed.

Despite these limitations, to the best of our knowledge, this is the first systematic review that investigates both biofeedback and neurofeedback applications in the treatment of EDs and EDs-related symptoms. In conclusion, the results of the present review suggest that, although future studies are needed in order to draw definitive conclusions, feedback-based techniques may be useful in the treatment of several dysfunctional eating behaviors (e.g., food craving, binge eating) operating both on top-down and bottom-up individual coping strategies.

Author Contributions: C.I.: study design, literature searches, data extraction, manuscript writing; M.M.: literature searches, data extraction, manuscript editing; G.D.M.: supervision, manuscript writing; E.M.V.: data extraction; B.F.: study design, supervision, manuscript writing.

Acknowledgments: We thank the Atena Onlus Foundation for assistance and support.

References

1. Treasure, J.; Claudino, A.M.; Zucker, N. Eating disorders. *Lancet* **2010**, *375*, 583–593. [CrossRef]
2. Hudson, J.I.; Hiripi, E.; Pope, H.G., Jr.; Kessler, R.C. The prevalence and correlates of eating disorders in the national comorbidity survey replication. *Biol. Psychiatry* **2007**, *61*, 348–358. [CrossRef] [PubMed]
3. Smink, F.R.; Van Hoeken, D.; Hoek, H.W. Epidemiology of eating disorders: Incidence, prevalence and mortality rates. *Curr. Psychiatry Rep.* **2012**, *14*, 406–414. [CrossRef] [PubMed]
4. Kaplan, A.S.; Garfinkel, P.E. Difficulties in treating patients with eating disorders: A review of patient and clinician variables. *Can. J. Psychiatry* **1999**, *44*, 665–670. [CrossRef] [PubMed]
5. American Psychiatric Association. *Diagnostic and Statistical Manual of Mental Disorders-DSM-5*, 5th ed.; American Psychiatric Publishing: Arlington, TX, USA, 2013.
6. Erzegovesi, S.; Bellodi, L. Eating disorders. *CNS Spectr.* **2016**, *21*, 304–309. [PubMed]
7. Hoek, H.W. Classification, epidemiology and treatment of dsm-5 feeding and eating disorders. *Curr. Opin. Psychiatry* **2013**, *26*, 529–531. [CrossRef] [PubMed]
8. Benjasuwantep, B.; Chaithirayanon, S.; Eiamudomkan, M. Feeding problems in healthy young children: Prevalence, related factors and feeding practices. *Pediatr. Rep.* **2013**, *5*, 38–42. [CrossRef] [PubMed]
9. Swanson, S.A.; Crow, S.J.; Le Grange, D.; Swendsen, J.; Merikangas, K.R. Prevalence and correlates of eating disorders in adolescents. Results from the national comorbidity survey replication adolescent supplement. *Arch. Gen. Psychiatry* **2011**, *68*, 714–723. [CrossRef] [PubMed]
10. Lindvall Dahlgren, C.; Wisting, L.; Ro, O. Feeding and eating disorders in the dsm-5 era: A systematic review of prevalence rates in non-clinical male and female samples. *J. Eat. Disord.* **2017**, *5*, 56. [CrossRef] [PubMed]
11. Weingarten, H.P.; Elston, D. The phenomenology of food cravings. *Appetite* **1990**, *15*, 231–246. [CrossRef]
12. Weingarten, H.P.; Elston, D. Food cravings in a college population. *Appetite* **1991**, *17*, 167–175. [CrossRef]
13. White, M.A.; Whisenhunt, B.L.; Williamson, D.A.; Greenway, F.L.; Netemeyer, R.G. Development and validation of the food-craving inventory. *Obes. Res.* **2002**, *10*, 107–114. [CrossRef] [PubMed]
14. Lafay, L.; Thomas, F.; Mennen, L.; Charles, M.A.; Eschwege, E.; Borys, J.M.; Basdevant, A. Gender differences in the relation between food cravings and mood in an adult community: Results from the fleurbaix laventie ville sante study. *Int. J. Eat. Disord.* **2001**, *29*, 195–204. [CrossRef]
15. Gendall, K.A.; Sullivan, P.F.; Joyce, P.R.; Bulik, C.M. Food cravings in women with a history of anorexia nervosa. *Int. J. Eat. Disord.* **1997**, *22*, 403–409. [CrossRef]
16. Moreno, S.; Rodriguez, S.; Fernandez, M.C.; Tamez, J.; Cepeda-Benito, A. Clinical validation of the trait and state versions of the food craving questionnaire. *Assessment* **2008**, *15*, 375–387. [CrossRef] [PubMed]
17. Van der Ster Wallin, G.; Norring, C.; Holmgren, S. Binge eating versus nonpurged eating in bulimics: Is there a carbohydrate craving after all? *Acta Psychiatr. Scand.* **1994**, *89*, 376–381. [CrossRef] [PubMed]
18. Waters, A.; Hill, A.; Waller, G. Bulimics' responses to food cravings: Is binge-eating a product of hunger or emotional state? *Behav. Res. Ther.* **2001**, *39*, 877–886. [CrossRef]
19. Moreno, S.; Warren, C.S.; Rodriguez, S.; Fernandez, M.C.; Cepeda-Benito, A. Food cravings discriminate between anorexia and bulimia nervosa. Implications for "success" versus "failure" in dietary restriction. *Appetite* **2009**, *52*, 588–594. [CrossRef] [PubMed]
20. White, M.A.; Grilo, C.M. Psychometric properties of the food craving inventory among obese patients with binge eating disorder. *Eat. Behav.* **2005**, *6*, 239–245. [CrossRef] [PubMed]
21. Fabbricatore, M.; Imperatori, C.; Pecchioli, C.; Micarelli, T.; Contardi, A.; Tamburello, S.; Innamorati, M.; Tamburello, A. Binge eating and bis/bas activity in obese patients with intense food craving who attend weight control programs. *Obes. Metab.* **2011**, *7*, e21–e27.
22. Delahanty, L.M.; Meigs, J.B.; Hayden, D.; Williamson, D.A.; Nathan, D.M. Diabetes Prevenion Program Research Group. Psychological and behavioral correlates of baseline bmi in the diabetes prevention program (DPP). *Diabetes Care* **2002**, *25*, 1992–1998. [CrossRef] [PubMed]
23. Franken, I.H.; Muris, P. Individual differences in reward sensitivity are related to food craving and relative body weight in healthy women. *Appetite* **2005**, *45*, 198–201. [CrossRef] [PubMed]

24. Meule, A.; Hermann, T.; Kubler, A. A short version of the food cravings questionnaire-trait: The fcq-t-reduced. *Front. Psychol.* **2014**, *5*, 190. [CrossRef] [PubMed]
25. Meule, A.; Lutz, A.; Vogele, C.; Kubler, A. Food cravings discriminate differentially between successful and unsuccessful dieters and non-dieters. Validation of the food cravings questionnaires in german. *Appetite* **2012**, *58*, 88–97. [PubMed]
26. Meule, A.; Westenhofer, J.; Kubler, A. Food cravings mediate the relationship between rigid, but not flexible control of eating behavior and dieting success. *Appetite* **2011**, *57*, 582–584. [CrossRef] [PubMed]
27. Sitton, S.C. Role of craving for carbohydrates upon completion of a protein-sparing fast. *Psychol. Rep.* **1991**, *69*, 683–686. [PubMed]
28. Boswell, R.G.; Kober, H. Food cue reactivity and craving predict eating and weight gain: A meta-analytic review. *Obes. Rev.* **2016**, *17*, 159–177. [CrossRef] [PubMed]
29. Goossens, L.; Soenens, B.; Braet, C. Prevalence and characteristics of binge eating in an adolescent community sample. *J. Clin. Child Adolesc. Psychol.* **2009**, *38*, 342–353. [CrossRef] [PubMed]
30. Heriseanu, A.I.; Hay, P.; Corbit, L.; Touyz, S. Grazing in adults with obesity and eating disorders: A systematic review of associated clinical features and meta-analysis of prevalence. *Clin. Psychol. Rev.* **2017**, *58*, 16–32. [CrossRef] [PubMed]
31. Goldschmidt, A.B.; Loth, K.A.; MacLehose, R.F.; Pisetsky, E.M.; Berge, J.M.; Neumark-Sztainer, D. Overeating with and without loss of control: Associations with weight status, weight-related characteristics, and psychosocial health. *Int. J. Eat. Disord.* **2015**, *48*, 1150–1157. [CrossRef] [PubMed]
32. Hay, P.; Chinn, D.; Forbes, D.; Madden, S.; Newton, R.; Sugenor, L.; Touyz, S.; Ward, W. Royal australian and new zealand college of psychiatrists clinical practice guidelines for the treatment of eating disorders. *Aust. N. Z. J. Psychiatry* **2014**, *48*, 977–1008. [CrossRef] [PubMed]
33. Herpertz-Dahlmann, B. Treatment of eating disorders in child and adolescent psychiatry. *Curr. Opin. Psychiatry* **2017**, *30*, 438–445. [CrossRef] [PubMed]
34. Amianto, F.; Ottone, L.; Abbate Daga, G.; Fassino, S. Binge-eating disorder diagnosis and treatment: A recap in front of dsm-5. *BMC Psychiatry* **2015**, *15*, 70. [CrossRef] [PubMed]
35. Lee, D.J.; Elias, G.J.B.; Lozano, A.M. Neuromodulation for the treatment of eating disorders and obesity. *Ther. Adv. Psychopharmacol.* **2018**, *8*, 73–92. [CrossRef] [PubMed]
36. Bartholdy, S.; Musiat, P.; Campbell, I.C.; Schmidt, U. The potential of neurofeedback in the treatment of eating disorders: A review of the literature. *Eur. Eat. Disord. Rev.* **2013**, *21*, 456–463. [CrossRef] [PubMed]
37. Musiat, P.; Hoffmann, L.; Schmidt, U. Personalised computerised feedback in e-mental health. *J. Ment. Health* **2012**, *21*, 346–354. [CrossRef] [PubMed]
38. Yucha, C.; Montgomery, D. *Evidence-Based Practice in Biofeedback and Neurofeedback*; Association for Applied Psychophysiology and Biofeedback: Wheat Ridge, CO, USA, 2008.
39. Schoenberg, P.L.; David, A.S. Biofeedback for psychiatric disorders: A. systematic review. *Appl. Psychophysiol. Biofeedback* **2014**, *39*, 109–135. [CrossRef] [PubMed]
40. McKee, M.G. Biofeedback: An overview in the context of heart-brain medicine. *Clevel. Clin. J. Med.* **2008**, *75*, S31–S34. [CrossRef]
41. Weiskopf, N. Real-time fmri and its application to neurofeedback. *Neuroimage* **2012**, *62*, 682–692. [CrossRef] [PubMed]
42. Brunoni, A.R.; Amadera, J.; Berbel, B.; Volz, M.S.; Rizzerio, B.G.; Fregni, F. A systematic review on reporting and assessment of adverse effects associated with transcranial direct current stimulation. *Int. J. Neuropsychopharmacol.* **2011**, *14*, 1133–1145. [CrossRef] [PubMed]
43. Lansbergen, M.M.; Van Dongen-Boomsma, M.; Buitelaar, J.K.; Slaats-Willemse, D. Adhd and eeg-neurofeedback: A double-blind randomized placebo-controlled feasibility study. *J. Neural Transm. (Vienna)* **2011**, *118*, 275–284. [CrossRef] [PubMed]
44. Thatcher, R.W. Advances in assessment and treatment of ADHD using network analyses. *Biofeedback* **2014**, *42*, 58–67. [CrossRef]
45. Sherlin, L.H.; Arns, M.; Lubar, J.; Heinrich, H.; Kerson, C.; Strehl, U.; Sterman, M.B. Neurofeedback and basic learning theory: Implications for research and practice. *J. Neurother.* **2011**, *15*, 292–304. [CrossRef]
46. La Vaque, T.J.; Hammond, D.C.; Trudeau, D.; Monastra, V.; Perry, J.; Lehrer, P.; Matheson, D.; Sherman, R. Template for developing guidelines for the evaluation of the clinical efficacy of psychophysiological interventions. *Appl. Psychophysiol. Biofeedback* **2002**, *27*, 273–281. [CrossRef]

47. Fielenbach, S.; Donkers, F.C.L.; Spreen, M.; Visser, H.A.; Bogaerts, S. Neurofeedback training for psychiatric disorders associated with criminal offending: A. review. *Front. Psychiatry* **2017**, *8*, 313. [CrossRef] [PubMed]
48. Cepeda-Benito, A.; Gleaves, D.H.; Williams, T.L.; Erath, S.A. The development and validation of the state and trait food-cravings questionnaires. *Behav. Ther.* **2000**, *31*, 151–173. [CrossRef]
49. Fairburn, C.G.; Beglin, S.J. Assessment of eating disorders: Interview or self-report questionnaire? *Int. J. Eat. Disord.* **1994**, *16*, 363–370. [PubMed]
50. Gearhardt, A.N.; Corbin, W.R.; Brownell, K.D. Preliminary validation of the Yale food addiction scale. *Appetite* **2009**, *52*, 430–436. [CrossRef] [PubMed]
51. Stunkard, A.J.; Messick, S. The three-factor eating questionnaire to measure dietary restraint, disinhibition and hunger. *J. Psychosom. Res.* **1985**, *29*, 71–83. [CrossRef]
52. Legenbauer, T.; Vocks, S.; Schütt-Strömel, S. Dysfunctional cognitions in eating disorders: Which contents areas can be discriminated? *J. Clin. Psychol. Psychother.* **2007**, *36*, 207–215.
53. Rosen, J.C.; Srebnik, D.; Saltzberg, E.; Wendt, S. Development of a body image avoidance questionnaire. *Psychol. Assess.* **1991**, *3*, 32–37. [CrossRef]
54. Nijs, I.M.; Franken, I.H.; Muris, P. The modified trait and state food-cravings questionnaires: Development and validation of a general index of food craving. *Appetite* **2007**, *49*, 38–46. [CrossRef] [PubMed]
55. Ihssen, N.; Sokunbi, M.O.; Lawrence, A.D.; Lawrence, N.S.; Linden, D.E.J. Neurofeedback of visual food cue reactivity: A potential avenue to alter incentive sensitization and craving. *Brain Imaging Behav.* **2017**, *11*, 915–924. [CrossRef] [PubMed]
56. Imperatori, C.; Valenti, E.M.; Della Marca, G.; Amoroso, N.; Massullo, C.; Carbone, G.A.; Maestoso, G.; Quintiliani, M.I.; Contardi, A.; Farina, B. Coping food craving with neurofeedback. Evaluation of the usefulness of alpha/theta training in a non-clinical sample. *Int. J. Psychophysiol.* **2017**, *112*, 89–97. [CrossRef] [PubMed]
57. Meule, A.; Freund, R.; Skirde, A.K.; Vogele, C.; Kubler, A. Heart rate variability biofeedback reduces food cravings in high food cravers. *Appl. Psychophysiol. Biofeedback* **2012**, *37*, 241–251. [CrossRef] [PubMed]
58. Schmidt, J.; Martin, A. Neurofeedback reduces overeating episodes in female restrained eaters: A randomized controlled pilot-study. *Appl. Psychophysiol. Biofeedback* **2015**, *40*, 283–295. [CrossRef] [PubMed]
59. Schmidt, J.; Martin, A. Neurofeedback against binge eating: A randomized controlled trial in a female subclinical threshold sample. *Eur. Eat. Disord. Rev.* **2016**, *24*, 406–416. [CrossRef] [PubMed]
60. Lackner, N.; Unterrainer, H.F.; Skliris, D.; Shaheen, S.; Dunitz-Scheer, M.; Wood, G.; Scheer, P.J.; Wallner-Liebmann, S.J.; Neuper, C. Eeg neurofeedback effects in the treatment of adolescent anorexia nervosa. *Eat. Disord.* **2016**, *24*, 354–374. [CrossRef] [PubMed]
61. Pop-Jordanova, N. Psychological characteristics and biofeedback mitigation in preadolescents with eating disorders. *Pediatr. Int.* **2000**, *42*, 76–81. [CrossRef] [PubMed]
62. Barba, E.; Burri, E.; Accarino, A.; Malagelada, C.; Rodriguez-Urrutia, A.; Soldevilla, A.; Malagelada, J.R.; Azpiroz, F. Biofeedback-guided control of abdominothoracic muscular activity reduces regurgitation episodes in patients with rumination. *Clin. Gastroenterol. Hepatol.* **2015**, *13*, 100–106.e1. [CrossRef] [PubMed]
63. Halland, M.; Parthasarathy, G.; Bharucha, A.E.; Katzka, D.A. Diaphragmatic breathing for rumination syndrome: Efficacy and mechanisms of action. *Neurogastroenterol. Motil.* **2016**, *28*, 384–391. [CrossRef] [PubMed]
64. Fattahi, S.; Naderi, F.; Asgari, P.; Ahadi, H. Neuro-feedback training for overweight women: Improvement of food craving and mental health. *NeuroQuantology* **2017**, *15*, 232–238. [CrossRef]
65. Leong, S.L.; Vanneste, S.; Lim, J.; Smith, M.; Manning, P.; De Ridder, D.A. Randomised, double-blind, placebo-controlled parallel trial of closed-loop infraslow brain training in food addiction. *Sci. Rep.* **2018**, *8*, 11659. [CrossRef] [PubMed]
66. Spetter, M.S.; Malekshahi, R.; Birbaumer, N.; Luhrs, M.; Van der Veer, A.H.; Scheffler, K.; Spuckti, S.; Preissl, H.; Veit, R.; Hallschmid, M. Volitional regulation of brain responses to food stimuli in overweight and obese subjects: A real-time fmri feedback study. *Appetite* **2017**, *112*, 188–195. [CrossRef] [PubMed]
67. Teufel, M.; Stephan, K.; Kowalski, A.; Kasberger, S.; Enck, P.; Zipfel, S.; Giel, K.E. Impact of biofeedback on self-efficacy and stress reduction in obesity: A randomized controlled pilot study. *Appl. Psychophysiol. Biofeedback* **2013**, *38*, 177–184. [CrossRef] [PubMed]

68. Higgins, J.P.T.; Altman, D.G.; Sterne, J.A.C. Chapter 8: Assessing risk of bias in included studies. In *Cochrane Handbook for Systematic Reviews of Interventions Version 5.1.0*; Higgins, J.P.T., Green, S., Eds.; The Cochrane Collaboration: London, UK, 2011.
69. Marzbani, H.; Marateb, H.R.; Mansourian, M. Neurofeedback: A comprehensive review on system design, methodology and clinical applications. *Basic Clin. Neurosci.* **2016**, *7*, 143–158. [PubMed]
70. Andersen, S.B.; Moore, R.A.; Venables, L.; Corr, P.J. Electrophysiological correlates of anxious rumination. *Int. J. Psychophysiol.* **2009**, *71*, 156–169. [CrossRef] [PubMed]
71. Gruzelier, J.H. Eeg-neurofeedback for optimising performance. Ii: Creativity, the performing arts and ecological validity. *Neurosci. Biobehav. Rev.* **2014**, *44*, 142–158. [CrossRef] [PubMed]
72. Imperatori, C.; Della Marca, G.; Amoroso, N.; Maestoso, G.; Valenti, E.M.; Massullo, C.; Carbone, G.A.; Contardi, A.; Farina, B. Alpha/theta neurofeedback increases mentalization and default mode network connectivity in a non-clinical sample. *Brain Topogr.* **2017**, *30*, 822–831. [CrossRef] [PubMed]
73. Lewer, M.; Bauer, A.; Hartmann, A.S.; Vocks, S. Different facets of body image disturbance in binge eating disorder: A review. *Nutrients* **2017**, *9*. [CrossRef] [PubMed]
74. Lewer, M.; Kosfelder, J.; Michalak, J.; Schroeder, D.; Nasrawi, N.; Vocks, S. Effects of a cognitive-behavioral exposure-based body image therapy for overweight females with binge eating disorder: A pilot study. *J. Eat. Disord.* **2017**, *5*, 43. [CrossRef] [PubMed]

17

Shared Concerns and Opportunity for Joint Action in Creating a Food Environment that Supports Health

Kendrin R. Sonneville [1,*] and Rachel F. Rodgers [2]

1 Department of Nutritional Sciences, University of Michigan School of Public Health, Ann Arbor, MI 48109, USA
2 Department of Applied Psychology, Bouve College of Health Sciences, Northeastern University, Boston, MA 02115, USA; R.Rodgers@northeastern.edu
* Correspondence: kendrins@umich.edu

Abstract: The food industry is a for-profit industry with high relevance to universal eating disorders prevention. To date, policy which targets the food industry and food environment has been underutilized in efforts to decrease the incidence of eating disorders and associated risk factors. In contrast, food policy has been extensively leveraged with the aim of reducing the incidence of obesity. While philosophical misalignments with these later efforts may have constituted an obstacle to identifying the food environment as a key target for eating disorders prevention, food policy is an area where shared interests can be found. Specifically, a shared goal of obesity and eating disorders prevention efforts is creating a food environment that supports health, while minimizing the influence of the food industry that profits from the sale of highly palatable, processed foods and "diet" foods and from increasing portions of foods served and eaten.

Keywords: eating disorders; obesity; prevention; food industry; food environment; food policy

---

1. Introduction

Eating disorders are a significant public health issue and affect people of all backgrounds [1–4]. Approximately 5% of individuals in the U.S. will have an eating disorder at some point in their lives [2] and many more will struggle with sub-threshold symptoms [5–7], putting them at risk for substantial psychiatric comorbidities [8] and serious medical complications [9]. As evidence emerges for sociocultural drivers of eating disorder risk, recognition of the need to identify population-level approaches to eating disorders prevention has increased [10]. For-profit industries that benefit when people have an unhealthy relationship with food and their bodies (e.g., the diet, fashion, and beauty industries) have been implicated as important targets for macro-level intervention for eating disorders prevention [11,12]. The food industry, which includes food and beverage companies and quick-serve restaurants, is another such for-profit industry with high relevance to universal eating disorders prevention. To date, however, it has been neglected in efforts to decrease the incidence of eating disorders and associated risk factors [13]. In contrast, policy related to the food industry has been leveraged with the aim of reducing the incidence of obesity [14–16]. In this way, food policy is an area where shared interests can be found with the goal of creating a food environment that supports health. While food policy encompasses a heterogeneous set of policies involving many sectors that impact how food is produced, processed, distributed, marketed, purchased, and consumed [17], we will specifically focus on policy which targets practices of the food industry related to the processing, distribution, and marketing of foods. The aim here is to outline the rationale for leveraging food policy as an approach to eating disorders prevention. We will examine ways in which this lens would benefit ongoing efforts to regulate the food environment that largely aim to reduce individuals' intake and will reflect upon the challenges to finding common ground in working towards informing food policy.

2. The Relevance of the Food Industry to Universal Eating Disorders Prevention Efforts

Eating disorders are characterized by an intense preoccupation with weight and shape, engagement in behaviors that aim to alter weight and shape, and/or the experience of loss of control while eating. In particular, restrictive-type eating disorders include efforts to eat less often, consume smaller quantities, and choose foods that are lower in caloric density [18]. These efforts frequently result in strict food rules and certain foods being thought of as permitted, while others are forbidden. In addition, binge-type eating disorders are characterized by the consumption of large amounts of food in a short amount of time, with an accompanying experience of loss of control [19]. These episodes may be followed by compensatory behaviors, including self-induced vomiting, fasting, over-exercise, or the use or diuretics and laxatives in an effort to offset or eliminate the calories consumed. Individuals who experience binge-eating behaviors have reported experiencing strong cravings for certain foods that may precipitate the eating episode [20]. Furthermore, avoidance of certain foods (i.e., restriction) has been shown to increase the risk for binge-eating behaviors [21]. We will discuss how practices, including the processing, distribution, and marketing of foods, employed by the food industry may be related to eating disorder symptoms, such as preoccupation with weight and shape, dietary restriction, binge-eating behaviors, and cravings. These practices include the ways in which products are developed, ("engineering" of foods), packaged (serving size and portion), and marketed ("diet" foods and "health halo") (Figure 1). This suggests that it is important to consider the food environment as a context that could increase the risk for eating disorders.

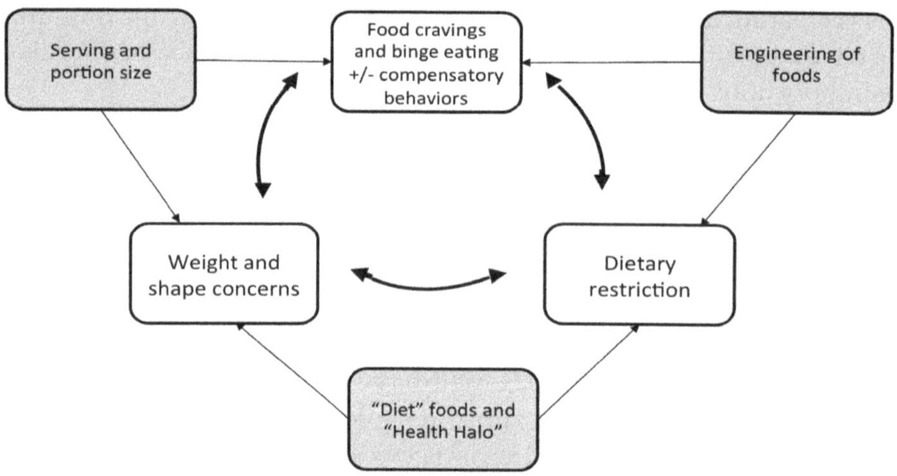

Figure 1. Food industry practices and eating disorder risk.

3. "*Engineering*" of Foods

In recent decades, the food industry has focused its resources on developing highly palatable, processed foods that are engineered to be as rewarding as possible to their target audience by combining levels of sugar, fat, and salt [22–24]. This has included research on the non-linear relationships between sweetness and the appeal of a food to identify the optimal sweetness for different foods. In particular, foods marketed specifically to children, such as children's breakfast foods, have been developed on the basis of their preference for markedly sweeter foods [25]. In addition, the food industry has paid increasing attention to developing foods that minimize satiety, such as liquids that possess a lower satiating capacity compared to solid foods [26]. The result of these practices is a range of foods that have been perfected in their capacity not only to appeal but also to fail to be satiating, so as to maximize consumption.

The engineering of foods in this manner is relevant to eating disorders prevention efforts in several ways and emerging data confirm the association between the consumption of these foods and eating disorder risk. Firstly, foods that are "engineered in ways that appear to surpass the rewarding properties of traditional foods" [24] may disturb the processes of appetite regulation. [27] Consistent with this, highly-processed foods, containing refined sugars and added fats, have been identified as being most associated with loss of control eating [28–30]. Furthermore, evidence from animal models of binge eating has supported the role of highly palatable, processed foods in triggering binge eating [31–34]. Relatedly, the capacity for these foods to disrupt the development of self-regulated eating processes in children has also been questioned. The role of reward in driving these eating behaviors has led researchers to draw parallels between the effects of these foods and those of addictive substances [35–37].

4. Serving and Portion Size

The contemporary Western food environment, through practices related to the presentation, packaging, and selling of food, has been linked to increasingly large serving and portion sizes of foods (e.g., [38,39]). Examples of these practices include normalizing large portion sizes through servings in restaurants, pricing scales designed to sell larger portions, displaying foods in stores in ways that increase purchasing, and selling foods in portions or packaging that exceed a typical serving size [40,41]. These practices could increase consumption [42–44] and thus potentiate profits, which may explain their perpetuation. Larger serving and portion sizes could also theoretically increase the risk for binge eating. Consistent with this, preliminary evidence supports the fact that the effects of large portion sizes on increased consumption are strongest among youth who experience loss of control eating or binge eating [45,46]. In addition, a food-rich environment, in conjunction with social appearance ideals of thinness/leanness and the stigmatization of larger bodies, may place some individuals under increased pressure to restrict their intake [47]. Thus, large serving and portion sizes may be associated with either binge-type eating pathology, or restriction, through different pathways and thus increase risk for eating disorders.

5. The Creation of "Diet" Foods and the "Health Halo"

The rising preoccupation with weight control and discourse identifying individual eating behaviors as determinants of health has been accompanied by the creation of numerous "diet" foods (e.g., reduced-calorie or "light" food products). These products have been developed to contain low-calorie artificial sweeteners in place of sugar, reduced levels of fat, or other reformulations of nutrients. For example, the food industry profited from dietary guidelines that emphasized reducing total fat in the diet by creating numerous low-fat, high-carbohydrate, high-sugar products [48,49]. In addition, the food industry has been described as manipulating perceptions of the health benefits of their products through the use of various claims about foods [50]. Importantly, while these claims may assist individuals in their food choices, they may also be misleading [51].

The increasing availability and marketing of "diet" foods may be relevant to eating disorders through a number of pathways. These products may be marketed as assisting in weight control and therefore attractive to individuals with weight concerns. Meta-analytic findings have confirmed that health-related claims on foods have a substantial effect on food choices and increased purchasing [50,52], which may particularly affect those with weight and shape concerns. However, consumption of "diet" or "health" products is unlikely to alleviate weight and shape concerns, or be helpful in terms of establishing eating patterns that are regulated by internal cues. Instead, consuming artificially-sweetened beverages rather than sugar-sweetened ones has been shown to be associated with increased levels of restrained and emotional eating [53,54]. Furthermore, consuming these products may increase cravings and loss of control eating through the process of cognitive restraint [55]. In addition, "diet' and "health" foods might substitute consumption of less processed foods, that are more helpful to appetite regulation [28]. Finally, at the macro-level, the proliferation of such foods and their intense marketing serves to increase weight-related pressures and contributes to the sociocultural discourse that promotes disordered eating [56]. In summary, the food environment may increase risk for eating disorders via multiple pathways and is therefore an important target for universal prevention efforts, particularly through policy and regulation.

6. Food Policy for the Prevention of Obesity

Efforts to leverage policy for the prevention of obesity are widespread and largely aim to reduce individuals' overall intake. Public policy strategies related to obesity prevention in the U.S. and abroad have focused on a wide range of environments, including those related to child care, health care, and schools, [14] and are designed to increase the availability, affordability, and acceptability of healthy food and beverage choices in various settings (e.g., schools, workplace, community), while decreasing the availability of less healthy options in these settings [15]. While many of these policy efforts could have relevance to eating disorders and their prevention, these potential intersections have been underexplored.

Policy efforts aimed at limiting portion sizes are an example of a food policy for obesity prevention that also has relevance for eating disorders prevention. Based on the body of research linking portion size to greater consumption [57], a number of initiatives have been undertaken, ranging from voluntary pledges to regulations [58]. In the U.S., the Food and Drug Administration (USDA) already requires a statement regarding portion sizes on the labels of foods. Furthermore, the USDA is currently in the process of implementing changes to the description of portion sizes to better reflect the amount generally consumed in the nutritional information included on the labels. These changes intend to ensure that food package labels provide a more easily interpretable estimation of the energy and nutrition provided by foods. However, because portion size signals a norm about what should be consumed, these changes could ultimately influence food consumption [43,59,60]. How such practices and the resultant policies affect eating disorders and associated risk factors warrants further investigation.

An additional example within the U.S. is regulation that requires calorie labeling in restaurants in an effort to guide consumers towards lower-calorie options [61]. While such policies are viewed positively for increasing food industry transparency, the impact of such policies on calorie consumption has been limited [62–64]. Moreover, a number of concerns have been expressed regarding the ways in which such labeling might impact individuals with eating concerns, who experience high levels of preoccupation around calorie content. Indeed, recent data suggest that individuals with disordered eating behaviors [65] and those with eating disorders [66] may be particularly vulnerable to unintended negative effects of calorie labels on menus. Given the limited efficacy of these policies and their potential for unintended negative effects, greater involvement from those with expertise in eating disorders prevention during the development of such policies is warranted.

A final example of a food policy related to obesity prevention involves the levying of sugar-taxes and the regulation of serving sizes, particularly in the context of sugar-sweetened beverages [67]. It has been suggested that the increase of sugar-related taxes would have a significant positive public health impact, as well as a number of economic benefits [68]. Similarly, unsuccessful efforts made by the New York City Board of Health to regulate the size of sugar-sweetened beverages sold in that state were considered to have a strong potential for positive impact on public health [69]. However, concern regarding other unintended harmful effects, such as increases in alcohol consumption and the disproportionate impact on low-income groups, have been voiced [70]. Furthermore, in the context of eating disorders, such policies may contribute to maintaining the focus on weight as opposed to health and thus perpetuate appearance-related pressures [56]. Thus, again, the inclusion of eating disorders prevention perspectives in the development of such policies is critical.

Broadly, efforts to regulate the food environment that have aimed to prevent obesity have targeted aspects of the food environment that are of relevance to the prevention of eating disorders, namely, the lack of transparency of the industry with regard to the nutritional content of foods, as well as the selling and marketing practices that aim to increase profit. As described above, these practices are those through which the food environment may increase risk for eating disorders. Therefore, policies that are capable of altering these practices could serve eating disorders prevention efforts.

7. Challenges to Integrating Eating Disorders and Obesity Prevention Policy

Common to obesity prevention and eating disorders prevention efforts is the desire to improve public health and reduce factors that drive disparities in health. As such, a shared goal of these prevention efforts would include access to a food environment that promotes health, while minimizing the influence of the food industry that profits from the sale of highly palatable, processed foods and "diet" foods, and from increasing portions sizes. Several challenges to targeting the food industry exist that relate to philosophical misalignments between the perspectives of eating disorders and obesity prevention efforts, however.

The first challenge relates to the extent to which weight is a primary indicator of health and as the primary rationale for changing food policy. Obesity prevention efforts are designed to reduce the prevalence of obesity using a definition based on body mass index (BMI). Using this framing to justify policy changes implies that weight gain is inherently unhealthy and crudely categorizes smaller bodies as "healthy" and larger bodies and "unhealthy" or "diseased." Weight stigma scholars and fat advocates generally reject the term obesity for this reason—that it pathologizes fat bodies, ignores natural size diversity, and, by relying solely on BMI, fails to measure health more holistically [71,72]. Within eating disorders prevention, experts generally reject the idea that weight gain is unhealthy (indeed, weight gain is a necessary and healthy part of recovery for many people with eating disorders, irrespective of weight), yet the erratic and disordered eating habits and/or binge eating behavior that may be associated with weight gain should be considered problematic. To the extent that the food industry contributes to and profits from this type of eating, eating disorders prevention must target their practices, while also advocating for weight-neutral approaches and advocating against weight bias.

A second challenge relates to the types of policy changes that are proposed. Many obesity prevention policy efforts focus on specific foods (e.g., sugar sweetened beverages, fast food, etc.). This approach is seemingly incompatible with evidence-based eating disorders frameworks based on moderation and trusting one's own internal cues of hunger, taste, and fullness (e.g., Health at Every Size®, intuitive eating, mindful eating, etc.) [73–75]. Many individuals with eating disorders assign "good" or "bad" labels to foods or have "forbidden foods" that they avoid eating out of fear or guilt. Learning to eat these in moderation has been shown to be a key element of successful treatment [76]. As such, eating disorders prevention messaging often adopts a "no good/bad foods" mantra. This perspective represents a substantial barrier to joining efforts to limit access to or penalize certain foods. Importantly, the food environment has changed considerably in the last few decades. Accordingly, a more nuanced perspective on food quality may better reflect the current reality of the food environment, and may need to be incorporated into approaches for the prevention of eating disorders. Individuals who are at risk for developing eating disorders may be particularly vulnerable to the presence in the food environment of foods that are designed to appeal to hedonic drives and override homeostatic drives. As such, the prevention of eating disorders includes the criticism of tactics used by the food industry that may capitalize on this vulnerability.

Philosophical differences and key concerns with messaging underlying obesity prevention policies do present an obstacle to integrating eating disorders prevention perspectives into existing efforts that target the food industry. These differences have contributed to the absence of efforts to leverage food policy as a means of the universal prevention of eating disorders. By steering clear of these efforts, however, the considerations that are unique and critical to efforts to prevent eating disorders are left out of the larger conversation related to the regulation of the food environment. Thus, the food industry benefits from minimal oversight related to their contribution to eating disorder risk.

8. Conclusions

The food industry is a key player in the creation of a food environment, characterized by the over-abundance and aggressive marketing of engineered foods that may increase risk for eating disorders or negatively impact their remission. Developing and implementing effective policy approaches to limit the food industry's capacity to continue shaping the food environment in this way is emerging as a critical goal for universal prevention efforts. However, the capacity for these efforts to pathologize larger bodies or vilify specific foods has constituted an obstacle to considering how the broader goal of obesity prevention efforts (i.e., creating a food environment that supports health) may also serve eating disorders prevention. An unintended consequence of this position may be the proliferation of food industry practices that might increase eating disorder risk. Meanwhile, those who are highly susceptible to the presence of these foods or food industry practices may suffer. Eating disorders experts have a crucial part to play in informing policies targeting the food industry to ensure that such policies do no harm. Furthermore, policy efforts targeting the food industry should be considered as a means of improving universal prevention and decreasing an important environmental risk for eating disorders.

Author Contributions: K.R.S. and R.F.R. conceived of the presented idea and contributed to the writing of the manuscript.

Financial Disclosure: The authors have no financial relationships relevant to this article to disclose.

References

1. Swanson, S.A.; Crow, S.J.; Le Grange, D.; Swendsen, J.; Merikangas, K.R. Prevalence and correlates of eating disorders in adolescents: Results from the national comorbidity survey replication adolescent supplement. *Arch. Gen. Psychiatry* **2011**, *68*, 714–723. [CrossRef] [PubMed]
2. Hudson, J.I.; Hiripi, E.; Pope, H.G., Jr.; Kessler, R.C. The prevalence and correlates of eating disorders in the national comorbidity survey replication. *Biol. Psychiatry* **2007**, *61*, 348–358. [CrossRef]
3. Lipson, S.K.; Sonneville, K.R. Eating disorder symptoms among undergraduate and graduate students at 12 U.S. Colleges and universities. *Eat. Behav.* **2017**, *24*, 81–88. [CrossRef] [PubMed]
4. Sonneville, K.R.; Lipson, S.K. Disparities in eating disorder diagnosis and treatment according to weight status, race/ethnicity, socioeconomic background, and sex among college students. *Int. J. Eat. Disord.* **2018**, *51*, 518–526. [CrossRef] [PubMed]
5. Field, A.E.; Sonneville, K.R.; Micali, N.; Crosby, R.D.; Swanson, S.A.; Laird, N.M.; Treasure, J.; Solmi, F.; Horton, N.J. Prospective association of common eating disorders and adverse outcomes. *Pediatrics* **2012**, *130*, e289–e295. [CrossRef] [PubMed]
6. Field, A.E.; Sonneville, K.R.; Crosby, R.D.; Swanson, S.A.; Eddy, K.T.; Camargo, C.A.; Horton, N.J.; Micali, N. Prospective associations of concerns about physique and the development of obesity, binge drinking, and drug use among adolescent boys and young adult men. *JAMA Pediatrics* **2014**, *168*, 34–39. [CrossRef] [PubMed]
7. Haines, J.; Hannan, P.J.; van den Berg, P.; Eisenberg, M.E.; Neumark-Sztainer, D. Weight-related teasing from adolescence to young adulthood: Longitudinal and secular trends between 1999 and 2010. *Obesity* **2013**, *21*, E428–E434. [CrossRef] [PubMed]
8. Chamay-Weber, C.; Narring, F.; Michaud, P.-A. Partial eating disorders among adolescents: A review. *J. Adolesc. Health* **2005**, *37*, 416–426. [CrossRef]
9. Rosen, D. Identification and management of eating disorders in children and adolescents. *Pediatrics* **2010**, *126*, 1240–1253. [CrossRef]
10. Austin, S.B. A public health approach to eating disorders prevention: It's time for public health professionals to take a seat at the table. *BMC Public Health* **2012**, *12*. [CrossRef]
11. Bell, M.J.; Rodgers, R.F.; Paxton, S.J. Towards successful evidence-based universal eating disorders prevention: The importance of zooming out. *Eat. Behav.* **2017**, *25*, 89–92. [CrossRef]

12. Austin, S.B. Accelerating progress in eating disorders prevention: A call for policy translation research and training. *Eat. Disord.* **2016**, *24*, 6–19. [CrossRef] [PubMed]
13. Rodgers, R.; Sonneville, K. Research for leveraging food policy in universal eating disorder prevention. *Int. J. Eat. Disord.* **2018**, *51*, 503–506. [CrossRef] [PubMed]
14. Chriqui, J.F. Obesity prevention policies in u.S. States and localities: Lessons from the field. *Curr. Obes. Rep.* **2013**, *2*, 200–210. [CrossRef]
15. Zhang, Q.; Liu, S.; Liu, R.; Xue, H.; Wang, Y. Food policy approaches to obesity prevention: An international perspective. *Curr. Obes. Rep.* **2014**, *3*, 171–182. [CrossRef] [PubMed]
16. Hawkes, C.; Smith, T.G.; Jewell, J.; Wardle, J.; Hammond, R.A.; Friel, S.; Thow, A.M.; Kain, J. Smart food policies for obesity prevention. *Lancet* **2015**, *385*, 2410–2421. [CrossRef]
17. Duncan, J.; Lambek, N. *Why We Need to Talk about Food Policy*; Committee on World Food Security: Rome, Italy, 2016.
18. Williamson, D.A.; White, M.A.; York-Crowe, E.; Stewart, T.M. Cognitive-behavioral theories of eating disorders. *Behav. Modif.* **2004**, *28*, 711–738. [CrossRef]
19. Corwin, R.L.; Buda-Levin, A. Behavioral models of binge-type eating. *Physiol. Behav.* **2004**, *82*, 123–130. [CrossRef]
20. Ng, L.; Davis, C. Cravings and food consumption in binge eating disorder. *Eat. Behav.* **2013**, *14*, 472–475. [CrossRef]
21. Stice, E.; Agras, W.S.; Telch, C.F.; Halmi, K.A.; Mitchell, J.E.; Wilson, T. Subtyping binge eating-disordered women along dieting and negative affect dimensions. *Int. J. Eat. Disord.* **2001**, *30*, 11–27. [CrossRef]
22. Martínez Steele, E.; Raubenheimer, D.; Simpson, S.J.; Baraldi, L.G.; Monteiro, C.A. Ultra-processed foods, protein leverage and energy intake in the USA. *Public Health Nutr.* **2017**, *21*, 114–124. [CrossRef] [PubMed]
23. Gearhardt, A.N.; Davis, C.; Kuschner, R.; Brownell, K.D. The addiction potential of hyperpalatable foods. *Curr. Drug Abus. Rev.* **2011**, *4*, 140–145. [CrossRef] [PubMed]
24. Gearhardt, A.N.; Grilo, C.M.; DiLeone, R.J.; Brownell, K.D.; Potenza, M.N. Can food be addictive? Public health and policy implications. *Addiction* **2011**, *106*, 1208–1212. [CrossRef] [PubMed]
25. Moskowitz, H.R. Relative importance of perceptual factors to consumer acceptance: Linear vs quadratic analysis. *J. Food Sci.* **1981**, *46*, 244–248. [CrossRef]
26. De Graaf, C.; Kok, F.J. Slow food, fast food and the control of food intake. *Nat. Rev. Endocrinol.* **2010**, *6*, 290–293. [CrossRef] [PubMed]
27. Erlanson-Albertsson, C. How palatable food disrupts appetite regulation. *Basic Clin. Pharmacol. Toxicol.* **2005**, *97*, 61–73. [CrossRef] [PubMed]
28. Schulte, E.M.; Avena, N.M.; Gearhardt, A.N. Which foods may be addictive? The roles of processing, fat content, and glycemic load. *PLoS ONE* **2015**, *10*, e0117959. [CrossRef]
29. Yanovski, S.Z.; Leet, M.; Yanovski, J.A.; Flood, M.; Gold, P.W.; Kissileff, H.R.; Walsh, B.T. Food selection and intake of obese women with binge-eating disorder. *Am. J. Clin. Nutr.* **1992**, *56*, 975–980. [CrossRef]
30. Rosen, J.C.; Leitenberg, H.; Fisher, C.; Khazam, C. Binge-eating episodes in bulimia nervosa: The amount and type of food consumed. *Int. J. Eat. Disord.* **1986**, *5*, 255–267. [CrossRef]
31. Hagan, M.M.; Chandler, P.C.; Wauford, P.K.; Rybak, R.J.; Oswald, K.D. The role of palatable food and hunger as trigger factors in an animal model of stress induced binge eating. *Int. J. Eat. Disord.* **2003**, *34*, 183–197. [CrossRef]
32. Boggiano, M.M.; Artiga, A.I.; Pritchett, C.E.; Chandler-Laney, P.C.; Smith, M.L.; Eldridge, A.J. High intake of palatable food predicts binge-eating independent of susceptibility to obesity: An animal model of lean vs obese binge-eating and obesity with and without binge-eating. *Int. J. Obes.* **2007**, *31*, 1357–1367. [CrossRef] [PubMed]
33. Corwin, R.L.; Avena, N.M.; Boggiano, M.M. Feeding and reward: Perspectives from three rat models of binge eating. *Physiol. Behav.* **2011**, *104*, 87–97. [CrossRef] [PubMed]
34. Oswald, K.D.; Murdaugh, D.L.; King, V.L.; Boggiano, M.M. Motivation for palatable food despite consequences in an animal model of binge eating. *Int. J. Eat. Disord.* **2011**, *44*, 203–211. [CrossRef] [PubMed]
35. Gearhardt, A.N.; Corbin, W.R.; Brownell, K.D. Food addiction: An examination of the diagnostic criteria for dependence. *J. Addict. Med.* **2009**, *3*, 1–7. [CrossRef] [PubMed]
36. Schulte, E.M.; Joyner, M.A.; Schiestl, E.T.; Gearhardt, A.N. Future directions in "food addiction": Next steps and treatment implications. *Curr. Addict. Rep.* **2017**, *4*, 165–171. [CrossRef]

37. Ahmed, S.H.; Guillem, K.; Vandaele, Y. Sugar addiction: Pushing the drug-sugar analogy to the limit. *Curr. Opin. Clin. Nutr. Metab. Care* **2013**, *16*, 434–439. [CrossRef] [PubMed]
38. Hill, J.O.; Peters, J.C. Environmental contributions to the obesity epidemic. *Science* **1998**, *280*, 1371–1374. [CrossRef]
39. Economos, C.D.; Hatfield, D.P.; King, A.C.; Ayala, G.X.; Pentz, M.A. Food and physical activity environments: An energy balance approach for research and practice. *Am. J. Prev. Med.* **2015**, *48*, 620–629. [CrossRef]
40. Benton, D. Portion size: What we know and what we need to know. *Crit. Rev. Food Sci. Nutr.* **2015**, *55*, 988–1004. [CrossRef]
41. Nestle, M. Increasing portion sizes in american diets: More calories, more obesity. *J. Am. Diet. Assoc.* **2003**, *103*, 39–40. [CrossRef]
42. Birch, L.L.; Savage, J.S.; Fisher, J.O. Right sizing prevention. Food portion size effects on children's eating and weight. *Appetite* **2015**, *88*, 11–16. [CrossRef] [PubMed]
43. Herman, C.P.; Polivy, J.; Pliner, P.; Vartanian, L.R. Mechanisms underlying the portion-size effect. *Physiol. Behav.* **2015**, *144*, 129–136. [CrossRef] [PubMed]
44. Steenhuis, I.; Poelman, M. Portion size: Latest developments and interventions. *Curr. Obes. Rep.* **2017**, *6*, 10–17. [CrossRef] [PubMed]
45. English, L.; Lasschuijt, M.; Keller, K.L. Mechanisms of the portion size effect. What is known and where do we go from here? *Appetite* **2015**, *88*, 39–49. [CrossRef] [PubMed]
46. Mirch, M.C.; McDuffie, J.R.; Yanovski, S.Z.; Schollnberger, M.; Tanofsky-Kraff, M.; Theim, K.R.; Krakoff, J.; Yanovski, J.A. Effects of binge eating on satiation, satiety, and energy intake of overweight children. *Am. J. Clin. Nutr.* **2006**, *84*, 732–738. [CrossRef] [PubMed]
47. Harriger, J.A.; Thompson, J.K. Psychological consequences of obesity: Weight bias and body image in overweight and obese youth. *Int. Rev. Psychiatry* **2012**, *24*, 247–253. [CrossRef] [PubMed]
48. La Berge, A.F. How the ideology of low fat conquered america. *J. Hist. Med. Allied Sci.* **2008**, *63*, 139–177. [CrossRef] [PubMed]
49. Willett, W. *Eat, Drink, and be Healthy: The Harvard Medical School Guide to Healthy Eating*; Simon and Schuster: New York, NY, USA, 2001.
50. Chandon, P.; Wansink, B. The biasing health halos of fast-food restaurant health claims: Lower calorie estimates and higher side-dish consumption intentions. *J. Consum. Res.* **2007**, *34*, 301–314. [CrossRef]
51. Mariotti, F.; Kalonji, E.; Huneau, J.F.; Margaritis, I. Potential pitfalls of health claims from a public health nutrition perspective. *Nutr. Rev.* **2010**, *68*, 624–638. [CrossRef]
52. Kaur, A.; Scarborough, P.; Rayner, M. A systematic review, and meta-analyses, of the impact of health-related claims on dietary choices. *Int. J. Behav. Nutr. Phys. Act.* **2017**, *14*, 93. [CrossRef]
53. Elfhag, K.; Tynelius, P.; Rasmussen, F. Sugar-sweetened and artificially sweetened soft drinks in association to restrained, external and emotional eating. *Physiol. Behav.* **2007**, *91*, 191–195. [CrossRef]
54. Lavin, J.; French, S.; Read, N. The effect of sucrose-and aspartame-sweetened drinks on energy intake, hunger and food choice of female, moderately restrained eaters. *Int. J. Obes.* **1997**, *21*, 37–42. [CrossRef]
55. Yang, Q. Gain weight by "going diet?" artificial sweeteners and the neurobiology of sugar cravings: Neuroscience 2010. *Yale J. Biol. Med.* **2010**, *83*, 101–108. [PubMed]
56. Rodgers, R.F. The role of the "healthy weight" discourse in body image and eating concerns: An extension of sociocultural theory. *Eat. Behav.* **2016**, *22*, 194–198. [CrossRef] [PubMed]
57. Vermeer, W.M.; Steenhuis, I.H.M.; Poelman, M.P. Small, medium, large or supersize? The development and evaluation of interventions targeted at portion size. *Int. J. Obes.* **2014**, *38*, S13–S18. [CrossRef] [PubMed]
58. Crino, M.; Sacks, G.; Wu, J.H. A review of population-level actions targeting reductions in food portion sizes to address obesity and related non-communicable diseases. *Curr. Nutr. Rep.* **2016**, *5*, 323–332. [CrossRef]
59. Kerameas, K.; Vartanian, L.R.; Herman, C.P.; Polivy, J. The effect of portion size and unit size on food intake: Unit bias or segmentation effect? *Health Psychol.* **2015**, *34*, 670–676. [CrossRef]
60. Marchiori, D.; Papies, E.K.; Klein, O. The portion size effect on food intake. An anchoring and adjustment process? *Appetite* **2014**, *81*, 108–115. [CrossRef]
61. Burton, S.; Kees, J. Flies in the ointment? Addressing potential impediments to population-based health benefits of restaurant menu labeling initiatives. *J. Public Policy Mark.* **2012**, *31*, 232–239. [CrossRef]
62. Swartz, J.J.; Braxton, D.; Viera, A.J. Calorie menu labeling on quick-service restaurant menus: An updated systematic review of the literature. *Int. J. Behav. Nutr. Phys. Act.* **2011**, *8*, 135. [CrossRef]

63. Sinclair, S.E.; Cooper, M.; Mansfield, E.D. The influence of menu labeling on calories selected or consumed: A systematic review and meta-analysis. *J. Acad. Nutr. Diet.* **2014**, *114*, 1375–1388. [CrossRef] [PubMed]
64. Long, M.W.; Tobias, D.K.; Cradock, A.L.; Batchelder, H.; Gortmaker, S.L. Systematic review and meta-analysis of the impact of restaurant menu calorie labeling. *Am. J. Public Health* **2015**, *105*, e11–e24. [CrossRef] [PubMed]
65. Larson, N.; Haynos, A.F.; Roberto, C.A.; Loth, K.A.; Neumark-Sztainer, D. Calorie labels on the restaurant menu: Is the use of weight-control behaviors related to ordering decisions? *J. Acad. Nutr. Diet.* **2018**, *118*, 399–408. [CrossRef] [PubMed]
66. Haynos, A.F.; Roberto, C.A. The effects of restaurant menu calorie labeling on hypothetical meal choices of females with disordered eating. *Int. J. Eat. Disord.* **2017**, *50*, 275–283. [CrossRef] [PubMed]
67. Brownell, K.D.; Frieden, T.R. Ounces of prevention—The public policy case for taxes on sugared beverages. *N. Engl. J. Med.* **2009**, *360*, 1805–1808. [CrossRef] [PubMed]
68. Andreyeva, T.; Chaloupka, F.J.; Brownell, K.D. Estimating the potential of taxes on sugar-sweetened beverages to reduce consumption and generate revenue. *Prev. Med.* **2011**, *52*, 413–416. [CrossRef] [PubMed]
69. Pomeranz, J.L.; Brownell, K.D. Can government regulate portion sizes? *N. Engl. J. Med.* **2014**, *371*, 1956–1958. [CrossRef] [PubMed]
70. Brown, A.W.; Allison, D.B. Unintended consequences of obesity-targeted health policy. *Virtual Mentor* **2013**, *15*, 339–346.
71. Tylka, T.L.; Annunziato, R.A.; Burgard, D.; Danielsdottir, S.; Shuman, E.; Davis, C.; Calogero, R.M. The weight-inclusive versus weight-normative approach to health: Evaluating the evidence for prioritizing well-being over weight loss. *J. Obes.* **2014**, *2014*, 983495. [CrossRef]
72. Meadows, A.; Daníelsdóttir, S. What's in a word? On weight stigma and terminology. *Front. Psychol.* **2016**, *7*. [CrossRef]
73. Tylka, T.L.; Kroon Van Diest, A.M. The intuitive eating scale–2: Item refinement and psychometric evaluation with college women and men. *J. Couns. Psychol.* **2013**, *60*, 137–153. [CrossRef] [PubMed]
74. Tylka, T.L.; Calogero, R.M.; Daníelsdóttir, S. Is intuitive eating the same as flexible dietary control? Their links to each other and well-being could provide an answer. *Appetite* **2015**, *95*, 166–175. [CrossRef]
75. Hepworth, N.S. A mindful eating group as an adjunct to individual treatment for eating disorders: A pilot study. *Eat. Disord.* **2010**, *19*, 6–16. [CrossRef] [PubMed]
76. Coelho, J.S.; Wilson, S.; Winslade, A.; Thaler, L.; Israel, M.; Steiger, H. Over-evaluation of thoughts about food: Differences across eating-disorder subtypes and a preliminary examination of treatment effects. *Int. J. Eat. Disord.* **2014**, *47*, 302–309. [CrossRef]

Permissions

All chapters in this book were first published by MDPI; hereby published with permission under the Creative Commons Attribution License or equivalent. Every chapter published in this book has been scrutinized by our experts. Their significance has been extensively debated. The topics covered herein carry significant findings which will fuel the growth of the discipline. They may even be implemented as practical applications or may be referred to as a beginning point for another development.

The contributors of this book come from diverse backgrounds, making this book a truly international effort. This book will bring forth new frontiers with its revolutionizing research information and detailed analysis of the nascent developments around the world.

We would like to thank all the contributing authors for lending their expertise to make the book truly unique. They have played a crucial role in the development of this book. Without their invaluable contributions this book wouldn't have been possible. They have made vital efforts to compile up to date information on the varied aspects of this subject to make this book a valuable addition to the collection of many professionals and students.

This book was conceptualized with the vision of imparting up-to-date information and advanced data in this field. To ensure the same, a matchless editorial board was set up. Every individual on the board went through rigorous rounds of assessment to prove their worth. After which they invested a large part of their time researching and compiling the most relevant data for our readers.

The editorial board has been involved in producing this book since its inception. They have spent rigorous hours researching and exploring the diverse topics which have resulted in the successful publishing of this book. They have passed on their knowledge of decades through this book. To expedite this challenging task, the publisher supported the team at every step. A small team of assistant editors was also appointed to further simplify the editing procedure and attain best results for the readers.

Apart from the editorial board, the designing team has also invested a significant amount of their time in understanding the subject and creating the most relevant covers. They scrutinized every image to scout for the most suitable representation of the subject and create an appropriate cover for the book.

The publishing team has been an ardent support to the editorial, designing and production team. Their endless efforts to recruit the best for this project, has resulted in the accomplishment of this book. They are a veteran in the field of academics and their pool of knowledge is as vast as their experience in printing. Their expertise and guidance has proved useful at every step. Their uncompromising quality standards have made this book an exceptional effort. Their encouragement from time to time has been an inspiration for everyone.

The publisher and the editorial board hope that this book will prove to be a valuable piece of knowledge for researchers, students, practitioners and scholars across the globe.

List of Contributors

Kamila Czepczor-Bernat
Faculty of Psychology in Katowice, SWPS University of Social Sciences and Humanities, 40-326 Katowice, Poland

Anna Brytek-Matera
Institute of Psychology, University of Wroclaw, 50-527 Wroclaw, Poland

Paweł Matusik
School of Medicine in Katowice, Department of Pediatrics and Pediatric Endocrinology, Medical University of Silesia, 40-752 Katowice, Poland

Araceli Muñoz-Garach and Francisco J. Tinahones
Department of Endocrinology and Nutrition, Virgen de la Victoria Hospital, Málaga University, Málaga 29010, Spain
CIBER Fisiopatologia Obesidad y Nutricion (CIBEROBN), Instituto de Salud Carlos III, Madrid 28029, Spain

Isabel Cornejo-Pareja
Department of Endocrinology and Nutrition, Virgen de la Victoria Hospital, Málaga University, Málaga 29010, Spain

Priyanka Thapliyal and Phillipa Hay
Translational Health Research Institute, School of Medicine, Western Sydney University, Building 3.G.P9, Locked Bag 1797, Penrith NSW 2751, Australia

Deborah Mitchison
Centre for Emotional Health, Department of Psychology, Macquarie University, Sydney 2109, Australia

Manuela Jaramillo and Marian Tanofsky-Kraff
Section on Growth and Obesity, Eunice Kennedy Shriver National Institute of Child Health and Human Development (NICHD), National Institutes of Health (NIH), DHHS, 10 Center Drive, Bethesda, MD 20892-1103, USA
Department of Medical and Clinical Psychology, Uniformed Services University of the Health Sciences (USUHS), 4301 Jones Bridge Road, Bethesda, MD 20814, USA

Natasha L. Burke
Department of Psychology, Fordham University, 411 East Fordham Road, Bronx, NY 10458, USA

Lauren B. Shomaker
Department of Human Development and Family Studies, Colorado State University, 303 Behavioral Sciences Building, 1570 Campus Delivery, Fort Collins, CO 80523, USA

Sheila M. Brady and Jack A. Yanovski
Section on Growth and Obesity, Eunice Kennedy Shriver National Institute of Child Health and Human Development (NICHD), National Institutes of Health (NIH), DHHS, 10 Center Drive, Bethesda, MD 20892-1103, USA

Merel Kozlosky
Nutrition Department, Clinical Center, NIH, DHHS, 10 Center Drive, Bethesda, MD 20892, USA

Sarah Barakat and Stephen Touyz
School of Psychology, University of Sydney, Sydney, NSW 2006, Australia

Sarah Maguire, Blagica Miceska and Kirsty Fromholtz
Centre for Eating and Dieting Disorders, Boden Institute, University of Sydney, Sydney, NSW 2006, Australia

Lois Surgenor
Department of Psychological Medicine, University of Otago at Christchurch, Christchurch 8140, New Zealand

Brooke Donnelly
Sydney Local Health District, Sydney, NSW 2006, Australia

Janice Russell
School of Medicine, University of Sydney, Sydney, NSW 2006, Australia

Francesco Savino, Allegra Sardo, Lorenza Rossi, Stefania Benetti and Andrea Savino
Department of Pediatrics, Regina Margherita Children's Hospital, Città della Salute e della Scienza di Torino, Piazza Polonia 94, Torino I-10126, Italy

Leandra Silvestro
Department of Public Health and Pediatric Sciences, University of Turin I-10126, Italy

Therese Fostervold Mathisen and Jorunn Sundgot-Borgen
Department of Sports Medicine, Norwegian School of Sport Sciences; Sognsvegen 220, 0806 Oslo, Norway

Jan H. Rosenvinge
Department of Psychology, Faculty of Health Sciences, UiT- the Arctic University of Norway, N-9037 Tromsø, Norway

Solfrid Bratland-Sanda
Department of Sports and Physical Education and Outdoor Sciences, University of South-Eastern Norway, N-3800 Bø in Telemark, Norway

Clare E. Collins and Melinda J. Hutchesson
Nutrition and Dietetics, School of Health Sciences, Faculty of Health and Medicine, The University of Newcastle, Callaghan, NSW 2308, Australia
Priority Research Centre in Physical Activity and Nutrition, The University of Newcastle, Callaghan, NSW 2308, Australia

Philip J. Morgan
Priority Research Centre in Physical Activity and Nutrition, The University of Newcastle, Callaghan, NSW 2308, Australia
School of Education, Faculty of Education and Arts, The University of Newcastle, Callaghan, NSW 2308, Australia

Christopher Oldmeadow and Daniel Barker
Clinical Research Design, IT and Statistical Support Unit, Hunter Medical Research Institute, Level 3 Pod, HMRI building Lot 1, Kookaburra Circuit, New Lambton Heights, NSW 2305, Australia
School of Medicine and Public Health, Faculty of Health and Medicine, The University of Newcastle, Callaghan, NSW 2308, Australia

Robin Callister
Priority Research Centre in Physical Activity and Nutrition, The University of Newcastle, Callaghan, NSW 2308, Australia
School of Biomedical Sciences and Pharmacy, Faculty of Health and Medicine, The University of Newcastle, Callaghan, NSW 2308, Australia

Ricarda Schmidt, Caroline Sebert, Christine Kösling, Anja Hilbert, Claudia Hübner and Lisa Schäfer
Integrated Research and Treatment Center Adiposity Diseases, Department of Medical Psychology and Medical Sociology and Psychosomatic Medicine and Psychotherapy, Leipzig University Medical Center, 04103 Leipzig, Germany

Martin Grunwald
Haptic-Research Laboratory, Paul-Flechsig-Institute for Brain Research, University of Leipzig, 04103 Leipzig, Germany

Kim Anh Nguyen, Nasheeta Peer and Andre Pascal Kengne
Non-Communicable Diseases Research Unit, South African Medical Research Council, Cape Town 7505, South Africa
Department of Medicine, University of Cape Town, Cape Town 7935, South Africa

Anniza de Villiers
Non-Communicable Diseases Research Unit, South African Medical Research Council, Cape Town 7505, South Africa

Barbara Mukasa
United Nations Population Fund (UNFPA), Mildmay Uganda, Lweza, Uganda

Tandi E. Matsha
Department of Biomedical Sciences, Faculty of Health and Wellness Science, Cape Peninsula University of Technology, Cape Town 7535, South Africa

Edward J. Mills
Global Evaluation Science, Vancouver, BC V6H 3X4, Canada

Marly Amorim Palavras
Eating Disorders Program (PROATA), Department of Psychiatry, Universidade Federal de São Paulo (UNIFESP), São Paulo 04017030, Brazil
Translational Health Research Institute, School of Medicine, Western Sydney University, Sydney 2751, Australia

Angélica Claudino
Eating Disorders Program (PROATA), Department of Psychiatry, Universidade Federal de São Paulo (UNIFESP), São Paulo 04017030, Brazil

Camilla Lindvall Dahlgren and Kristin Stedal
Regional Department for Eating Disorders, Division of Mental Health and Addiction, Oslo University Hospital, Ullevål HF, 0424 Oslo, Norway

Wei Yang, Jian-Ping Li, Yan Zhang, Fang-Fang Fan and Yong Huo
Department of Cardiology, Peking University First Hospital, Beijing 100034, China

Xi-Ping Xu, Bin-Yan Wang, Xin Xu and Xian-Hui Qin
National Clinical Research Center for Kidney Disease, State Key Laboratory for Organ Failure Research, Renal Division, Nanfang Hospital, Southern Medical University, Guangzhou 510515, China

Hou-Xun Xing, Gen-Fu Tang and Zi-Yi Zhou
Institute for Biomedicine, Anhui Medical University, Hefei 230032, China

Dong-Feng Gu
State Key Laboratory of Cardiovascular Disease, Fuwai Hospital, National Center for Cardiovascular Diseases, Chinese Academy of Medical Sciences and Peking Union Medical College, Beijing 100037, China

Dong Zhao
Department of Epidemiology, Beijing Anzhen Hospital, Capital Medical University, Beijing Institute of Heart, Lung and Blood Vessel Diseases, Beijing 100029, China

Caitlyn G. Edwards and Sharon V. Thompson
Division of Nutritional Sciences, University of Illinois, Urbana, IL 61801, USA

Anne M. Walk and Sean P. Mullen
Department of Kinesiology and Community Health, University of Illinois, Urbana, IL 61801, USA

Hannah D. Holscher
Division of Nutritional Sciences, University of Illinois, Urbana, IL 61801, USA
Department of Kinesiology and Community Health, University of Illinois, Urbana, IL 61801, USA
Department of Food Science and Human Nutrition, University of Illinois, Urbana, IL 61801, USA

Naiman A. Khan
Division of Nutritional Sciences, University of Illinois, Urbana, IL 61801, USA
Department of Kinesiology and Community Health, University of Illinois, Urbana, IL 61801, USA
Neuroscience Program, University of Illinois, Urbana, IL 61801, USA

Claudia Harper
The Boden Institute of Obesity, Nutrition, Exercise and Eating Disorders, Sydney Medical School, The University of Sydney, Level 2, Charles Perkins Centre, John Hopkins Drive, Camperdown, NSW 2006, Australia

Judith Maher
Faculty of Science, Health, Education and Engineering, University of the Sunshine Coast, 90 Sippy Downs Dr, Sippy Downs, QLD 4556, Australia

Claudio Imperatori, Miranda Mancini and Benedetto Farina
Department of Human Sciences, European University of Rome, Via degli Aldobrandeschi 190, 00163 Roma, Italy

Giacomo Della Marca
Sleep Disorders Unit, Institute of Neurology, Catholic University, 00153 Rome, Italy

Enrico Maria Valenti
Department of Human Sciences, European University of Rome, Via degli Aldobrandeschi 190, 00163 Roma, Italy
Department of Dynamic and Clinical Psychology, Sapienza University of Rome, 00185 Rome, Italy

Kendrin R. Sonneville
Department of Nutritional Sciences, University of Michigan School of Public Health, Ann Arbor, MI 48109, USA

Rachel F. Rodgers
Department of Applied Psychology, Bouve College of Health Sciences, Northeastern University, Boston, MA 02115, USA

Index

www.ingramcontent.com/pod-product-compliance
Lightning Source LLC
LaVergne TN
LVHW060520210926
848485LV00005B/1114